# Basic Histopathology

## A COLOUR ATLAS AND TEXT

D0126812

**Paul Wheater**
BA Hons (York), BMed Sci Hons (Nott), BM BS (Nott)
Queen's Medical Centre, University of Nottingham

**George Burkitt**
BDSc Hons (Queensland), MB BChir (Cantab), MMed Sci (Nott), FRACDS
School of Clinical Medicine, University of Cambridge

**Alan Stevens**
MB BS (Lond) FRCPath
Senior Lecturer in Pathology, University of Nottingham
Honorary Consultant Pathologist, Trent Regional Health Authority (T)

**James Lowe**
B Med Sci Hons (Nott), BM BS (Nott), MRCPath
Lecturer in Pathology, University of Nottingham

Prepared in the Department of Pathology,
University of Nottingham


*Foreword by*

**Ian M. P. Dawson** MA MD, FRCP, FRCPath
Professor of Pathology
University of Nottingham (retired)

## Churchill Livingstone
EDINBURGH LONDON MELBOURNE AND NEW YORK 1985

CHURCHILL LIVINGSTONE
Medical Division of Longman Group UK Limited

Distributed in the United States of America by Churchill
Livingstone Inc., 1560 Broadway, New York, N.Y. 10036,
and by associated companies, branches and representatives
throughout the world.

© Longman Group Limited 1985

All rights reserved. No part of this publication may be
reproduced, stored in a retrieval system, or transmitted in any
form or by any means, electronic, mechanical, photocopying,
recording, or otherwise, without the prior permission of the
publishers (Churchill Livingstone, Robert Stevenson House,
1-3 Baxter's Place, Leith Walk, Edinburgh EH1 3AF).

First published 1985
  Reprinted 1986 (twice)
  Reprinted 1987
  Reprinted 1988

ISBN 0 443 02252 6

British Library Cataloguing in Publication Data
Basic histopathology.
  1. Histology, Pathological
  I. Wheater, Paul R.
  611'.018  RB25

Library of Congress Cataloging in Publication Data
Basic histopathology.
  Includes index.
  1. Histology, Pathological — Atlases. I. Wheater,
Paul R. [DNLM: 1. Histology — atlases. 2. Pathology —
atlases. QZ 17 B311]
RB22.B26  1984 611'.018  84-14212

Produced by Longman Group (FE) Ltd
Printed in Hong Kong

*Cover photograph:* Renal tuberculosis (HM)

# Foreword

Were it not that they appear to enjoy life, one might feel sorry for present-day medical students. The elastic bounds of knowledge are for ever stretching and, as those who sit on Faculty Boards and Curriculum Committees know only too well, no-one is more adept than a Head of Department in insisting that *his* subject is more important than that of any of his colleagues, that it can in no way be reduced in content and that, anyway, a quart of knowledge can be force-fed into a pint pot of student time if one really tries.

As regards the first premise it is true that pathology, like the Pope, is, in importance, at least first among equals, being the basis of medicine on which others build. The interpretation of the symptoms with which the patient presents, the signs which one can elicit and the investigations to which one can then subject him all depend on an accurate appreciation of what is happening in the tissues. It is also true that histopathology provides the simplest and easiest means of learning and remembering what is going on at structural, microscopical and ultrastructural levels.

So far, so good; the case for a sound knowledge of pathology can be made and defended but the problem of the quart and the pint pot remains; the former is steadily increasing to a 2-litre bottle and the latter is shrinking to a wine glass. Most students now learn their histopathology from class slides, supplemented by colour TV demonstrations and the use of slide–tape programmes. There is little opportunity for class revision and a good deal of learning and experience must now be acquired in that mythical period known as 'one's spare time', when no tutor is available. For students thus engaged, good books on histology and histopathology are indispensable. Two of the authors have already produced the former; *Functional Histology* has been an enormous success and *Basic Histopathology* is a companion volume for the student in pathology, who, one hopes, will already possess the former. Both books can be used together in the study of class slides, alongside a standard textbook of pathology or on their own. Almost 40 years of teaching pathology have convinced me that when it is properly presented students find it fascinating; a book as well illustrated as this — the colour reproductions are superb — and not overburdened with unhelpful detail is exactly what is needed in a crowded curriculum. There is no need to write more; a good wine needs no bush and I have no doubts as to its future. It will be widely used and deserves to be.

Nottingham, 1985                                                                                                         I.M.P.D.

# Preface

Histopathology is an essential component of pathology teaching in all medical and dental courses, nevertheless the scope, content and emphasis on microscopy vary considerably between different centres. Adding to this diversity are the different stages in the preclinical and/or clinical years when the subject matter is presented. This book has been designed to meet as closely as possible the requirements of these many differing courses. We believe that practical microscopy is an important part of pathology teaching, and therefore we have chosen to centre our discussion around appropriate colour photo-micrographs as might be done in the lecture room or microscope laboratory. The text has been designed as a series of amplified captions explaining not only the features visible in the labelled colour plates, but also providing some background text in order to relate the subject matter to the theoretical and clinical implications of the pathological processes. Consequently this book should not be regarded as a copiously illustrated introductory textbook of pathology, but rather it is intended as a histopathology companion to any of the many excellent standard pathology textbooks; the text, though more than normally found in an atlas, is thus by no means comprehensive.

The subject matter has been divided into two sections, the first covering basic pathological processes and the second encompassing the common diseases encountered in systems pathology. In general, our material has been taken from both surgical and necropsy specimens of common clinical conditions. Uncommon conditions have been included only where they illustrate important pathological principles. The haematoxylin and eosin staining method has mainly been employed as is standard practice in pathology laboratories, but special staining methods have been occasionally used where appropriate. Rather than specifying numerical magnification factors, each micrograph has been designated as low power, medium power or high power by the abbreviations LP, MP and HP respectively as this is probably more relevant to student needs.

It is our hope that this book will be useful both as a guide in formal practical classes, as well as assisting the student in private study. Although the book is primarily aimed at preclinical and clinical medical and dental students, it would also prove useful for other groups such as veterinary science students, medical laboratory scientists specialising in histopathology, and candidates for post-graduate examinations in surgery and pathology.

P.R.W.
H.G.B.
A.S.
J.S.L.

Nottingham, 1985

# Acknowledgements

In a book such as this, the illustrations which finally appear represent only a minute fragment of the photographs taken and of the vast number of microscope slides which have been prepared for review and selection prior to photography. Our biggest debt of gratitude, therefore, is owed to Janet Palmer and Anne and Ian Wilson who, between them, skilfully sectioned an enormous number of paraffin blocks, often at many levels, staining the sections with a number of different haemotoxylin and eosin schedules, to meet our frequently inordinate demands. Their skill, industry and patience have played an important part in the successful outcome of this enterprise. Mr Stan Terras developed and printed the electron micrographs and Jane Watson prepared the resin sections of bone.

We are most grateful to our many colleagues who helped us by providing suitable material from their own collections: in particular Professors Ian Dawson and D. R. Turner, Dr Peter James, Dr Alasdair Mackay and Dr Peter Smith of University Hospital, Nottingham; Dr David Howell of Derby Royal Infirmary. Dr Roy Reeve, Professor Roger Cotton; Dr Stephen Jones of the City Hospital, Nottingham and Dr George Hall kindly gave us access to a personal index file of outstanding material and to the paraffin block stores at the General Hospital, Nottingham.

The text (with its many revisions) was typed by Christine Stevens and Isabella Streeter, to whom we would like to express our thanks. Finally, all the colour illustrations were photographed by one of the authors (PRW) using a Leitz vario-orthomat photomicroscope and Agfachrome 50L film.

# Contents

# PART 1

# Basic Pathological Processes

# 1. Cellular responses to injury

## Introduction

The cellular environment is constantly changing and as a consequence cells have to make continuous adjustments to accommodate these changes. The cell has a great capacity for adaptation to its environment and is able to respond to changes in the internal and external environments by alterations in both cellular structure and function. For example, adipose tissue cells respond to prolonged excessive food intake by increasing their synthesis of storable fat; this is reflected by an increase in the size of adipocytes due to the presence of large globules of triglyceride in the cytoplasm. Another physiological example of cellular adaptation is seen in the epithelium lining the uterus; under the influence of hormones, this epithelium undergoes cyclical changes during the menstrual cycle which involve both changes in morphology and function.

Certain environmental changes lie outside an acceptable physiological range. Such adverse environmental changes may be termed *pathological stimuli*. Cells may respond to pathological stimuli by extending their normal physiological adaptative processes. These adaptive processes include:

(a) **Increased cellular activity**
    (i) Increase in cell size (*hypertrophy,* see Fig. 5.1)
    (ii) Increase in cell number (*hyperplasia,* see Fig. 5.2)
    (iii) Enzyme or metabolic induction.

(b) **Decreased cellular activity**
    (i) Reduced cell size (*cell atrophy,* see Fig. 5.4)
    (ii) Reduced number of cells (*tissue* or *organ atrophy*).
    (iii) Diminished cellular metabolic function.

(c) **Change in morphology and function of mature cell type**
Modification and transformation to a cell type more suited to the changed environment (*metaplasia,* see Fig. 5.5)

Examples of these adaptive responses are as follows:

Skeletal muscle fibres increase in size in response to increased work load as seen in athletes; this is an example of *physiological hypertrophy.* Similarly, cardiac muscle fibres undergo hypertrophy in response to increased work demands when the aortic valve outlet is narrowed as a result of disease; this is an example of *pathological hypertrophy.* During pregnancy there is an increase in the number and size of secretory cells in the breast lobules as a result of hormonal stimulation; this is an example of *physiological hyperplasia.* There is an increase in the size and number of thyroid acinar cells in the presence of an abnormal immunoglobulin (LATS) which mimics the effects of thyroid stimulating hormone; this is an example of *pathological hyperplasia.* The reduced size of skeletal muscle fibres in the elderly or the immobile is an example of *physiological atrophy.* In contrast, the reduced size of skeletal muscle fibres after denervation due to spinal cord disease such as polio is an example of *pathological cell atrophy.* Organ atrophy may occur as a result of atrophy of all the individual cells of which the organ is composed, e.g. endometrial atrophy after the menopause, or as a result of loss of one component of the tissue only, e.g. death of cerebral cortical neurones in senile dementia which leads to organ atrophy of the brain. In some instances, the lost component may be replaced by a nonfunctional element such as fat or fibrous tissue; organ size may be preserved, but the organ becomes physiologically atrophic. An example is the fat replacement of the parathyroid gland in older age (see Fig. 19.6a); parathyroid size is normal but the active cells are greatly reduced in number. Finally, an example of metaplasia is the change of the bladder mucosa from transitional epithelium to squamous epithelium in response to the chronic trauma of a bladder stone or chronic infection by parasites. A more detailed account of such adaptive responses is provided in Chapter 5.

## Failure of cellular adaptation

Cells which are intrinsically unable to adapt, or which have reached their limit of adaptability, begin to show structural changes which indicate their failure to withstand the changed environment. For example, susceptible cells which are exposed to prolonged hypoxia begin to show cytoplasmic changes as a manifestation of organelle failure; these ultrastructural changes are shown in Fig. 1.1. At the light microscopic level, these changes have been variously termed *cloudy swelling* and *hydropic degeneration*, and are described in Fig. 1.2. Other cells may respond to hypoxia or toxins by failure to metabolize fatty acids normally; this results in the accumulation of intracytoplasmic lipid vacuoles and hence the descriptive term *fatty change* (see Fig. 1.3). This feature is found particularly in liver cells, cardiac muscle cells and renal cortical tubular epithelial cells, since all of these cell types are dependent on fatty acids as metabolic substrates. Both hydropic and fatty degeneration are potentially reversible if the deleterious stimulus is short lived. If adverse conditions persist however, or if the initial pathological stimulus was severe, then these processes continue and progress into a sequence of events leading to cell death (*cell necrosis*). The onset of this irreversible cell change is heralded by distinct morphological changes in the cell cytoplasm and the cell nucleus which are illustrated in Figs 1.4 and 1.5.

Under certain conditions, pathological stimuli may cause the loss of the normal responsiveness of cells to the factors which control their rate of growth and degree of maturation. Such cells may divide more rapidly than normal and fail to reach their fully differentiated state; this phenomenon is known as *dysplasia* and is discussed in Chapter 5. Other pathological stimuli may damage the genetic material of cells such that the cells proliferate in an uncontrolled manner. Such an autonomous mass of cells is known as a *neoplasm* and may give rise to a progressively enlarging tumour. Neoplastic disease forms the basis of Chapter 6 where further examples are given. Neoplasia may be considered as a maladaptive response to an abnormal environmental stimulus, although in many cases the precise stimulus cannot be identified.

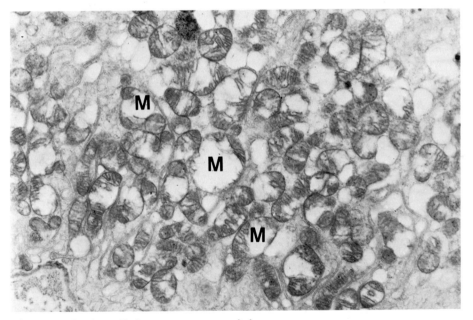

## Fig. 1.1 Early cellular responses to injury (EM)

The initial response of cells to injury is manifest at a subcellular level by morphological changes in the various cytoplasmic organelles. Membrane enzyme systems such as those constantly engaged in maintaining ionic gradients and membrane transport are particularly vulnerable to pathological influences. One of the earliest consequences is a loss of efficiency of the sodium pump permitting ingress of sodium ions and water, resulting in swelling of the cell. In this high power electron micrograph of a renal tubular cell damaged by hypoxia, mitochondrial membranes have been damaged producing swelling of the mitochondria **M**. This change is potentially reversible if the noxious stimulus is insufficient to

cause cell death. Further damage leads to increased mitochondrial swelling and loss of cristae. There is also dilatation of endoplasmic reticulum with detachment of ribosomes from rough endoplasmic reticulum (not seen in this micrograph). The nucleus remains relatively unchanged at this stage. If the cell sustains irreversible damage, mitochondria become more swollen and disruption of oxidative phosphorylation deprives the cell of aerobic metabolism. The resulting collapse of many intracellular homeostatic mechanisms leads to progressive disintegration of nuclear and cytoplasmic organelles and release of lysosomal enzymes, leading to autodigestion of the cell.

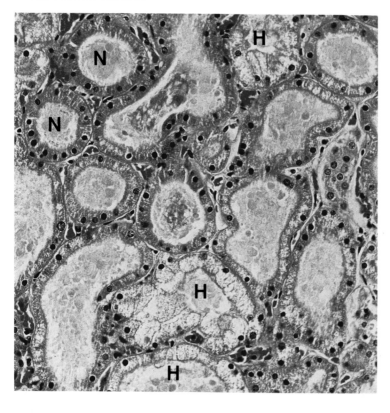

## Fig. 1.2 Hydropic degeneration: renal tubular cells (HP)

With light microscopy, one of the earliest discernible manifestations of metabolic disruption becomes evident when swelling of intracellular organelles and detachment of ribosomes leads to a loss of normal cytoplasmic basophilia and the cytoplasm assumes a pale staining appearance. This early, subtle change is known as *cloudy swelling* or *hydropic change* and is considered to be reversible. With further damage there is marked disruption of organelles and the cytoplasm becomes waterlogged. With the light microscope the cytoplasm appears swollen, pale and apparently vacuolated a condition described as *hydropic degeneration.*

This micrograph shows a section of renal cortex which has been exposed to hypoxia resulting in a condition known as *acute tubular necrosis.* Not all the tubules are equally affected; note in the same microscopic field some relatively normal looking renal tubules **N** exhibiting the usual degree of cytoplasmic basophilia, and those which are undergoing hydropic degeneration **H** showing cytoplasmic vacuolation, and consequent pallor, but with relatively intact nuclei.

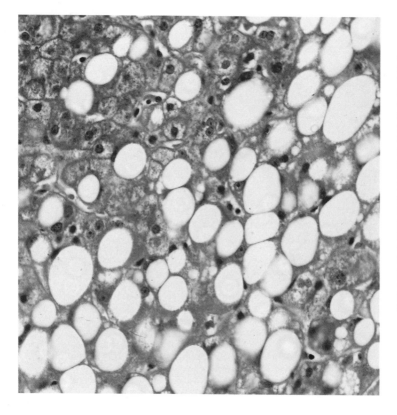

## Fig. 1.3 Fatty change: liver (HP)

*Fatty change* is another light microscopic manifestation of sublethal, usually chronic, metabolic derangement; this is most often seen in the liver, as in this example, but also occurs in the myocardium and the kidney. Hypoxia, toxins (particularly alcohol and halogenated organic solvents such as carbon tetrachloride) and diabetes are common causes. The cellular injury may be reversible if not too severe. Impaired lipid metabolism leads to intracellular accumulation of fat in the form of triglyceride droplets. Routine slide preparation techniques lead to removal of lipids before staining, thus lipid droplets are represented by unstained areas or so-called *vacuoles.* Fatty change in liver cells can be seen in alcoholic liver disease (see Fig. 13.2). Note the fat vacuolation often pushing the hepatocyte nucleus to one side. Not all cells are equally affected.

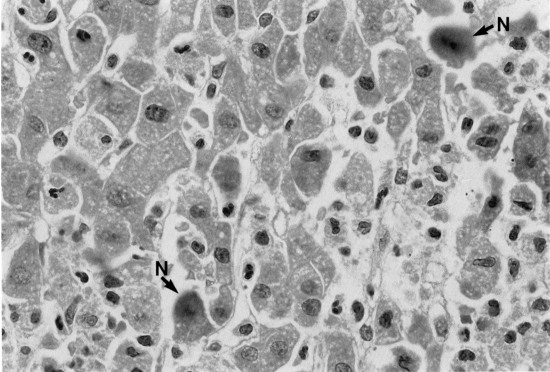

(a)

## Fig. 1.4 Cell necrosis
**(a) liver** (HP)
**(b) renal cortex** (HP)

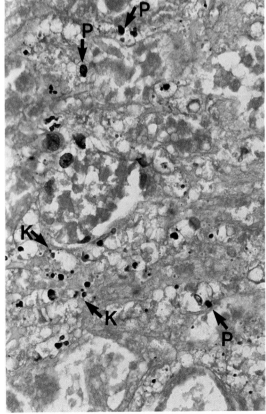

(b)

When a cell has sustained irreversible damage, a succession of morphological changes occur which are grouped under the term *cell necrosis*.

Micrograph (a) illustrates a section of liver severely damaged by an exogenous toxin. Most of the hepatocytes exhibit signs of early cloudy swelling, however several cells show the features of frank necrosis **N**. The dead cells have a homogenous eosinophilic (pink) cytoplasm when compared with the living cells. This cytoplasmic appearance is due to loss of basophilic RNA from the damaged rough endoplasmic reticulum, disorganization of mitochondria and exposure of increased numbers of acidophilic groups from breakdown of structural protein. The nuclei of the dead cells are smaller, more darkly stained and less well defined. This condensed nuclear appearance which is known as *pyknosis* is the end result of changes in which the nuclear chromatin becomes progressively clumped, possibly due to the low pH from anaerobic metabolism.

This nuclear change is also seen in micrograph (b) which is a portion of necrotic kidney; a pyknotic nucleus stands out as an intact rounded dark staining body **P**. Following this nuclear change there is breakdown of the nuclear membrane with fragmentation of the abnormally condensed and denatured nuclear chromatin. At first this is into several small dark staining bodies which represent pieces of denatured nuclear material. This is termed *karyorrhexis* **K**.

Further breakdown of nuclear material by intracellular enzymes leads to loss of the chemical groups which take up the purple haematoxylin dye. This process is termed *karyolysis*; when karyolysis is complete the dead cell is seen as an anucleate homogeneous mass of pink stained protein.

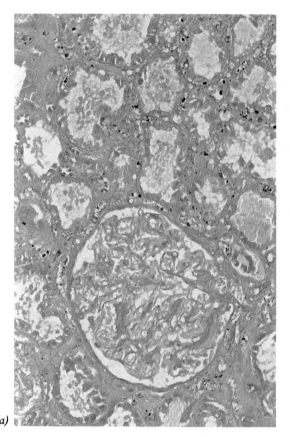

(a)

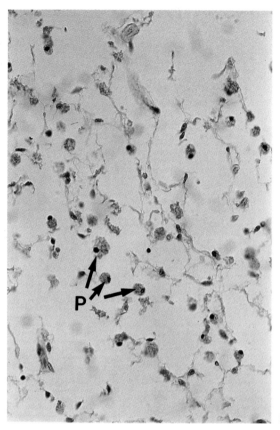

(b)

## Fig. 1.5   Patterns of tissue necrosis
## (a) coagulative necrosis of kidney (MP)
## (b) colliquative necrosis in brain (HP)

Traditionally, three main patterns of tissue necrosis have been recognized: *coagulative, colliquative* and *caseous.*

Caseous necrosis is a pattern where cells die and form a homogeneous pink staining mass of proteinaceous material in which no elements of former cell structure are discernible. This pattern is typically seen in tuberculosis.

In coagulative necrosis much of the original cell outline can be discerned in the necrotic areas although all the cell components are dead.

Colliquative necrosis was the term coined to describe the gross appearance of infarction in the brain at a stage when the dead area was replaced by semiliquid material. The terms 'coagulative' and 'colliquative' necrosis are archaic and of little relevance today. Increasing knowledge of the changes occurring in dead tissues indicates that there is an initial coagulative-like phase in all tissues, cell organization and outline being preserved although all cells are dead. This is even true of brain infarcts which are traditionally described as being colliquative. In brain, where extracellular structural proteins such as collagen and reticulin are minimal, cell death is rapidly followed by loss of architecture and formation of a semiliquid

mass of dead cells, fluid exudate, and reactive phagocytic cells. Thus the colliquative phase of cerebral infarction is really a phenomenon of organisation and healing, not the process of necrosis *per se.* Liquification of dead tissue in organs other than the brain is not common except in areas of necrosis which are associated with pyogenic bacteria such as in an abscess (see Fig. 2.13).

Micrograph (a) shows an area of necrotic kidney from the centre of a recent renal infarct. Note that the architecture can be still recognized although all tissues are dead and there is virtually no nuclear staining; the residual purple staining structures are pyknotic nuclei. Examples of caseous necrosis can be seen in many tuberculous lesions (see Figs 3.6 to 3.17). The early coagulative necrosis of brain is seen in Fig. 22.2(a) and the later colliquative phase in micrograph (b) above. Here at high power, no residual evidence of brain structure is present. The infarcted area is composed of phagocytic cells **P** which have engulfed debris from dead brain tissue. Wisps of pink proteinaceous material are seen representing fibres from astrocytic cells in the infarcted area.

# 2. Acute inflammation and sequelae

## Introduction

Living tissues may sustain injury from a wide variety of physical, chemical, microbial or immunological causes, and the usual response in dealing with resulting tissue damage or destruction is known as *inflammation*. Whatever the cause or type of tissue involved, the initial series of processes which classically ensues is described as *acute inflammation* and is directed towards neutralizing the injurious agents and to restoration of the tissue to useful function.

The characteristic feature of acute inflammation is the formation of an *inflammatory exudate* which has three principal constituents: fibrin, serum and leucocytes, predominantly neutrophils. The formation of the inflammatory exudate involves three vascular phenomena:

   (i) dilation of local blood vessels leading to engorgement with blood (*hyperaemia*);
   (ii) increased capillary permeability permitting plasma proteins to pass into the tissue;
   (iii) migration of leucocytes from blood vessels into the area of injured tissue.

The various stages in the evolution of the acute inflammatory response are shown in Figs 2.1 and 2.2 and typical examples are shown in Figs 2.3 to 2.5.

## Possible sequelae of acute inflammation

The outcome of acute inflammation depends on three major factors: the degree of tissue injury, the nature of the injurious agent and the type of tissue involved. When tissue damage is minimal, the exudate is reabsorbed into nearby vessels leaving no subsequent evidence of injury; this process is known as *resolution* and usually occurs after for example pneumonia (see Fig. 2.12) or a very minor burn such as sunburn. More frequently, the exudate undergoes a process called *organization and repair* in which dead tissue is removed by phagocytosis (see Fig. 2.6) and the defect is filled by a highly vascular connective tissue called *granulation tissue* (see Fig. 2.7); this then progressively undergoes *fibrous repair* with the formation of a dense fibrous scar at the site of the original tissue destruction (see Figs 2.8 to 2.10).

Depending on the type of tissue damage, there may also be some degree of *regeneration* of original tissue which depends on the ability of cells of mature tissue to undergo division. The most common example of regeneration is the proliferation of epithelium across a healing skin or mucous membrane wound. Another common example is the repair of a bone fracture (see Fig. 2.11). More surprising is the ability of liver hepatocytes to regenerate after major liver damage. Axons may also 'regenerate' after injury, however this only occurs if their cell bodies remain undamaged; since mature neurones cannot divide, this is not a true example of regeneration. When tissue damage is caused by certain types of bacteria such as staphylococci, then large numbers of dead and dying neutrophils accumulate with the fibrin and fluid of the acute inflammatory exudate to form a localized collection of *pus* known as an *acute abscess*.

In some circumstances, an injurious agent persists over a prolonged period causing continuing tissue destruction whilst at the same time the body is attempting to deal with previous tissue damage by the processes of acute inflammation, organization and repair; in such a case the damaged area may exhibit tissue necrosis, acute inflammatory exudate, granulation tissue and fibrous scar tissue concurrently. This process is known as *chronic inflammation* and is described in Chapter 3. The features of acute inflammation and its sequelae are summarized in Fig. 2.14.

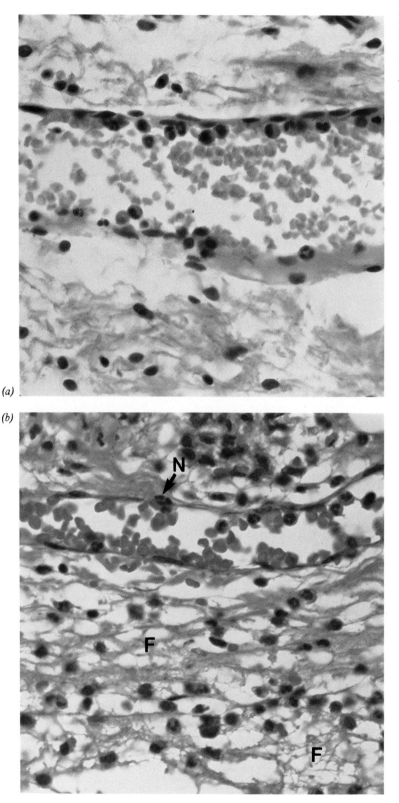

*(a)*

*(b)*

## Fig. 2.1   Stages in exudate formation
## (a) early vascular changes (HP)
## (b) early exudate formation (HP)

*Acute inflammation,* the classic response of tissue to injury, is characterized by the production of a protein-rich fluid exudate infiltrated by neutrophils. The process begins shortly after an area of tissue has been damaged when capillaries and postcapillary venules in adjacent healthy tissue become dilated and blood flow within them slows. The permeability of the vessel walls increases markedly causing plasma to leak out into the surrounding tissue, thus producing localized *oedema.* At the same time, neutrophils move to the periphery of the vessels and tend to become adherent to the endothelium; this process is known as *margination* and is best seen in micrograph (a). Note also in this illustration, the looseness and swelling of the connective tissue around the vessel due to the plasma exudate.

One of the plasma proteins which leaks from the vessels is fibrinogen. Once in the tissues, this normally soluble protein polymerizes to produce the insoluble fibrillar protein, *fibrin*; this forms an interwoven meshwork of fine strands **F**, which stain bright pink with the H & E stain as seen in micrograph (b). The marginated neutrophils pass through the vessel walls by first insinuating themselves through the gaps between adjacent endothelial cells, and then breaking through the underlying basement membrane. A neutrophil **N** in the process of passing through a vessel wall is seen in micrograph (b). Once outside the vessels, neutrophils migrate to the area of tissue damage. Later they are followed by monocytes, local macrophages (see Fig. 2.6) and some lymphocytes.

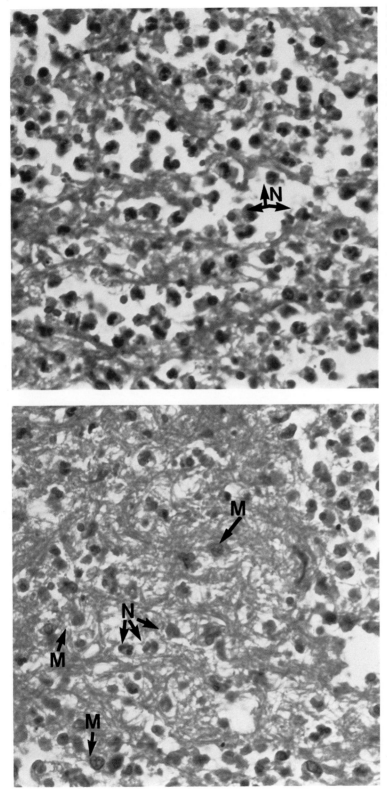

*(a)*

*(b)*

## Fig. 2.2  Acute inflammatory exudates
### (a) highly fluid exudate (HP)
### (b) highly fibrinous exudate (HP)

The predominant element of the acute inflammatory exudate may vary considerably depending on the state and nature of the injured tissues and the type of noxious agent involved. These two micrographs show established acute inflammatory exudates differing from one another in numbers of neutrophils **N** and amounts of fibrin present; the pink stained fibrin is relatively sparse in micrograph (a) but abundant in micrograph (b).

Once out in the extravascular tissues, neutrophils engulf necrotic fragments of damaged tissue, breaking them down with their lysosomal enzymes. When tissue damage is caused by living bacteria (e.g. as in lobar pneumonia seen in Fig. 2.5), neutrophils also phagocytose and destroy the bacteria. The activity of neutrophils is, however, limited by their inability to regenerate their lysosomal enzymes and after a burst of phagocytosis the neutrophils degenerate; nevertheless their numbers are sustained for some time by new arrivals from the circulation. Degenerate neutrophils can be recognized by the condensation (pyknosis) or fragmentation (karyorrhexis) of their nuclei and cytoplasmic disintegration; this is best demonstrated in micrograph (b).

The phagocytic role of neutrophils is later augmented by the arrival of macrophages, many derived from blood monocytes migrating from vessels in a similar manner to the neutrophils. Macrophages **M**, a few of which can be seen in micrograph (b), continue the phagocytic work begun by neutrophils and ultimately mop up the degenerate neutrophils and fibrin strands. Unlike neutrophils, macrophages can regenerate their lysosomal enzymes and are thus capable of sustained activity.

The fate of the acute inflammatory exudate depends upon a variety of factors including the nature and destructability of the injurious agent, the extent of tissue damage and the properties of the tissue in which the damage has occurred. The process of acute inflammation may proceed to one of four main possible outcomes: resolution, organization and repair, abscess formation or chronic inflammation.

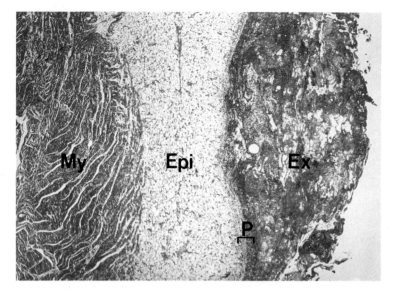

### Fig. 2.3    Acute pericarditis (LP)

When an acute inflammatory exudate forms on a serosal surface, the exudate is often dominated by the presence of large amounts of fibrin, producing a visible rough shaggy layer on the formerly smooth surface. This is seen commonly in acute pericarditis (as demonstrated here), acute pleurisy and acute peritonitis.

In this micrograph taken at low magnification, the exudate **Ex** is well established and is largely composed of dense masses of pink-staining fibrin with comparatively few neutrophils seen here as purple stained areas. On the extreme left is the myocardium **My** and in the centre is the epicardial fat **Epi**. The thickened pericardium **P** will show the early changes associated with organization of the exudate (see Figs 2.6 and 2.7).

### Fig. 2.4    Acute meningitis (LP)

Under other circumstances, very little fibrin is formed, and the exudate is almost entirely composed of oedema fluid and neutrophils. An example is acute meningitis as shown here, where the presence of pathogenic bacteria beneath the arachnoid excites the formation of an exudate rich in neutrophils but low in fibrin. This type of exudate most commonly occurs in response to a bacterial infection and is often described as *purulent* because of the mass of neutrophils.

In this micrograph, note the predominantly neutrophil exudate **Ex** lying between the brain tissue **B** and the arachnoid **A**, and in the sulcus between adjacent convolutions of the cerebral cortex, but not extending into the brain tissue. The small blood vessels **V** are markedly dilated and may be congested with blood.

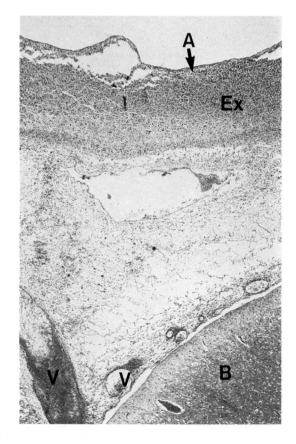

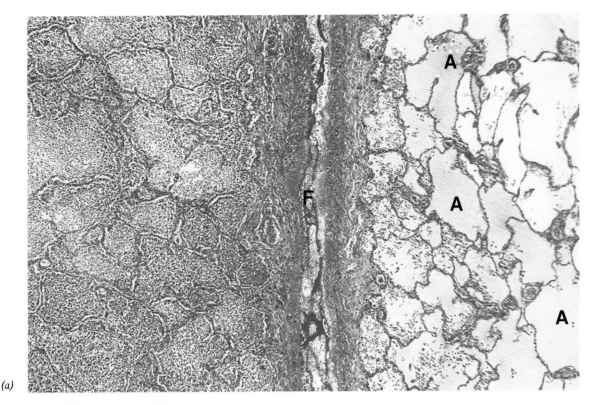

*(a)*

*(b)*

## Fig. 2.5   Lobar pneumonia
**(a)** (MP)
**(b)** (HP)

Lobar pneumonia describes a pattern of acute inflammation of
the lung where a whole lobe becomes solidified due to a
massive outpouring of fluid, fibrin and neutrophils into the
alveolar spaces. This pattern of pneumonia is most commonly
caused by the pneumococcus.

In micrograph (a) a portion of lung is shown with an
interlobar fissure **F** running vertically. The lung tissue on the
left shows obliteration of alveolar spaces by dark staining
masses of inflammatory cells and fibrin; this is termed
*consolidation*. Alveolar walls can just be discerned. The dense
inflammatory exudate is sharply limited by the interlobar
fissure. The lung on the right shows the earliest changes of
inflammation with engorged alveolar wall vessels and pale
pink-staining fluid in alveoli **A** representing an early serous
exudate. This pattern of pulmonary infection spreads through
the lung via alveoli and their interconnecting pores. Infection
is usually limited at interlobar fissures but in this case direct
extension is just beginning across the adjacent pleural surfaces.

At higher power in micrograph (b), alveolar walls are seen
with capillaries **C** engorged with blood. The alveolar spaces
are obliterated by a dense exudate of neutrophils and wispy
pink staining strands of fibrin. Occasional larger, pale
histiocytic cells **H** (macrophages) are present but these are few
in the acute phase of the disease.

If untreated there may be three consequences. Death may
occur, as in this patient. Complete resolution may occur with
restoration of normal structure and function (Fig. 2.12) or, less
commonly, the inflammatory exudate may become organized
with consequent fibrosis in the lungs.

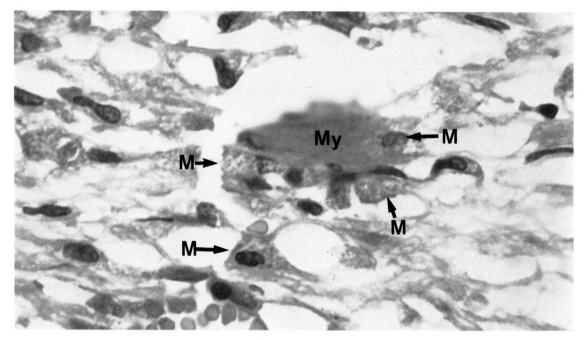

## Fig. 2.6   Macrophage accumulation (HP)

Under favourable conditions, the most common outcome of
acute inflammation is organization of the exudate by ingrowth
of highly vascular tissue and subsequent repair by fibrous
connective tissue. Once the acute inflammatory exudate is well
established, macrophages gradually migrate into the damaged
area and take over the phagocytic duties of neutrophils and
proceed to remove cell debris, dead neutrophils and fibrin.
Eventually all neutrophils and fibrin strands are cleared and
the space formerly occupied by damaged tissue is occupied by
macrophages and fluid; a variable number of lymphocytes and
plasma cells are also present reflecting an immune response to
any introduced antigens.

This micrograph shows an area of cardiac muscle which has
undergone necrosis following abrupt cessation of its arterial
supply. The acute inflammatory response to the damaged
tissue has almost run its course and the neutrophils and fibrin
predominant in the earlier stages have been removed by
macrophages. All that remains is a soft, loose tissue containing
a few necrotic myocardial remnants **My**, one of which is
shown here being engulfed by macrophages **M**; the
macrophages are usually identified by the brownish granules of
previously engulfed debris in their cytoplasm. Further details
of the sequence of changes in this particular lesion (myocardial
infarction) are shown in Fig. 9.3.

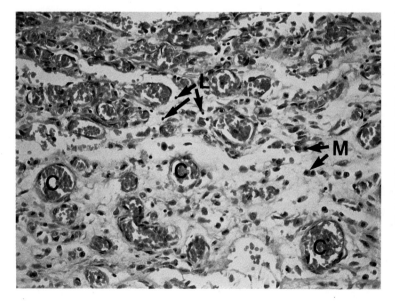

## Fig. 2.7   Vascular granulation tissue (HP)

The former site of tissue damage and
acute inflammation, now cleared of
debris, comes to be occupied by a highly
vascular tissue called *vascular granulation
tissue*. This is produced by ingrowth of
an extensive interconnecting capillary
network **C** as a result of budding and
proliferation of vessels in adjacent
undamaged tissue. Spaces between the
vascular channels are occupied by
residual macrophages **M** and
lymphocytes **L** most of which gradually
pass back into the lumina of the new
capillaries to re-enter the general
circulation.

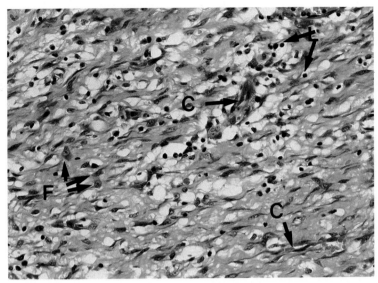

## Fig. 2.8  Fibrous granulation tissue (HP)

The spaces in the vascular meshwork vacated by the macrophages are now invaded by plump spindle-shaped fibroblasts growing in from the margins of the damaged area. The fibroblasts continue to proliferate forming collagen fibres and the capillary network undergoes progressive atrophy, eventually leaving only a few scattered vessels. The tissue is now known as *fibrous granulation tissue*.

In this micrograph, note the plump spindle-shaped appearance of active fibroblasts **F**, a few capillaries **C** persisting from the vascular granulation stage, and occasional lingering lymphocytes **L**.

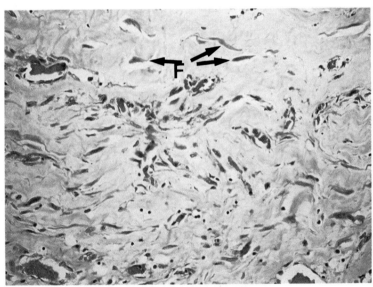

## Fig. 2.9  Fibrous scar tissue (HP)

Over a period of some weeks, fibroblasts in fibrous granulation tissue progressively lay down collagen fibres which become appropriately oriented to meet the functional stresses to which the new tissue is being subjected. Eventually, large amounts of collagen fill the tissue defect and the formerly plump, active fibroblasts became contracted, elongated and attenuated **F**, reflecting a relatively inactive state.

Thus the area of formerly damaged tissue becomes replaced by a *fibrous scar* composed of collagenous connective tissue and a few residual vessels. This micrograph shows a fibrous scar in the myocardium following tissue necrosis resulting from arterial occlusion (see also Fig. 9.4).

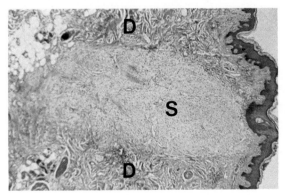

## Fig. 2.10  Skin scar (LP)

This micrograph illustrates a moderately recent but fully formed scar in skin after healing of a simple incision. Note the cellular fibroblastic tissue forming recent pale scar **S** replacing the normal coarse pink staining collagen bundles of the dermis **D**. At this stage of wound healing the epidermis has proliferated to cover the dermal scar. Note that there are no skin appendages present in the scar tissue. During the ensuing months and years the scar slowly contracts so that after many years the scar may be almost undetectable; this process, the result of interdigitation of parallel collagen fibres, is often referred to as *cicatrization*.

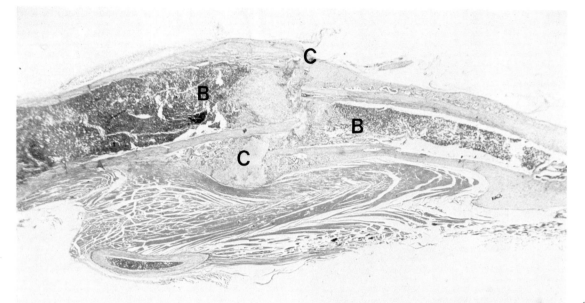

*(a)*

## Fig. 2.11   Specialized repair: repair of fractured bone

**(a)** (LP)
**(b)** (HP)

In most tissues, fibrous scar forms a functionally adequate albeit unspecialized replacement for damaged tissues. In certain circumstances however, the replacement of damaged tissue by fibrous scar is particularly inadequate for restoration of even partial function. In most damaged tissues, restoration of the original tissue type is rarely achievable and the healing process leads to scar formation. The repair of bone fractures is an important exception as the final product is not fibrous scar but refashioned new bone.

Following a fracture there is usually considerable bleeding into the bone. Acute inflammatory changes are usually inconspicuous and the main feature is the mass of coagulated blood termed a *haematoma*. The haematoma undergoes the process of organization in much the same way as described earlier with formation of vascular granulation tissue.

In the specific example of bone fracture, the granulation tissue is called *provisional callus* **C** and forms around the fractured ends of the bones **B** loosely uniting them; this is seen at low magnification in micrograph (a). Instead of producing large amounts of collagen, the fibroblastic cells in the fibrovascular granulation tissue **G**, shown in micrograph (b), differentiate into osteoblasts **O** which lay down pink staining osteoid **Os**; note that each island of osteoid is surrounded by a rim of active osteoblasts. On calcification, this forms the *bony callus* firmly uniting the bone ends. Extensive remodelling of this haphazardly formed new bone later leads to restoration of that bony architecture best adapted to resist local functional stresses. The regaining of full normal structure and function is known as *restitution*.

If the fracture site is not immobilized, this process cannot occur. Osteoid is then not formed, and healing occurs by the usual process of fibrous scar formation with dense collagen deposition. This is termed *fibrous non-union* and the result is unstable.

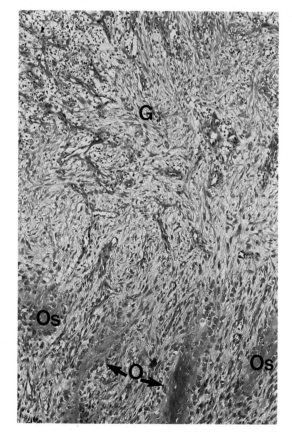

*(b)*

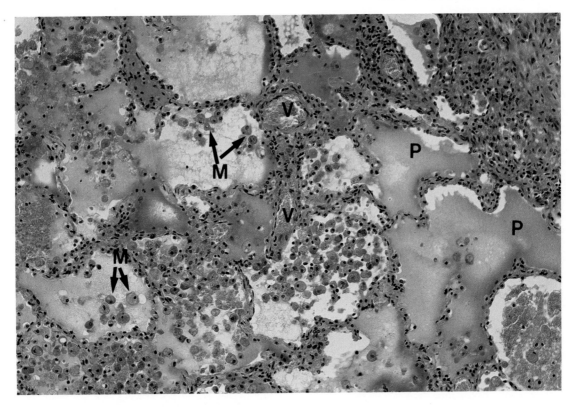

## Fig. 2.12  Resolution: lobar pneumonia (HP)

Occasionally, a potentially damaging stimulus may excite an acute inflammatory response even though the amount of tissue damage is minimal. In such circumstances, the process of *resolution* of the exudate may occur without proceeding to organization and repair and leaving no residual tissue scarring.

This phenomenon occurs in lobar pneumonia in which a florid acute inflammatory exudate fills the alveolar space of a lung lobe in response to the presence of bacteria, most commonly pneumococci, in the alveoli spaces (see Fig. 2.5). The bacteria are engulfed by neutrophils of the inflammatory exudate and fibrin strands are broken down by fibrinolysins derived from the plasma and neutrophil lysosomes. Macrophages **M** follow to mop up and destroy necrotic neutrophils, erythrocytes and other debris. Fluid and degraded proteins **P**, together with the macrophages, are then reabsorbed into the circulation via alveolar wall vessels **V** and interstitial lymphatics, leaving the alveoli clear for resumption of gaseous exchange. Regeneration of any damaged alveolar lining epithelium completes the return to normal structure and function. In this way a consolidated lung lobe may be restored to normal function in a matter of hours.

### Fig. 2.13   Abscess formation: lung (LP)

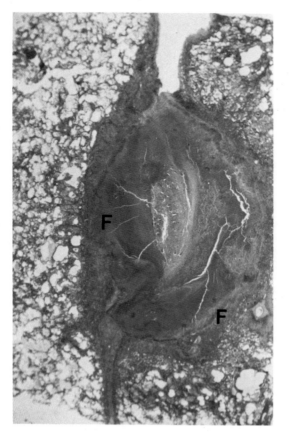

An abscess is a localized collection of pus, which usually develops following extensive tissue damage by one of the group of pyogenic (pus-forming) bacteria, such as *Staphylococcus aureus*; such organisms excite an inflammatory exudate in which neutrophils predominate. In these circumstances vast numbers of neutrophils die and release their lysosomal enzymes which autolyse the cells; the resulting viscous fluid, *pus*, contains dead and dying neutrophils, necrotic tissue debris and the fluid component of the inflammatory exudate with a little fibrin. Pyogenic bacteria often remain viable within the purulent contents of an abscess cavity and may cause persistent tissue damage leading to progressive enlargement of the lesion, which at this stage is described as an *acute abscess*. Usually at an early stage however, attempts are made to limit expansion of the lesion and minimize further tissue damage by the processes of organization and repair at the margins of the abscess. Thus the abscess may become walled off, isolating the bacteria-containing pus from adjacent tissue and preventing further tissue damage; an abscess with fibrous granulation tissue in its wall is known as a *chronic abscess*. On the other hand, if the bacteria are highly virulent and present in large numbers, such attempts at organization and repair may be overwhelmed, and expansion of the abscess continues by progressive tissue destruction at the periphery of the lesion. This coexistence of continuing tissue damage and attempts at organization and repair are an example of the process known as chronic inflammation, the subject of Chapter 3. Common examples of abscesses are boils, lung abscesses and renal cortical abscess in acute pyelonephritis.

The micrograph shows an abscess in a lung. The centre is composed of a purple staining mass of pus. At its margin with relatively intact lung is a pink staining zone of fibrin **F**. The lung immediately adjacent shows some consolidation but as yet there is little evidence of organization at the margins of the abscess; this therefore represents an acute abscess.

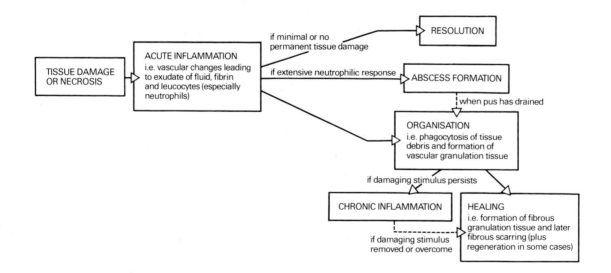

### Fig. 2.14   Acute inflammation and its sequelae

# 3. Chronic inflammation

## Introduction

In the previous chapter, the sequence of changes which follows an episode of tissue damage is described. An acute inflammatory reaction to the tissue damage or the presence of the injurious agent is usually followed by organization of the acute inflammatory exudate to form granulation tissue which fills the defect left by removal of the damaged tissue. This granulation tissue is gradually replaced by fibrous tissue which ultimately produces a fibrous scar at the site of damage. In most cases the injurious agent is destroyed or neutralized in the earliest stages of the acute inflammatory reaction, and the rest of the changes follow in sequence. Sometimes, however, the damaging stimulus persists despite the tissue responses directed at destroying or neutralizing it, and further episodes of tissue destruction may result. In such cirumstances the changes of tissue damage, acute inflammation, granulation tissue formation and attempts at fibrous repair may all proceed concurrently instead of sequentially as they do when the injurious agent is eliminated early in the sequence. This phenomenon is known as *chronic inflammation* and it most commonly follows previous acute inflammation where that process has failed to eradicate the damaging stimulus. The process is well demonstrated in chronic peptic ulceration (see Fig. 3.1), bronchiectasis (see Fig. 3.3) and ulcerative colitis (see Fig. 3.4).

Chronic inflammation also follows many acute abscesses; bacteria frequently survive and proliferate in the pus at the centre of the abscess cavity and are not easily accessible to endogenous or therapeutic bacteriocidal substances. The wall of a chronic abscess is composed of fibrous granulation tissue, with an inner zone of acute inflammatory exudate bordering the pus-filled cavity.

## Specific chronic inflammations

Less commonly, chronic inflammation occurs virtually *de novo* in response to specific damaging agents which are resistant to destruction by neutrophils during the acute inflammatory reaction or which fail to excite a strong acute reaction. Such noxious agents include microorganisms such as *Mycobacterium tuberculosis* (the causative organism of tuberculosis) and *Treponema pallidum* (the causative organism of syphilis), and foreign materials such as talc and beryllium; the tissue reactions which they provoke are collectively known as the *specific chronic inflammations*. When the damaging agent is not destroyed by neutrophils, the initial neutrophil response is usually sparse and short lived, and is quickly followed by a macrophage response which persists and dominates the histological picture. This local macrophage accumulation produces a discrete lesion called a *granuloma*, and the chronic inflammations characterized by this type of response e.g. tuberculosis, sarcoidosis etc are known as the *chronic granulomatous diseases*. Tuberculosis is of great pathological and clinical importance and its various manifestations are shown in Figs 3.6 to 3.17. Examples of sarcoidosis, syphilis and foreign body granulomata complete the chapter.

As the term implies, a notable feature of chronic inflammation is its prolonged course, reflecting a state of balance between recurrent tissue damage on the one hand, and continuing attempts to repair the damage by organization and repair on the other. The outcome of chronic inflammation thus depends on whether local and systemic factors favour the injurious agent (thereby leading to progressive tissue damage with enlargement of the lesion) or, alternatively, the attempts at healing and fibrous repair (resulting in shrinkage of the lesion and scar formation).

Since chronic inflammations are often of considerable duration, immunological mechanisms often play an important role, and infiltrations of lymphocytes and plasma cells are also a characteristic histological feature (see Fig. 3.2).

In summary, chronic inflammation is marked by continuing tissue damage, acute inflammatory exudation, organization and fibrous repair occurring concurrently rather than sequentially; the process is prolonged and is usually overlaid by immunological responses. It may be a result of inconclusive acute inflammation or may be a direct reaction to certain specific microorganisms or foreign bodies.

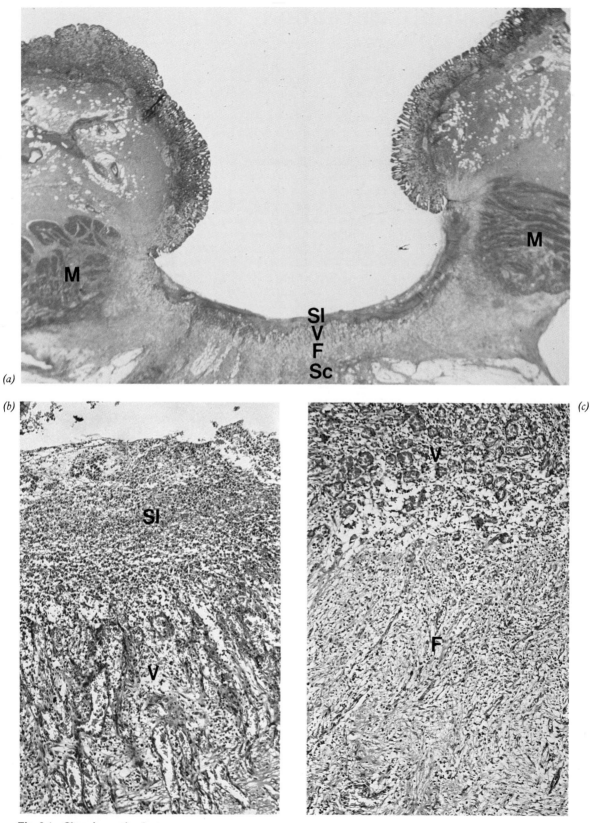

Fig. 3.1   Chronic peptic ulcer

## Fig. 3.1   Chronic peptic ulcer (illustrations opposite)
**(a) entire ulcer** (LP)
**(b) surface layers of the ulcer** (MP)
**(c) deep layers of the ulcer** (MP)

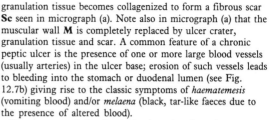

A common example which illustrates the principles of nonspecific chronic inflammation is the localized chronic ulceration of stomach, duodenum or lower oesophagus caused, in certain susceptible individuals, by the damaging effects of acidic gastric secretions; such lesions are collectively referred to as *chronic peptic ulcers.*

The lesion begins with initial breach of the surface mucous membrane which fails to heal rapidly; this allows access of the highly irritant gastric juices to the underlying submucosal tissues. Necrosis of the unprotected tissue then ensues, leading to the formation of an acute ulcer which progressively enlarges as deeper tissues become involved. Occasionally the process continues virtually unchecked through the full thickness of the gut wall causing perforation and escape of gastric or duodenal contents into the peritoneal cavity (see Fig. 12.7a). Most commonly however, the destructive process is checked by the formation of granulation tissue which then undergoes fibrous repair. Thus a temporary state of balance is reached in which the rate of granulation tissue formation (i.e. organization) and fibrous repair just keeps pace with the rate of tissue destruction by the gastric acid; this tenuous equilibrium may be maintained for months or even years.

A section through such a chronic ulcer is shown at low magnification in micrograph (a). The ulcerated surface is covered by a *slough* **Sl** composed of a pink staining thin layer of necrotic material mixed with the fibrin and leucocytes of an acute inflammatory exudate. Beneath the slough is a zone of predominantly vascular granulation tissue **V** which becomes progressively less vascular deeper in the wall where it merges with a zone of fibrous granulation tissue **F**; these features are seen at high magnification in micrograph (b). Micrograph (c) shows a deeper level of the ulcer floor where the vascular granulation tissue **V** gives way to more fibrous and less vascular, fibrous granulation tissue **F**. Deeper still, the fibrous

granulation tissue becomes collagenized to form a fibrous scar **Sc** seen in micrograph (a). Note also in micrograph (a) that the muscular wall **M** is completely replaced by ulcer crater, granulation tissue and scar. A common feature of a chronic peptic ulcer is the presence of one or more large blood vessels (usually arteries) in the ulcer base; erosion of such vessels leads to bleeding into the stomach or duodenal lumen (see Fig. 12.7b) giving rise to the classic symptoms of *haematemesis* (vomiting blood) and/or *melaena* (black, tar-like faeces due to the presence of altered blood).

The outcome of chronic peptic ulceration depends on whether local or systemic conditions favour the damaging stimulus i.e. gastric acid, or the reparative processes. In the latter case, fibrous tissue progressively fills the ulcer crater and, under favourable circumstances, mucosa regenerates from the ulcer margins to re-cover the surface thus protecting the underlying scar tissue from further attack by gastric acid. A healed peptic ulcer therefore consists of a localized area of fibrous scar replacing part or the full thickness of the muscular wall of the gut. Internally, the regenerated mucosa is usually puckered due to contraction of the underlying scarred muscular layer. Externally, the serosa may be thickened and exhibit fibrous adhesions to adjacent structures due to the organization of fibrinous exudate. The most important single factor which favours healing of a peptic ulcer is reduction of gastric acid; this may be achieved by ingestion of neutralizing solutions such as alkali, by diminishing mucosal gastric acid secretion by vagotomy, $H_2$ receptor antagonists or surgical resection of that part of the stomach containing the bulk of the acid-producing cells. Factors favouring the destructive process include excessive gastric acid secretion, which is difficult to reduce or neutralize (this is particularly relevant in duodenal ulceration), or diminished capacity for repair which may result from corticosteroid therapy.

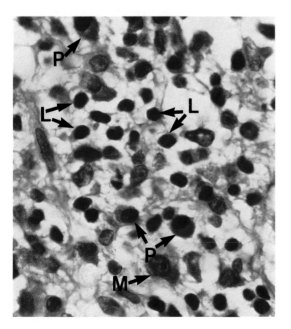

## Fig. 3.2   Chronic inflammatory cells (HP)

The term chronic inflammatory cells is used to indicate a cellular infiltrate composed of lymphocytes, plasma cells, and macrophages. In epithelial tissues such as in the gastro-intestinal tract and the nose, eosinophils are also commonly seen. Very occasional neutrophils may also be encountered.

This micrograph shows at high magnification, an inflammatory infiltrate in the stroma of a chronically inflamed uterine cervix. The cells are mainly plasma cells **P** with some lymphocytes **L** and occasional macrophages **M**.

A population of cells like this persists in an area of inflammation long after the active process of organization has occurred.

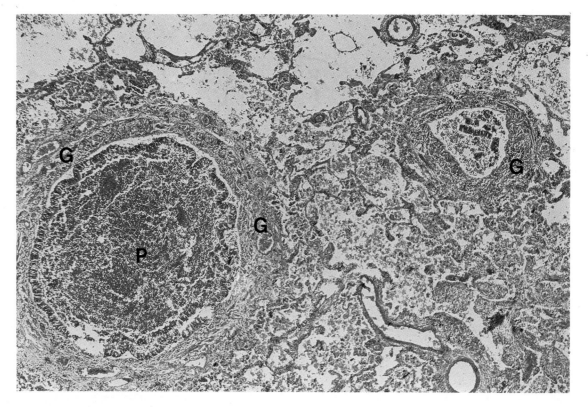

## Fig. 3.3 Bronchiectasis (LP)

*Bronchiectasis* is a chronic inflammation of the bronchi and bronchioles associated with permanent dilatation.

Repeated damage to the bronchial wall, usually the result of repeated episodes of bacterial infection, leads to progressive destruction of the normal elastic and muscular components of the airway wall. This is particularly likely to occur in airways which are partially or completely obstructed. The elastic and muscular components of the wall are replaced by fibrovascular granulation tissue and later by collagenous fibrous tissue; this process weakens the wall, leading to dilatation of the airway, which in turn predisposes to stagnation of secretions and further episodes of bacterial infection. In this micrograph note that the airway walls are formed by fibrovascular granulation tissue **G** in which there is heavy infiltration by small dark-staining chronic inflammatory cells, mainly lymphocytes. In the larger, more dilated bronchiole there is evidence of early bacterial infection, the lumen being filled with pus **P**.

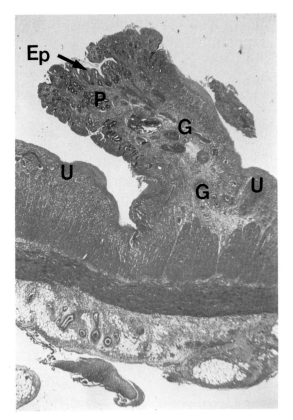

### Fig. 3.4  Ulcerative colitis (LP)

*Ulcerative colitis* is a chronic relapsing inflammatory disease of
the colon of unknown pathogenesis; it is characterised by
phases of relative quiescence punctuated by acute exacerbations
in which there is extensive mucosal and submucosal ulceration.
Between acute attacks the mucosa shows infiltration of its
lamina propria by chronic inflammatory cells (see Fig. 3.2).
During an acute attack, confluent areas of mucosal ulceration
**U** occur, leaving islands of chronically inflamed mucosa and
submucosa which may protrude, simulating small colonic
polyps. These so called pseudopolyps **P** bear remnants of
nonulcerated colonic epithelium **Ep**. The submucosa becomes
largely replaced by fibrovascular granulation tissue **G** with a
variable chronic inflammatory cell infiltrate. Ulcerative colitis
is illustrated in more detail in Fig. 12.13.

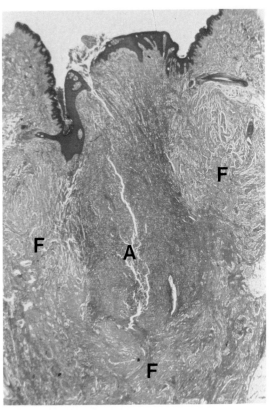

### Fig. 3.5  Pilonidal sinus (LP)

A common example of a chronic abscess is the *pilonidal sinus*.
In this condition a chronic subcutaneous abscess forms most
commonly in the sacrococcygeal area. Hair shafts, derived both
from locally destroyed follicles and possibly from shed body
hair, are present in the abscess and act as a nidus for persistent
chronic inflammation. Successful healing and repair are
hindered by the presence of foreign material which is resistant
to phagocytosis. Secondary infection may further complicate
the process. As part of the attempt at healing, epithelium
migrates from the skin surface and comes to line a track
leading down into the abscess cavity; such a track is known as
a *sinus*.

In this micrograph, note the subcutaneous abscess cavity **A**
the wall of which is formed by chronic inflammatory
granulation tissue heavily infiltrated by lymphocytes. There is
also marked surrounding fibrosis **F** in the dermis from the
continued attempts at fibrous repair.

A pilonidal sinus, like any other chronic inflammatory
lesion, will only heal if the source of persistent irritation is
removed; surgical excision often provides the only satisfactory
method in this situation.

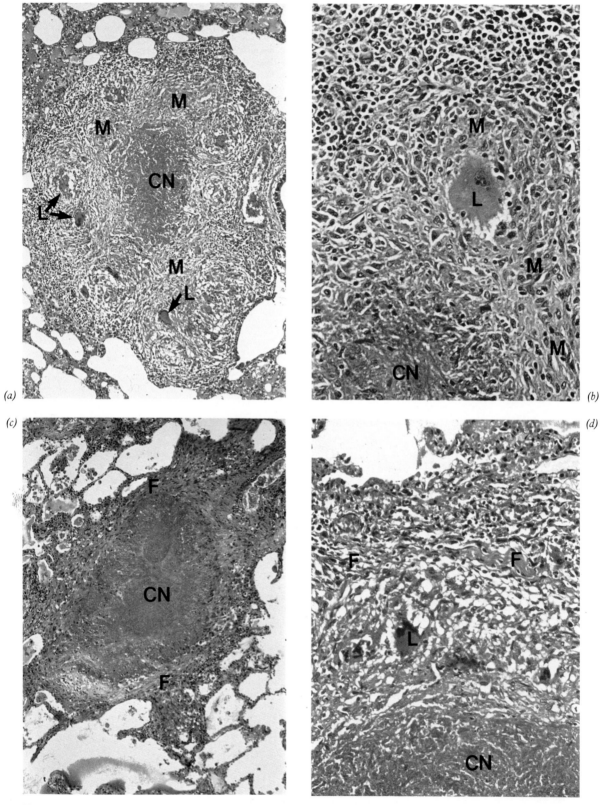

Fig. 3.6  **Early pulmonary tuberculosis**

## Fig. 3.6  Early pulmonary tuberculosis *(illustrations opposite)*
**(a) early tubercle** (MP)
**(b) early tubercle** (HP)
**(c) later tubercle** (MP)
**(d) later tubercle** (HP)

As described earlier, certain infecting organisms and foreign materials do not excite a full acute inflammatory reaction, but instead, almost from the outset, excite a response more typical of chronic inflammation. In this type of reaction, macrophages aggregate in the vicinity of the organisms to form a lesion traditionally called a *granuloma*. An example of this is tuberculosis, caused by the bacterium *Mycobacterium tuberculosis*; in this case the specific granuloma is known as a *tubercle*.

When tubercle bacilli gain access to the lungs by inhalation, they tend to localize in the periphery of the lung where they excite a transient and inconclusive neutrophil response. The organisms survive neutrophil enzyme activity, probably because of their thick and resistant glycolipid bacterial cell wall and the short life span of neutrophils. The tubercle bacilli are then ingested by macrophages although they may initially continue to divide within macrophage cytoplasm. The tubercle bacilli also antigenically stimulate some lymphocytes which thereby become 'sensitized'. The sensitized lymphocytes then produce various factors (lymphokines) which attract and 'activate' the macrophages, enhancing their ability to kill ingested tubercle bacilli. Such activated macrophages become large and develop granular eosinophilic cytoplasm and because of their supposed resemblance to epithelial cells, were formerly known as *epithelioid cells*. These cells form a major component of all granulomata including tubercles.

Micrograph (a) shows an entire tubercle at an early stage and (b) illustrates a sector of the same tubercle at higher magnification. At the centre of the tubercle is an area of caseous necrosis **CN** containing tubercle bacilli; these can only be demonstrated by specific staining methods for acid-fast bacilli. The caseous area is surrounded by a zone of plump macrophages **M** with abundant granular eosinophilic cytoplasm (epithelioid cells). Some of the macrophages fuse to produce large multinucleate giant cells called *Langhans' giant cells* **L**; a typical Langhans' giant cell is shown in more detail in Fig. 3.7. Peripheral to the macrophages, aggregation of lymphocytes occurs, indication of the involvement of immune mechanisms in the granulomatous response.

Progressive central caseous necrosis results in enlargement of the tubercle, although the zone of peripheral macrophages and lymphocytes becomes relatively thinner. These changes can be observed by comparing micrograph (a) with micrograph (c)

which shows a more advanced tubercle. With further development, spindle-shaped fibroblasts **F** appear in the peripheral lymphocytic zone of the tubercle where they begin to lay down collagen in the extracellular tissue; this process is evident in micrograph (c) and at higher magnification of the same specimen in (d).

At this stage, further changes in the tubercle can occur in one of two ways. If the tubercle bacilli are virulent and present in large numbers, and particularly if the body's resistence is low (as for example in a debilitated or immuno-suppressed patient), then the tubercle rapidly enlarges due to increasing caseous necrosis and the macrophage-lymphocyte-fibroblast defensive reaction is overwhelmed, failing to confine the infection; an example is seen in Fig. 3.10. On the other hand, if the balance of resistance and attacking factors is reversed, the macrophage-lymphocyte-fibroblast barrier resists enlargement of the tubercle, and proliferation of fibroblasts produces a firm shell confining the infection. Production of collagen by these fibroblasts further strengthens this capsule, imprisoning the necrotic tissue and its contained tubercle bacilli, and isolating the organisms from other susceptible tissue (see Fig. 3.8). Calcium salts may become deposited in the collagenous shell and necrotic centre. In the lung, carbon is also taken up by the macrophages of the granuloma.

In children, the initial tubercle in the lung is known as a *Ghon focus* and is usually situated in the subpleural area in the middle zone of the lung. This lesion rarely attains a large size and undergoes the process of fibrosis described above. Before the lung lesion is walled off however, tubercle bacilli pass via lymphatics to regional lymph nodes in the lung hilum where tubercles develop in a manner identical to the Ghon focus in the lung. The outcome of the infection depends on what happens to this tuberculous infection of the lymph nodes; possible outcomes are discussed in Figs 3.8 to 3.17.

In adults where previous exposure has afforded partial immunity, the pattern of infection is somewhat different. The initial lung lesion is usually located at the apex of the lung where it is known as an *Assmann focus*, and tends to enlarge and produce a cavitating abscess from whence further infection of the rest of the lungs may occur; regional lymph nodes are rarely involved. If host resistance is high, healing occurs by fibrosis in the same way as described above.

## Fig. 3.7  Langhans' giant cell (HP)

This micrograph illustrates a typical Langhans' giant cell formed by fusion of macrophages in a tuberculous granuloma. A ring of peripherally arranged nuclei characteristically encircles a faintly granular eosinophilic cytoplasm.

Although prominent in tuberculosis, similar multinucleate giant cells occur in other chronic inflammatory conditions such as leprosy and in response to the presence of certain nonlysable foreign bodies. In such conditions, the nonspecific term *foreign body giant cell* is usually applied.

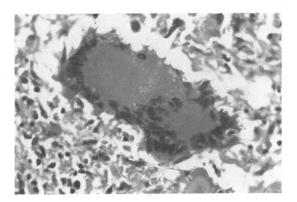

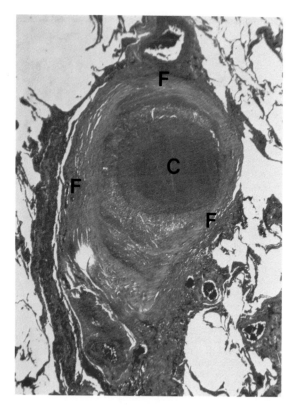

## Fig. 3.8 Fibrocaseous tuberculous nodule (LP)

In favourable circumstances, healing of tubercles occurs by proliferation of peripheral fibroblasts and deposition of an encircling wall of dense collagen (see Fig. 3.6). If the healing process is initiated at an early stage of tubercle formation as frequently occurs with a Ghon focus, then all that later remains is a small fibrous nodule often heavily calcified and containing little or no central caseous material. If the healing process supervenes at a later stage in tubercle development, then the fibrous shell often surrounds a mass of caseous material. Such a structure is called a *fibrocaseous tuberculous nodule* and is most frequently seen in healed, adult-pattern pulmonary tuberculosis where such nodules are usually located at the lung apices. Viable tubercle bacilli may remain dormant within the sequestered caseous material from which they may reinfect adjacent lung tissue should the restricting fibrous wall break down. This phenomenon, known as *reactivated fibrocaseous tuberculosis*, may occur when a patient becomes debilitated as in malnutrition or immunosuppressive therapy.

The fibrocaseous nodule illustrated here was taken from the lung apex of an adult whose pulmonary tuberculosis had been successfully treated by chemotherapy. A strong fibrous wall **F** completely encircles a mass of caseous necrotic material **C**. In this case there has been little calcium deposition.

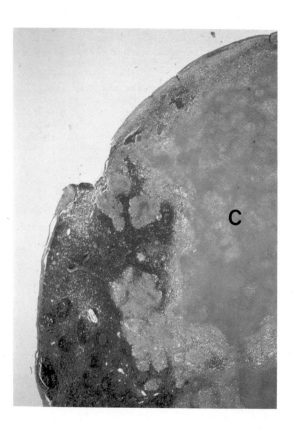

## Fig. 3.9 Tuberculous lymph node (LP)

With the formation of a Ghon focus in a child's lung, tubercle bacilli may pass via lung lymphatics to regional lymph nodes where they initiate caseous necrosis and tubercle formation similar to that in the lung. The combination of a Ghon focus in the lung and tuberculous regional (peribronchial) lymph nodes is called a *primary complex*.

The outcome of infection in a child depends on the fate of the lymph node lesion. If the child's defences are strong, healing of all the tubercles occurs by fibrosis as described previously; all that remains is a small fibrocalcific nodule in the lung periphery and similar lesions in the regional lymph nodes. On the other hand, if the patient's defence mechanisms are poor, the lymph node tubercle enlarges as a result of extensive caseous necrosis, tending to overwhelm the surrounding macrophage-lymphocyte-fibroblast reactions. The lymph node enlarges until its capsule is breached, then ruptures discharging caseous material, heavily populated by tubercle bacilli, into surrounding tissues. The enlarging node may ulcerate through nearby bronchial walls (see Fig. 3.10) or blood vessels (see Fig. 3.11) leading to extensive spread of the tubercle bacilli.

In this micrograph, the tubercle has greatly enlarged so that the lymph node has almost been destroyed by caseous necrosis **C** and the zone of cellular reaction around it is very thin and insignificant. The necrosis has almost reached the lymph node capsule; rupture is imminent.

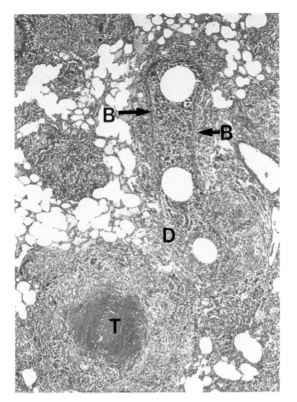

### Fig. 3.10    Tuberculous bronchopneumonia (MP)

When the wall of a bronchus is eroded by an enlarging tuberculous node or an apical Assmann focus, tubercle bacilli pass into the bronchial lumen from which they may be spread in various ways. If coughed up in sputum, the infection may be transmitted to other susceptible persons by droplet infection, sometimes infecting the patient's larynx (*tuberculous laryngitis*) on the way. Infected sputum may be swallowed and subsequently produce *tuberculous oesophagitis* or *ileitis*. Infected sputum may also gravitate to lower areas of the same or opposite lung where by destruction of a bronchiolar wall the organism may invade peribronchial lung tissue to form further caseating tubercles. This is called *tuberculous bronchopneumonia*.

In this example of an early lesion in tuberculous bronchopneumonia, note a segment of bronchiole containing infected material; the walls of the bronchiole are indicated by the arrows marked **B**. A segment of the bronchiolar wall has been destroyed **D** permitting access of bacilli which have initiated a caseating tubercle **T** in the nearby lung parenchyma. Large numbers of such lesions may form, merging with one another to produce a wide area of rapidly enlarging caseation usually in the lower lobes of the lungs. This is the pathogenesis of the once dreaded 'galloping consumption'.

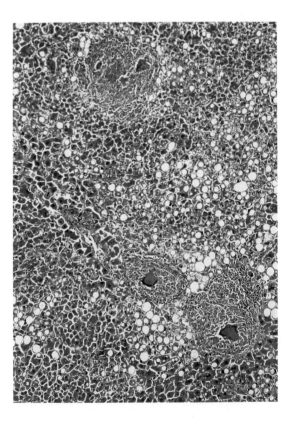

### Fig. 3.11    Miliary tuberculosis (MP)

If a ruptured tuberculous lymph node (or a rapidly enlarging Assmann focus in an adult) erodes a blood vessel wall, masses of tubercle bacilli are discharged into the circulation and may be carried along in the blood until they lodge in the microcirculation. When the eroded vessel is a branch of the pulmonary artery, the organisms are passed to other areas of the lung; when a pulmonary venous tributary is involved they are spread in the systemic circulation to many organs notably the liver, kidney and spleen. In this way, vast numbers of new tubercles may be produced throughout the body. Such multiple lesions rarely attain any great size because this occurrence usually produces rapid clinical deterioration and death; because the gross appearance of individual lesions resembles millet seeds, this condition is known as *miliary tuberculosis*.

In this illustration are three miliary tubercles in the liver, recently formed as a result of blood-borne spread from pulmonary tuberculosis. The centre of two of the new tubercles is formed by a Langhans' giant cell, and the third shows early central caseous necrosis.

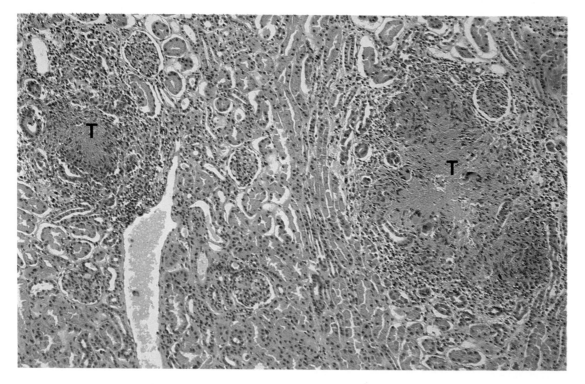

## Fig. 3.12  Renal tuberculosis (MP)

Most episodes of pulmonary tuberculous infection are well enough contained by local and systemic defence mechanisms that gross, blood-borne (miliary) tuberculosis does not occur, nevertheless it appears that a relatively small number of organisms can be disseminated via the bloodstream to a variety of other organs. For many reasons, probably including low bacterial virulence and high host resistance, most of these blood-borne bacilli are neutralized without initiating the formation of significant lesions in the organs in which they lodge. It seems that in certain tissues, some organisms remain viable but quiescent, only to become reactivated at a later date when the host's immune status is temporarily or permanently impaired; this is often long after the initial pulmonary lesion has completely healed. Active tuberculosis, with the formation of characteristic caseating granulomata, may then reappear in tissues remote from the original lesion and often many years

later. This phenomenon is known as *metastatic* or *isolated organ tuberculosis* and most commonly involves the kidneys, adrenals, meninges, bone, Fallopian tubes, endometrium and epididymis.

This micrograph illustrates renal involvement with the formation of small tubercles **T** in the renal cortex. The granulomata exhibit the classical central caseation of tuberculosis with larger tubercles tending to become confluent with adjacent lesions. Continuation of this process results in destruction of much of the renal cortex and medulla with eventual rupture of large confluent tubercles into the pelvicalyceal system which becomes distended with caseous material; this condition is known as *tuberculous pyonephrosis*. In more advanced cases, the infection spreads to involve the ureter and bladder. Renal tuberculosis is frequently bilateral and may result in renal failure.

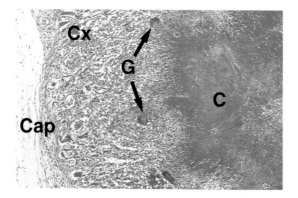

## Fig. 3.13  Adrenal tuberculosis (MP)

The adrenal glands are a common site of metastatic tuberculosis and bilateral caseous destruction of the adrenal cortex may be so extensive that the patient develops *Addison's disease* (adrenocortical insufficiency).

This micrograph illustrates part of an adrenal gland in which caseous material **C** occupies most of the cortex leaving only small surviving areas of cortical tissue **Cx** beneath the capsule **Cap**. Note the Langhans' giant cells **G** which are mainly seen near the margins of the lesion.

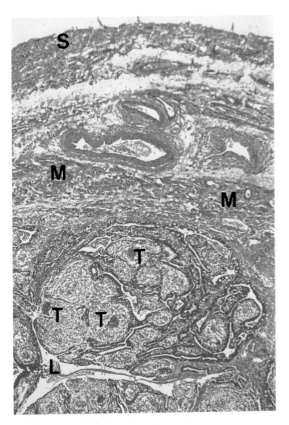

### Fig. 3.14   Tuberculous salpingitis (MP)

Tuberculous involvement of the Fallopian tubes is a common complication of pulmonary tuberculosis, particularly if this is contracted during adolescence. Tuberculous granulomata **T** develop in the mucosa of the Fallopian tube, producing gross thickening of the mucosa and encroachment upon the lumen **L**; the muscular wall **M** and serosa **S** in this example are relatively uninvolved. With healing, subsequent scarring often leads to distortion of the tube and obliteration of the tubal lumen, and tubal tuberculosis is thus an important cause of female infertility in some countries.

*Tuberculous salpingitis* is frequently accompanied by involvement of the endometrium and adjacent myometrium although *tuberculous endometritis* may also occur in isolation from salpingitis.

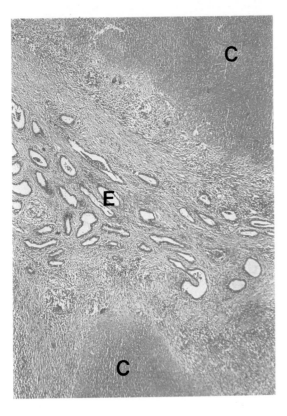

### Fig. 3.15   Epididymal tuberculosis (LP)

The male reproductive tract may also be infected by blood-borne spread of pulmonary tuberculosis; the epididymis is the most common site initially involved.

Enlargement of multiple tubercles leads to extensive areas of confluent caseation **C** leading to destruction and atrophy of epididymal tubules **E**; clinically, the epididymis may be thickened on palpation.

If untreated, epididymal infection may extend to involve adjacent areas of the testis. *Tuberculous epididymitis* is sometimes associated with tuberculous infection of the prostate and seminal vesicles; however these glands are more usually involved as an occasional complication of renal and urinary tract tuberculosis.

### Fig. 3.16   **Tuberculosis of bone** (MP)

Bone tuberculosis *(tuberculous osteomyelitis)* most frequently
affects the long bones and associated joints, and the vertebrae;
involvement of vertebrae often leads to spontaneous collapse
and is known as *Pott's disease.* In long bones, the infection
may produce a localized, painful, tumour-like swelling which
may drain to the skin to form a chronic sinus. Joint
involvement, *tuberculous arthritis*, is most common in children
and often affects the hips or joints associated with the
vertebrae *(tuberculous spondylitis)* as part of Pott's disease of the
spine.

As in other tissues, the characteristic tuberculous lesions are
caseating granulomata **G** which cause progressive destruction
of the bony trabeculae **B**. The infection tends to spread
extensively in the cancellous medullary bone leading to
necrosis of surrounding cortical bone.

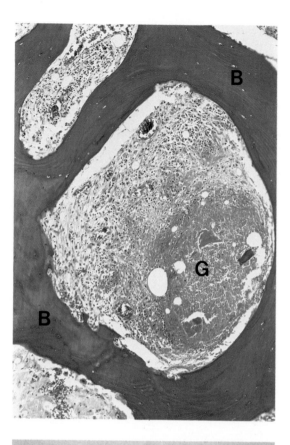

### Fig. 3.17   **Tuberculous meningitis** (MP)

Meningitis is a fatal although uncommon complication of
pulmonary tuberculosis; most commonly involved are the
meninges around the base of the brain and spinal cord.

Tuberculous granulomata **G** with characteristic central areas
of caseation develop in the leptomeninges and adjacent brain
tissue where they may damage cranial and spinal nerves.

Langhans' giant cells are relatively sparse in the granulomata
but a heavy infiltrate of lymphocytes is almost always present.
The presence of numerous lymphocytes in CSF obtained from
lumbar puncture is useful in distinguishing *tuberculous
meningitis* from purulent (bacterial) meningitis; in the latter
neutrophils are predominant.

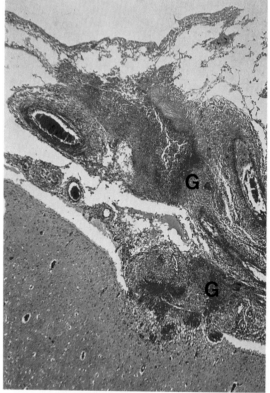

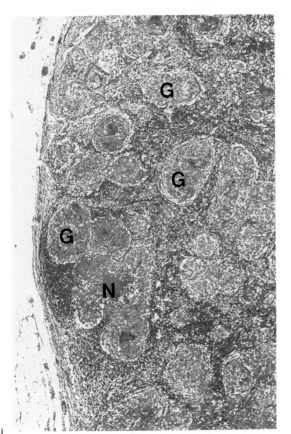

*(a)*

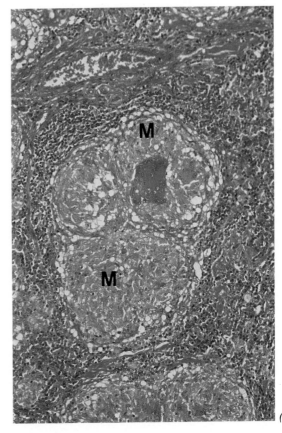

*(b)*

## Fig. 3.18 Sarcoidosis
### (a) sarcoidosis in a lymph node (MP)
### (b) sarcoid granulomata (HP)

*Sarcoidosis* is a chronic granulomatous inflammation of unknown aetiology characterized by the formation of multiple discrete granulomata similar in many respects to those of tuberculosis. In marked distinction to tuberculous granulomata, those of sarcoidosis do not typically undergo central caseation although small foci of necrosis may be seen in large granulomata. The sarcoid granuloma is largely composed of a broad zone of macrophages, but multinucleate giant cells are a feature of most of the granulomata. The cytoplasm of sarcoid giant cells may contain inclusion bodies of two types, star-shaped *asteroid bodies* or small laminated calcific concretions called *Schaumann's bodies*; in practice, these inclusion bodies are rarely seen. Although characteristic of sarcoid giant cells, such inclusion bodies are occasionally found in other chronic inflammatory granulomata.

Sarcoidosis may occur in any organ or tissue notably the spleen, liver, skin and lymph nodes but frequently also involves the lungs which may be peppered with numerous granulomata. In most cases of pulmonary sarcoidosis, the hilar lymph nodes are also grossly enlarged by masses of granulomata; such massive nodes are a useful diagnostic feature when visible on a chest radiograph.

Micrograph (a) illustrates part of a typical lymph node. Note the scattered noncaseating granulomata **G**; one larger granuloma exhibits a small area of necrosis **N**. Since there is no central mass of caseation, the sarcoid granuloma differs from the tuberculous granuloma by having a much broader zone of epithelioid macrophages. As in tuberculosis, sarcoid granulomata are surrounded by a zone of lymphocytic infiltration except that this feature is much less obvious in sarcoid lesions.

Micrograph (b) shows a typical sarcoid granuloma at high magnification. Note the broad zone of epithelioid macrophages **M** and prominent multinucleate giant cells.

Sarcoidosis is most commonly a chronic remitting disease often exhibiting no symptoms; in persistent cases the granulomata undergo progressive fibrosis although some giant cells still remain. In pulmonary sarcoidosis, the diffuse fibrosis may lead to chronic respiratory failure and its sequelae.

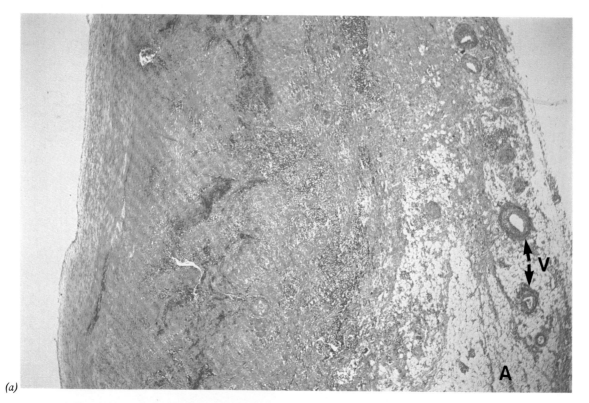

*(a)*

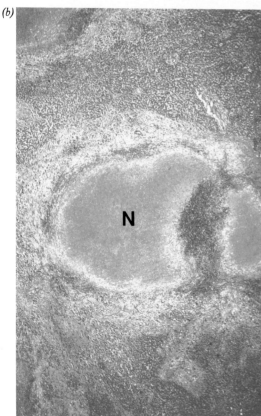

*(b)*

## Fig. 3.19 Syphilis
**(a) syphilitic aortitis** (MP)
**(b) syphilitic gumma of the liver** (LP)

Although now relatively uncommon, late stage syphilis is still regarded as one of the classic examples of specific chronic inflammation. The infecting organism, the spiral-shaped *Treponema pallidum*, resists usual tissue defences and excites a progression of fascinating pathological and clinical phenomena which represent typical chronic inflammatory responses with superimposed hypersensitivity reactions mounted by the immune system. Classically the condition proceeds through three stages extending over a long period.

In brief, the organism usually gains access to the body by penetrating the genital skin where it produces a single, small primary lesion known as a *chancre*. The chancre is a raised, reddened nodule caused by an intense local accumulation of plasma cells and lymphocytes in the subepithelial connective tissue. The chancre may ulcerate at this stage, but is often painless and may easily pass unnoticed. By the time the chancre has developed, the organism has multiplied extensively and has been disseminated via local lymphatics to regional lymph nodes and thence into the bloodstream causing a generalized bacteraemia. The chancre and concomitant bacteraemia (*primary syphilis*) are followed some weeks or months later by a transient *secondary stage* characterized by a widespread variable skin rash often with moist warty genital lesions and ulceration of the oral mucosa. These various mucosal lesions are histologically similar to the primary chancre and are full of spirochaetes. The syphilis is now at its most contagious yet the patient usually feels well and the only other evidence of a generalized infection is a widespread lymphadenopathy and positive serological findings.

In most untreated cases, the infection is effectively resolved by body defences and in many of these even serological evidence of previous infection disappears. Unfortunately, a proportion of untreated cases proceed from the secondary stage to the formation of *tertiary syphilis* after a variable interval of from one to many years. The lesions of tertiary syphilis may be either focal or diffuse and it is the focal lesion of tertiary syphilis, known as the *gumma*, which exhibits many of the features of a granulomatous inflammation. Tertiary lesions may occur in almost any organ or tissue and the clinical consequences vary enormously. The diffuse form of tertiary syphilis most notably involves the cardiovascular system, particularly the aorta, and less commonly the central nervous system; the well known tabes dorsalis and general paralysis of the insane are two of the manifestations of diffuse neurosyphilis. In the focal form of tertiary syphilis, gummata may develop in the liver, bone, testes and other sites, the clinical outcome depending on the nature and extent of local tissue destruction.

Micrograph (b) illustrates the classical appearance of a gumma. The active gumma has a central area of homogeneous coagulative necrosis **N** surrounded by a zone of cells typical of chronic granulomatous inflammation namely 'epithelioid' macrophages, lymphocytes, plasma cells and plump fibroblasts. Fibrous healing of liver gummata may produce a pattern of coarse deep scars dividing the liver surface into numerous irregular lobules; this condition is known as *hepar lobatum*.

Micrograph (a) illustrates *syphilitic aortitis*, the most common form of diffuse tertiary syphilitic lesion. The characteristic feature of diffuse tertiary syphilis, and also of primary and secondary syphilitic lesions, is a low grade chronic vasculitis of small vessels which exhibit thickening of the wall and a perivascular cuff of lymphocytes and plasma cells. In the aorta, the vasculitis affects the vasa vasorum **V** of the tunica

adventitia **A** and their smaller branches which extend into the tunica media; the blue stained areas in the tunica media represent lymphocytic cuffing around numerous small vessels. The smooth muscle and elastic fibres of the media undergo necrosis, probably due to ischaemia, and subsequent fibrous scarring. This leads to loss of elasticity and contractility in the aortic wall which becomes progressively stretched with the formation of an *aortic aneurysm*, usually in the ascending aorta or aortic arch.

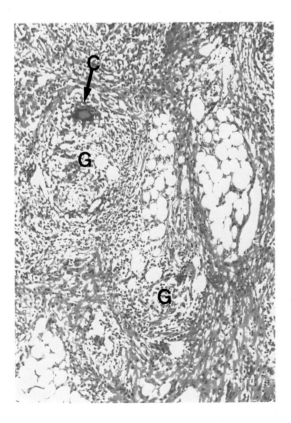

### Fig. 3.20 Talc granuloma (MP)

The presence of certain nonlysable foreign materials in the tissues may excite a chronic granulomatous inflammatory response similar to that seen in sarcoidosis. Common examples of such *foreign body reactions* are those produced by talc and starch (introduced into the tissues as glove powder during surgical procedures), suture material, wood, metal or glass splinters, and inorganic materials such as silica and beryllium inhaled deep into the lungs during industrial dust exposure. Inhaled materials are of particular clinical importance because of their tendency to produce progressive pulmonary fibrosis similar to that which may occur in sarcoidosis. Many of these foreign bodies are refractile when viewed with polarized light and can be identified within the granulomata or giant cells.

This micrograph illustrates granulomata **G** formed in the peritoneum in response to the introduction of talc particles during surgery. Foreign body giant cells **C** are a characteristic feature; the actual talc particles are too small to be seen. This trivial lesion was an incidental finding at autopsy.

# 4. Amyloidosis

## Introduction

Amyloidosis is a condition in which a homogeneous acellular material known as *amyloid* is deposited in a wide variety of tissues and organs. Early microscopists applied the term amyloid to this deposit in the mistaken belief that it was a form of starch, however it is now known that amyloid is protein in nature. In common H&E preparations, amyloid is uniformly eosinophilic (pink stained), and it stains orange-red with the dyes Congo and Sirius red; these latter methods are commonly employed in histological diagnosis.

Amyloidosis may involve almost any tissue, but most commonly affects the kidneys, spleen, liver, adrenals and heart. It is deposited almost exclusively in extracellular sites with a particular predilection for blood vessel walls. Continuing deposition may lead to partial or complete occlusion of vascular channels, and encroachment upon, and destruction of, parenchymal cells; such loss of functioning cells may have serious clinical consequences when vital organs are involved.

Electron microscopy has shown amyloid to be composed of masses of tangled unbranched fibrils, each fibril being 8–10 nm in diameter (see Fig. 4.1). Biochemical and immunochemical studies have shown that the fibrillar amyloid protein is composed of chains of amino acids arranged in a $\beta$-pleated sheet pattern. Recent work on the sequencing of the amino acid residues has suggested that distinct subtypes of amyloid may exist, and this forms the basis for a proposed chemical/immunochemical classification of amyloid. One subtype (*immunoamyloid*) contains sequences of amino acids which are almost identical to those seen in the variable region of the short chains of IgG molecules.

The following is a simple working classification of amyloid based on its clinical associations:

(i) *Amyloid associated with chronic inflammatory disorders*, both infective (e.g. tuberculosis, chronic osteomyelitis) and noninfective (e.g. rheumatoid arthritis)

(ii) *Tumour-associated amyloid.* Nearly 15% of all patients with the plasma cell tumour, myeloma (see Fig. 15.7), eventually develop amyloidosis. It occurs much less commonly in association with Hodgkin's disease and renal adenocarcinoma. An unusual association between tumour and amyloid occurs in medullary carcinoma of the thyroid (see Fig. 4.6).

(iii) *Heredofamilial amyloid;* for example, in association with familial Mediterranean fever, or in other familial amyloid syndromes such as cardiac amyloid (see Fig. 4.5).

(iv) *Senile amyloid,* mainly involving the heart.

Most examples of amyloidosis fall within one of the above groups, but a few remain in which there is no apparent clinical association; these cases are classified as *primary amyloid*, a category which is shrinking as more clinical associations are becoming recognized.

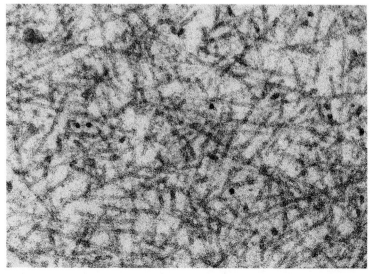

### Fig. 4.1 Amyloid ultrastructure: kidney (EM)

This electron micrograph shows amyloid in a renal glomerulus; it was present in capillary basement membranes and also within the mesangium.

The amyloid can be seen to have a fibrillar ultrastructure which is highly characteristic.

Electron microscopy provides a useful diagnostic aid particularly when the amyloid is present in small amounts or does not react with special stains used for its identification by light microscopy.

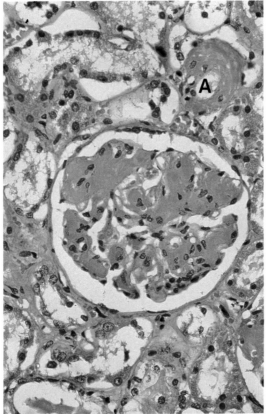

(a)

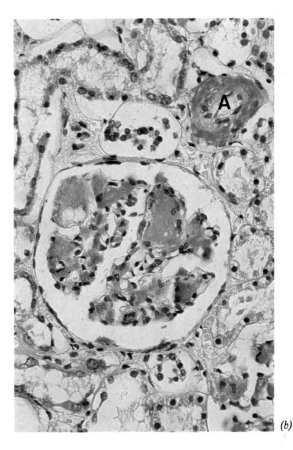

(b)

## Fig. 4.2   Renal amyloidosis
(a) H&E (HP)
(b) Sirius red (HP)

The kidneys are the organs most commonly involved by systemic amyloidosis and renal failure is one of the most serious clinical complications, accounting for the majority of deaths from the disease. These sections from the same glomerulus are from an autopsy specimen taken from a 58 year old woman with a 20 year history of rheumatoid arthritis; the sections have been stained with contrasting histological methods to illustrate the principal features.

Amyloid deposition usually begins in the glomerular mesangium and around glomerular capillary basement membranes, leading to progressive obliteration of capillary lumina, destruction of glomerular endothelial, mesangial and podocyte cells and eventually almost complete replacement of glomeruli by confluent masses of amyloid. Concurrently, the walls of renal arteries and arterioles **A** may become infiltrated

by amyloid, causing diminished blood supply and increasing renal ischaemia. Interstitial spaces between renal tubules may also become infiltrated further compromising already ischaemic tubules which undergo marked atrophy. With the H&E staining method as in micrograph (a) the amyloid is a homogeneous eosinophilic (pink stained) material difficult to distinguish from normal structures. Staining methods such as Congo red or Sirius red as in micrograph (b) readily distinguish the amyloid which stands out as red stained material, in this case in the glomerulus and afferent arteriole.

Amyloid of the kidney usually presents with proteinuria, often severe enough to produce the nephrotic syndrome. As increasing amyloid deposition leads to glomerular ischaemia and tubular atrophy, chronic renal failure supervenes.

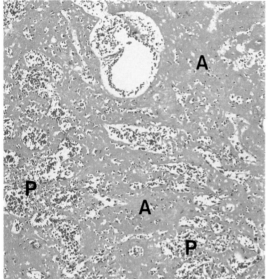

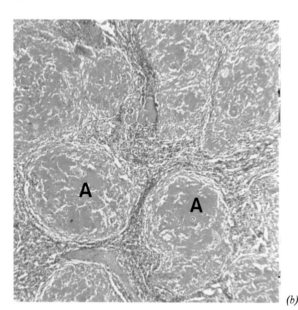

*(a)*                                                                                          *(b)*

## Fig. 4.3   Splenic amyloidosis
## (a) diffuse (lardaceous) type (MP)
## (b) 'Sago' spleen (MP)

There are two patterns of amyloid deposition seen in the
spleen described as either *diffuse* or *nodular*.

Micrograph (a) shows the more common diffuse pattern.
*Splenic amyloidosis* most commonly begins with deposition of
amyloid in the walls of splenic sinuses. With progressive
accumulation, the deposits coalesce to form large diffuse pink
staining amyloid masses **A**, leaving some intervening splenic
red pulp **P** and lymphoid tissue (white pulp, not seen in this
specimen). This form is sometimes termed *'lardaceous'* because

of the macroscopic waxy firmness of the spleen when cut.

Less commonly, amyloid deposition results in the formation
of the so called *'sago' spleen* as illustrated in micrograph (b). In
this pattern amyloid **A** becomes deposited within the
periarteriolar lymphoid sheaths (white pulp), giving the gross
appearance of discrete deposits on the cut surface. Note the
small vessels in the centre of the pink staining nodular amyloid
deposits.

## Fig. 4.4   Hepatic amyloidosis (HP)

In the liver, amyloid is initially deposited
in the space of Disse but progressively
extends to constrict the hepatic sinusoids
and compress the hepatic parenchymal
cells. As the condition becomes more
advanced as in this specimen (from the
same patient as the spleen in Fig. 4.3 (a)
above), ribbon-like pink staining deposits
of amyloid **A** are laid down in the
sinusoids. Hepatic cells become
compressed and undergo atrophy.

Even when liver involvement is severe
there is rarely significant clinical
evidence of impaired liver function
although the liver may be grossly
enlarged with a smooth surface and firm
consistency.

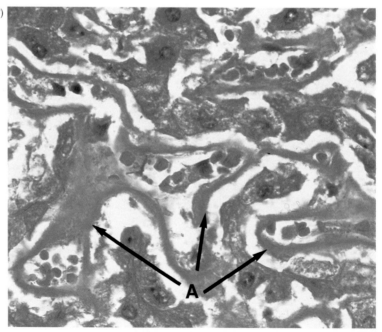

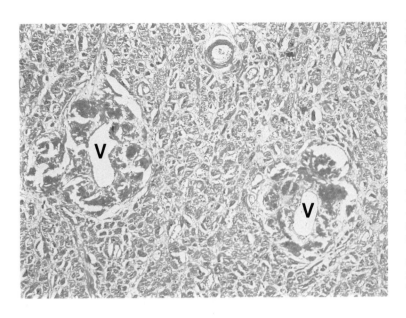

### Fig. 4.5   Cardiac amyloid: heredofamilial type (MP)

Amyloid involvement of the heart is discovered frequently as an incidental postmortem finding in the elderly, and in such cases it usually represents *senile amyloidosis*. The most severe form of cardiac involvement is seen in *heredofamilial amyloidosis* as illustrated in this micrograph; amyloid accumulates in the walls of vessels **V**, and may extend to form masses within the myocardium.

Myocardial involvement leads to reduction of effective myocardial tissue with subsequent intractable heart failure, whilst subendocardial amyloid may interfere with the conducting system causing arrythmias.

This specimen is from a 29 year old man who died of congestive cardiac failure; his father died at about the same age with similar symptoms.

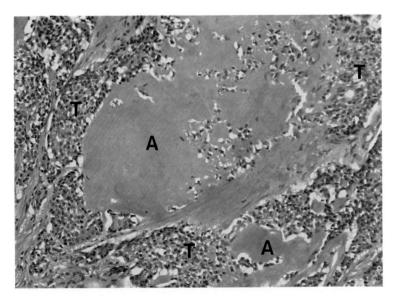

### Fig. 4.6   Medullary carcinoma of thyroid (MP)

Systemic amyloidosis involving various tissues may be associated with some tumours, particularly myeloma and renal adenocarcinoma. One particular tumour, the *medullary carcinoma of thyroid*, is of special interest in that masses of amyloid are found only within the tumour itself. Medullary carcinoma of thyroid is a tumour of thyroid 'C' (parafollicular) cells which secrete calcitonin and is an APUD tumour (see Chapter 6).

Histologically, the tumour is composed of tightly packed small cells **T** with masses of amyloid **A** in the interstitium.

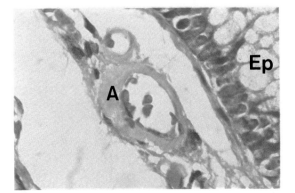

### Fig. 4.7   Vessel amyloid in rectal biopsy (HP)

The diagnosis of systemic amyloidosis can only be confirmed by positive tissue biopsy findings and in clinical practice the rectum is the most frequently biopsied site, although gingival biopsy is also employed in some centres.

In rectal biopsies, amyloid can be detected in the submucosal blood vessels in 60 to 75% of cases of generalized amyloidosis.

This micrograph, taken at very high magnification, shows rectal glandular epithelium **Ep** with a small blood vessel in the underlying lamina propria. Note that the vessel wall is thickened by homogeneous pink staining amyloid **A**. Amyloid in small vessels is a subtle feature in many cases. Confirmation of the diagnosis may be made by using a stain such as Congo red.

# 5. Disorders of growth

## Introduction

Cells respond to environmental changes in several fundamentally different ways depending on the nature of the stimulus. If the stimulus is overwhelming, then the cell may undergo degeneration or cell death (see Chapter 1). Many less noxious stimuli cause cells to adapt by changing their pattern of growth. Changes in growth pattern may involve change in the size of cells, change in the differentiation of cells, or change in the rate of cell division. Within an organ composed of several different types of cell, these processes may occur in only one of the constituent cell types thus altering the relative proportions of cells within the organ. The consequence of this adaptive response in an organ may be an alteration in structure and hence function. In many instances such changes in growth pattern are normal physiological events, as in the menstrual cycle, while in other instances these changes occur in response to abnormal pathological stimuli.

The normal pattern of cell growth in an organ depends on factors inherent in the cells as well as extrinsic environmental factors. Intrinsically, cells may be divided into three types by their capacity for cell division. Some cells, such as squamous cells in the epidermis, divide and replicate continuously. Others, such as liver cells, are capable of cell division in response to certain demands (such as partial hepatectomy) and are described as facultative dividers. Some cells, typified by neurones and cardiac muscle cells, are unable to divide and are described as nonreplicators. Thus the heart and brain have no capacity to regenerate further functional tissue. Extrinsic to the cell, factors such as blood supply, nervous innervation, hormonal stimulation, physical stress, or biochemical alterations will determine the normal pattern of cell growth in an organ or tissue. Depending on the intrinsic characteristics of a particular cell type, a change in environment may result in a change in the growth pattern.

## Increased cell mass

Certain organs may respond to environmental stimulation by an increase in functional cell mass. There are two mechanisms by which this occurs:

   (i)  increase in cell number as a consequence of cell division; this is termed *hyperplasia*.

   (ii)  increase in the volume of the existing cells; this is termed *hypertrophy*.

In practice, increase in functional cell mass is more often due to a combination of both hyperplasia and hypertrophy e.g. myometrium in pregnancy (Fig. 5.3). Hypertrophy occurs in skeletal muscle in response to exercise and in myocardial muscle in response to increased demand on cardiac function. Hypertrophy also occurs in the muscle of a viscus which is obstructed such as small bowel proximal to an obstructing tumour (see Fig. 5.1).

Hyperplasia occurs in the parathyroid gland in response to increased demand for parathormone in hypocalcaemia (see Fig. 19.6). Thickening of the epidermis in response to local trauma is due to hyperplasia of the squamous epithelium. Hyperplasia occurs most commonly in response to endocrine stimuli and in target endocrine glands in particular; a classic example is endometrial proliferation during the menstrual cycle (Fig. 5.2). For poorly understood reasons, the process of hyperplasia may not be uniform throughout an organ or tissue; in these instances, nodules of excessive cell growth arise in between areas of unaltered cell growth. This phenomenon, known as *nodular hyperplasia*, is seen in the thyroid gland (see Fig. 19.4), the adrenal gland (see Fig. 19.9), the prostate gland (see Fig. 18.5) and the breast (see Fig. 17.2).

A cardinal feature of the forms of increased cell mass described above is that following removal of the environmental stimulus, the altered pattern of growth ceases and usually the tissue reverts to its former state. Hypertrophy and hyperplasia can in many circumstances be regarded as normal physiological adaptations, as exemplified by exercise-induced skeletal muscle hypertrophy, and hyperplasia and hypertrophy of the pregnant myometrium. Many pathological stimuli on the other hand, may also invoke the responses of hypertrophy and hyperplasia.

## Reduction in functional cell mass

When the mass of functioning cells in a tissue is reduced, the tissue is then said to have undergone *atrophy*. The mechanisms of atrophy may involve reduction in cell volume or in cell number, both leading to a reduction in functional capacity. Grossly, the appearance of the tissue depends on whether the functional cell loss is replaced by other tissue. Commonly, when atrophy occurs, the lost cells are replaced by either adipose or fibrous tissue thus maintaining the overall size of the organ; when adipose or fibrous replacement does not occur then the overall size of the organ is reduced. Examples are the testis in the elderly (see Fig. 5.4) and the adrenal gland when suppressed by exogenous steroid administration (see Fig. 19.7b). Atrophy may occur as a physiological event, when it is usually termed *involution*. An example is the normal involution of the thymus gland during adolescence.

Atrophy must be distinguished from *hypoplasia*, a condition where there is incomplete growth of an organ, and *agenesis*, a condition where there is complete failure of growth of an organ during embryological development. In general, conditions opposite to those causing hypertrophy or hyperplasia cause atrophy. Thus disuse of skeletal muscle will result in a loss of cell mass. Removal of endocrine stimulation causes atrophy in target organs. Reduction in blood supply to a tissue may result in loss of functional cells; this is termed *ischaemic atrophy* and is seen commonly in the kidney.

In many atrophic tissues, a brown pigment accumulates within the shrunken cells which is termed *lipofuscin*. This is thought to represent degenerate lipid material produced by breakdown of the cellular constituents and taken up into secondary lysosomes. It accumulates particularly in the atrophic myocardial fibres of the hearts of elderly people and gives rise to the term *brown atrophy*.

## Change in cell differentiation

When cells adapt to a change in environment by altering their morphological appearance, this is termed *metaplasia*. Metaplasia is thought to be an adaptive response which produces cells better equipped to withstand a new environment. For example, in the bronchi, the respiratory epithelium may be replaced by squamous epithelium under the influence of chronic irritation by cigarette smoke (*squamous metaplasia*). Similarly, in the bladder, the normal transitional epithelium may be replaced by squamous epithelium in response to chronic irritation by, for example, bladder stones (see Fig. 5.5). Metaplasia may coexist with hyperplasia and hypertrophy.

Metaplasia most commonly occurs in epithelial tissues but may also be seen in mesodermal tissues; for example, areas of fibrous tissue exposed to chronic trauma may form bone (*osseous metaplasia*). A key feature of metaplastic transformation is that one mature, fully differentiated cell type takes on the morphology of a totally different fully differentiated cell type.

## Dysplasia

Cells may undergo a morphological transformation in which an increased rate of cell division is coupled with incomplete maturation of the resultant cells. This change is known as *dysplasia*. The cells of dysplastic tissues tend to exhibit a high nuclear to cytoplasmic ratio and there is an increased rate of mitotic cell division. The incomplete cellular maturation is often reflected by partial or complete loss of certain specialized cellular structures normally seen in that cell type, such as cilia or mucin vacuoles. Dysplastic tissues may also show loss of the normal architectural relationships between cells.

Like metaplasia, dysplasia is most frequently seen in epithelia subject to chronic irritation. Dysplasia is present to some degree in the regenerating epithelia of damaged tissues and in these instances it is associated with concomitant inflammatory and reparatory changes. In other instances, dysplasia occurs in the absence of obvious tissue damage or repair, and in such cases the cytological features of the dysplastic tissue may merge with those seen in neoplastic conditions (see Chapter 6). It is a well documented phenomenon that malignant neoplastic change commonly follows pre-existing dysplastic change. Dysplasia *per se* is not a neoplastic condition and removal of the adverse environmental stimulus will cause restoration of the normal cell growth pattern.

Dysplastic change may be seen in the squamous epithelium at the squamocolumnar junction of the uterine cervix and in the epidermis of the sun-exposed skin (see Fig. 5.6). Dysplastic changes in colonic and gastric mucosa are associated with chronic colitis and chronic gastritis respectively.

Because of the sinister association of dysplasia with the development of neoplasia, treatment of dysplastic conditions is undertaken to minimise the risk of subsequent development of a malignancy. Recognition of dysplastic changes by cytological examination of cervical smears forms the basis of surveillance for neoplasia of the cervix (see Fig. 16.5).

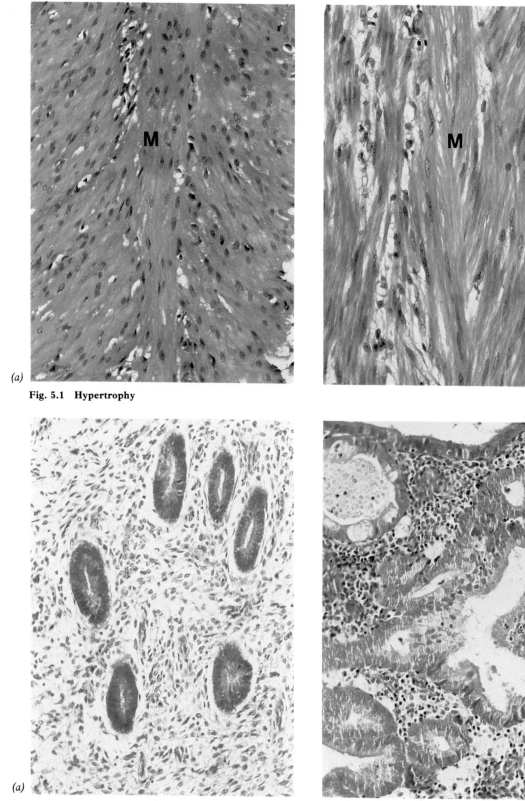

*(a)*

**Fig. 5.1   Hypertrophy**

*(b)*

*(a)*

**Fig. 5.2   Hyperplasia**

*(b)*

## Fig. 5.1    Hypertrophy *(illustrations opposite)*
## (a) normal small bowel muscle (HP)
## (b) hypertrophy of muscle of bowel wall (HP)

Pure hypertrophy without coexisting hyperplasia is virtually only seen in muscle where the stimulus is an increased demand for work. Micrograph (a) shows the muscle **M** of normal small bowel whilst micrograph (b) shows a portion of thickened muscle in small bowel proximal to an intestinal obstruction. Called upon to increase its peristaltic activity in order to overcome the obstruction, the muscle of the bowel wall responds by increasing cell mass by the process of hypertrophy. Note that the individual cells in micrograph (b) are larger than in the normal bowel photographed at the same magnification.

A similar type of change is seen in myocardial muscle when there is an increased demand on cardiac function caused by obstructed or incompetent valves or systemic hypertension. Skeletal muscle increases in bulk by hypertrophy in response to regular exercise. Prostatic obstruction of the bladder neck is followed by hypertrophy of the muscle of the bladder wall. In all the foregoing examples, when the stimulus for hypertrophy is removed the muscle cells will slowly return to their normal size.

## Fig. 5.2    Hyperplasia *(illustrations opposite below)*
## (a) normal late proliferative endometrium (HP)
## (b) hyperplasia of endometrium after excessive endocrine stimulation (HP)

Endometrial hyperplasia occurs when there is abnormal oestrogenic stimulation. Micrograph (a) shows the degree of endometrial hyperplasia which occurs under normal ovarian oestrogenic stimulation. In contrast, in micrograph (b), the endometrial glands are markedly hyperplastic and a few show some degree of cystic dilatation; this example is from a woman taking an oestrogen-containing preparation where the administered hormone causes persisting growth of the

endometrium. This may also be seen in the endometrium of women with oestrogen-secreting ovarian tumours. In such examples, removal of the abnormal oestrogenic stimulation causes restoration of the normal pattern of endometrial growth. The menstrual cycle can be regarded as a classic example of physiological endocrine-induced hyperplasia which normally occurs on a monthly cyclical basis under the control of ovarian hormones.

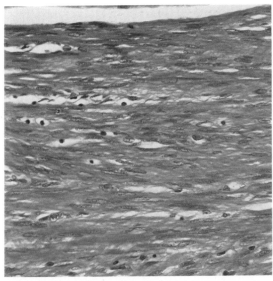

*(a)*

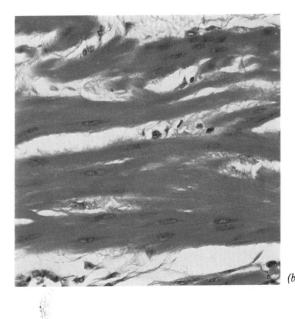

*(b)*

## Fig. 5.3    Hyperplasia with hypertrophy
## (a) normal myometrium (HP)
## (b) hyperplasia and hypertrophy in pregnant myometrium (HP)

Hypertrophy and hyperplasia commonly occur together in response to increased functional requirements. When compared to the normal myometrial fibres seen in micrograph (a), the fibres of the pregnant uterus, shown in micrograph (b) at the same magnification, are greatly enlarged; their larger nuclei reflect increased protein synthesis.

Within the uterus as a whole the number of cells is increased by hyperplasia. Occasionally in the uterus a mitotic figure may be seen where a myometrial cell is in the process of undergoing cell division. Following pregnancy, the uterus returns to normal size by physiological atrophy.

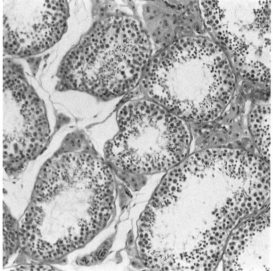

(a)

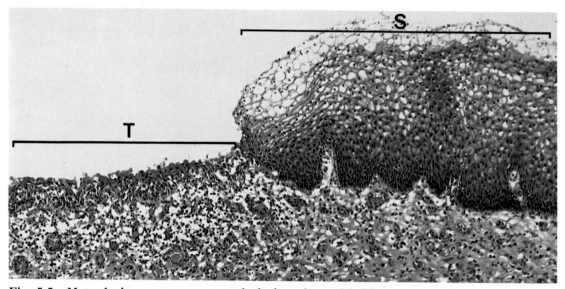

(b)

## Fig. 5.4  Atrophy
## (a) normal testis (HP)
## (b) atrophic testis (HP)

Micrograph (b) illustrates atrophy of the testis in a man aged 94; reduced secretion of trophic hormones may be responsible. When compared with the normal testis in micrograph (a) the seminiferous tubules of the atrophic testis show minimal spermatogenic activity. The tubular walls are thickened and pink stained, a process known as *hyalinization*, and the

interstitial tissue shows an increased deposition of fibrous tissue **F**.

Hyaline change is a common end result of atrophy or cell damage (see also end-stage kidney, Fig. 14.11) and is frequently accompanied by fibrosis.

## Fig. 5.5  Metaplasia: squamous metaplasia in urinary bladder (HP)

This micrograph illustrates the effects of chronic irritation upon the bladder mucosa by a bladder stone. The transitional epithelium **T** is inflamed and degenerate and squamous metaplasia has occurred in one area with the replacement of the native transitional epithelium by stratified squamous epithelium **S**. Note the coexisting acute and chronic

inflammatory change in the supporting connective tissue.

Squamous metaplasia also occurs in the bladder in chronic irritation by the parasitic infection, schistosomiasis. In these examples, the squamous epithelium is better suited to withstand the irritating environment.

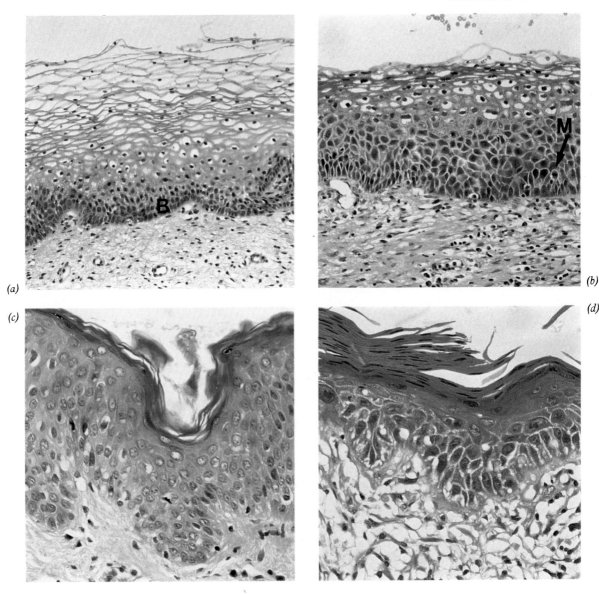

## Fig. 5.6 Dysplasia
**(a) normal cervix** (HP)  **(b) dysplasia in the cervix** (HP)
**(c) normal skin** (HP)  **(d) dysplastic skin** (HP)

Dysplasia is a morphological feature characterized by increased cellular proliferation with incomplete maturation of cells. It occurs commonly at the uterine cervix and in the skin and in both cases is thought to predispose to neoplastic change.

Micrograph (a) illustrates normal stratified squamous epithelium from the cervix. Cellular proliferation is confined to the basal layer **B** where the cells are small, uniform and darkly stained. As the cells migrate through various strata towards the surface, their cytoplasm expands and becomes more eosinophilic (pink stained), and towards the surface the cells become progressively flattened; the ratio of nucleus to cytoplasm diminishes as the cells pass from basal to surface layers. In contrast, micrograph (b) shows dysplastic cervical

epithelium where there is disruption of the normal orderly maturation sequence. Cells in the mid strata exhibit very large nuclei with prominent nucleoli and a mitotic figure **M** is seen above the basal layer; cells near the surface show a higher ratio of nucleus to cytoplasm. It is the presence of surface cells with large nuclei which alert the cytologist to underlying dysplasia in a cervical smear.

Micrographs (c) and (d) demonstrate similar differences between normal and dysplastic skin respectively. Note how the normal cellular stratification is disrupted in the dysplastic specimen by cells with large, darkly staining nuclei extending far up into the middle strata.

# 6. Neoplasia

## Introduction

In the preceding chapter the concept of hyperplasia was discussed and described as cellular proliferation in response to environmental stimulation. The key feature of hyperplastic cellular proliferation is that excessive growth ceases with removal of the promoting stimulus. In contrast, in the neoplastic state, cellular proliferation and growth persists in the absence of any continuing external stimulus. Thus the term neoplasia describes a state of uncontrolled cell division, and the resulting tissue mass is termed a *neoplasm*. In neoplastic cells and tissues, there is a failure of the mechanisms controlling cellular proliferation; this defect resulting in loss of control of cell division is transmitted to each new generation of cells, thus implying that the neoplastic transformation involves changes in genetic material.

Although causally related factors are known for several neoplasms, a great many are poorly understood and the majority unknown. Some neoplasms develop in the setting of another disturbed pattern of growth such as hyperplasia, metaplasia or dysplasia; these are discussed in Chapter 5.

By convention, a neoplastic mass of cells is termed a 'tumour'. The term, however, in its literal sense refers to any tissue swelling although this literal use has largely gone out of fashion.

## Characteristics of neoplasms

Neoplasms may be divided into two broad groups depending on how they behave. If the margins of the tumour are well defined and cell growth is entirely local, then the neoplasm is termed *benign*. If the margins of the neoplasm are poorly defined and the neoplastic cells extend into and destroy surrounding tissues, then the neoplasm is termed malignant. The property of growth into and at the expense of surrounding tissue is termed *invasion*. A further property of malignant neoplasms is distant spread of neoplastic cells away from the main neoplasm (the *primary tumour*) to form subpopulations of neoplastic cells which are not in continuity with the primary tumour. These detached neoplastic masses are termed *secondary tumours*, the property of distant spread of tumour is termed *metastasis*, and secondary tumours are often termed *metastases*.

In general terms, a benign tumour will behave in a relatively innocuous manner, and a malignant tumour will have deleterious effects often causing the death of the patient. There are, however, exceptions to these generalizations, and factors other than the biological growth pattern of a tumour may be important in influencing the outcome, for example, its location. A benign tumour of the brain stem may lead to rapid death whereas a malignant tumour of the skin may progress slowly over many years. Generalized symptoms such as weight loss, loss of appetite and general malaise frequently accompany malignant tumours; the cause in most cases is not understood. Some tumours, benign and malignant, retain the function of their organ of origin and if this happens to be an endocrine function then the tumour may exert harmful effects by secretion of excess hormone.

A feature of normal tissue growth is the maturation of constituent cells into a form adapted to a specific function; this adaptation may involve the acquisition of specialized structures such as mucin vacuoles, neurosecretory granules, microvilli or cilia. This process of structural and functional maturation is termed differentiation. A fully mature cell of any particular cell line is said to be highly differentiated, whereas its primitive precursor cells are described as being relatively undifferentiated. Thus in any given tissue, the normal cells have a characteristic state of differentiation. In contrast, neoplastic cells exhibit variable states of differentiation. In general, the cells of benign neoplasms are differentiated to a degree which fairly closely corresponds to that of the cells from which they were derived. In the case of malignant neoplasms there is a variable degree of differentiation. At one end of the spectrum the constituent cells may closely resemble the tissue of origin in which case the tumour is described as being a *well differentiated* malignant neoplasm; alternatively the constituent cells may bear little resemblance to the tissue of origin, in which case the neoplasm is described as being *poorly differentiated*. On the basis of clinical observation and pathological investigation, it has been shown that the degree of differentiation of a neoplasm is generally related to its behaviour. A poorly differentiated neoplasm tends to be more invasive and more aggressive than a well differentiated neoplasm.

Poorly differentiated neoplasms have a high ratio of nucleus to cytoplasm with numerous mitoses. In the poorly differentiated neoplasms there is also a greater variation in nuclear size between cells and a greater variation in overall cell size; this heterogeneity of size is termed *pleomorphism*. At the extreme end of the spectrum, neoplasms which exhibit no evidence of differentiation are termed *anaplastic neoplasms*; in such undifferentiated tumours it is not possible to identify the cell of origin on morphological grounds alone. The histological features which distinguish benign and malignant tumours are summarized in Fig. 6.1 and cytological features are shown in Figs 6.2 and 6.3.

## Modes of spread of malignant neoplasms

The main modes of tumour spread are as follows:

(i)   Spread by local invasion. Invasive tumours tend to spread into surrounding tissues by the most direct route (see Figs 6.4 and 6.5). Some tumours, however, spread along the line of least resistance such as naturally occurring tissue planes e.g. around and along nerve bundles.

(ii)  Via the lymphatics draining the site of the primary tumour; neoplastic cells are conducted to local lymph nodes where they become trapped and set up secondary tumours (see Figs 6.7 and 6.8).

(iii) Via the venules and veins draining the primary site; gut tumours tend to be conducted via the portal vein to the liver where secondary tumours are very frequently established. In the systemic circulation, neoplastic cells may be trapped in the capillaries of the lung to form pulmonary metastases (see Fig. 6.6).

(iv)  Directly across coelomic spaces, e.g. across the peritoneal or pleural cavities.

## In situ neoplasia

Occasionally, a neoplasm exhibits cytological features of malignancy i.e., cellular pleomorphism and increased mitotic activity, but is seen not to be invasive. This phenomenon is found commonly in epithelial tissues particularly in the squamous epithelium of the cervix (see Fig. 16.5) and the skin (see Figs 18.8 and 20.17). This type of lesion is termed *carcinoma in situ* since the cytological features are of a malignant epithelial neoplasm yet in terms of spread the basement membrane is not breached. Other examples of this phenomenon are seen in the breast where cytologically malignant cells may be confined within ducts (intraduct carcinoma) or within lobules (intralobular carcinoma, see Fig. 17.5). The diagnosis of in situ neoplasia is important as such lesions may progress to become invasive. Treatment at a preinvasive stage is often completely curative.

### Fig. 6.1   Histological features of neoplasms

|  | Benign | Malignant |
|---|---|---|
| *Behaviour* | Expansile growth only. Grows locally. | Expansile and invasive growth. May metastasize. |
| *Histology* | Resembles cell of origin (well differentiated) | May show loss of cellular differentiation |
|  | Few mitoses | Many mitoses some of which are abnormal forms. |
|  | Normal or slight increase in ratio of nucleus to cytoplasm | High nuclear to cytoplasmic ratio. |
|  | Cells are uniform through the tumour. | Cells vary in shape and size (cellular pleomorphism) or nuclei vary in shape and size (nuclear pleomorphism). |

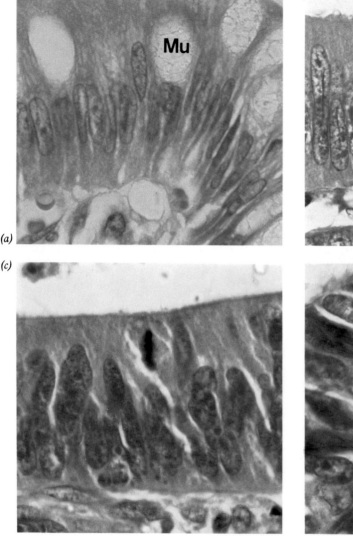

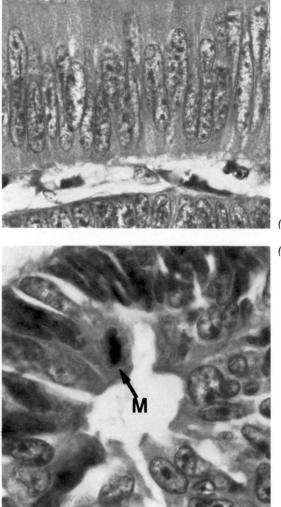

*(a)*

*(b)*

*(c)*

*(d)*

## Fig. 6.2   Degrees of tumour differentiation

**(a) normal colonic mucosa** (HP)
**(c) well differentiated malignant colonic neoplasm** (HP)

**(b) benign colonic neoplasm** (HP)
**(d) poorly differentiated colonic neoplasm** (HP)

This series of micrographs demonstrates the variable degree of differentiation that may be seen in tumours arising from the same cell of origin, in this case the mucus-secreting columnar epithelium of the colon.

Note the similarity between normal colonic mucosa in micrograph (a) and a benign colonic neoplasm in micrograph (b); in both cases the epithelial cells are tall, columnar and regular in form. The main points of difference are that the cells of the benign neoplasm contain no mucin **Mu** and their nuclei are more prominent. Note also that the nuclei of the benign neoplasm are more intensely stained with haematoxylin, a feature termed *hyperchromatism*.

The cells of the well differentiated malignant colonic neoplasm shown in micrograph (c) are also tall and columnar, but the nuclei are irregular in shape and arrangement and are

hyperchromatic; there is no mucin secretion, most of the cell being occupied by nucleus, ie. there is a high nuclear-cytoplasmic ratio. Despite these cytological changes, the cells still retain a reasonable semblance of the normal columnar arrangement.

In contrast, in the poorly differentiated colonic neoplasm shown in micrograph (d), the cells and their organisation bear less resemblance to the tissue of origin having lost most semblance of a columnar pattern. The cells show a great variability in size and nuclear shape, mitoses **M** are seen, and there is no evidence of mucin secretion.

All four micrographs illustrated here were prepared from minute samples of suspicious lesions in the rectal wall obtained by biopsy through a sigmoidoscope.

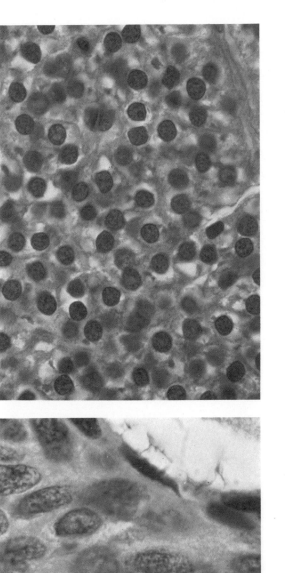

*(a)*

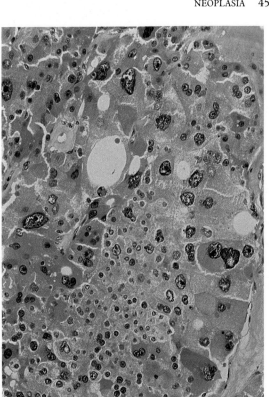

*(b)*

*(c)*

### Fig. 6.3    Pleomorphism, nuclear hyperchromicity and abnormal mitoses
**(a) benign neoplasm** (HP)
**(b) malignant neoplasm** (HP)
**(c) malignant neoplasm** (HP)

Pleomorphism, nuclear hyperchromicity and abnormal mitotic activity are features of malignant neoplasms and are not usually seen in benign neoplasms. In the benign neoplasm in (a), note the uniformity of cell and nuclear size and shape and the regular nuclear staining. The malignant tumour illustrated in (b) shows remarkable variation in cell size and shape (cellular pleomorphism) and nuclear size and shape (nuclear pleomorphism); in addition many nuclei are very darkly stained (nuclear hyperchromicity). Increased numbers of cells in mitosis are seen in many conditions in which there is excess cellular proliferation (eg. hyperplasia) but in malignant neoplasms many of the mitotic figures are abnormal; micrograph (c) shows an abnormal tripolar mitosis in a poorly differentiated malignant neoplasm.

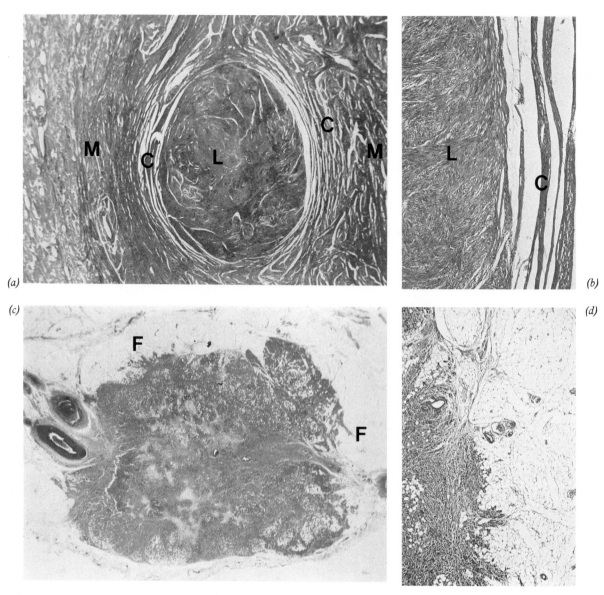

## Fig. 6.4   Invasiveness in solid organs
**(a) benign neoplasm of myometrium** (LP) **(b) margin of lesion in (a)** (MP)
**(c) malignant neoplasm of breast** (LP)     **(d) margin of lesion in (c)** (MP)

These micrographs compare the invasive behaviour of benign and malignant neoplasms within solid organs. Micrograph (a) shows a benign neoplasm of the uterine smooth muscle, a leiomyoma **L**, surrounded by normal myometrium **M**. The tumour margin is shown at higher magnification in micrograph (b). Note that the neoplasm is well circumscribed and shows no evidence of local invasion. This neoplasm has expanded symmetrically and compressed the supporting stroma of the myometrium to form a *pseudocapsule* **C**. Note in micrograph

(b), the similarity between neoplastic and the normal smooth muscle cells.

Micrograph (c) illustrates a malignant neoplasm of female breast epithelium; note that the neoplasm has an irregular outline with tongues of neoplastic cells invading the fatty tissue **F** of the breast. There is no tendency to form a capsule. The ill defined tumour margin is illustrated in micrograph (d) in which dark staining malignant cells can be seen infiltrating the surrounding adipose tissue.

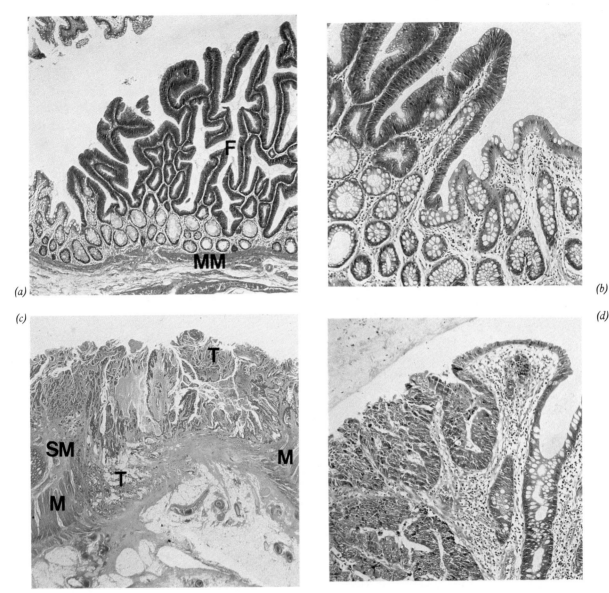

## Fig. 6.5   Invasive characteristics of surface neoplasms
**(a) non-invasive (benign) neoplasm of surface epithelium** (MP)   **(b) same lesion as in (a)** (HP)
**(c) invasive (malignant)  neoplasm of surface epithelium** (LP)   **(d) same lesion as in (c)** (HP)

Benign neoplasms of surface epithelia usually grow in the form of warty, papillary or nodular outgrowths from the surface and show no tendency to infiltrate downwards into the subepithelial connective tissue or submucosa. Micrograph (a) shows one form of benign neoplasm occuring in the colon; note that this benign epithelial tumour has grown into the lumen in the form of papillary fronds **F**. The underlying muscularis mucosae **MM** is intact and there is no downward invasion by the tumour; at higher magnification in micrograph (b) the differences between the normal and benign neoplastic epithelium are more readily seen.

Malignant neoplasms of surface epithelium not only grow outwards but also infiltrate across the epithelial basement membrane to spread into subepithelial connective tissues and further. In micrographs (c) and (d) of a malignant neoplasm of the colon, note that the tumour cells **T** have grown outwards into the lumen but have also broken through the epithelial basement membrane and are invading muscularis mucosae submucosa **SM** and the muscle **M** of the colon wall. Compare the cytological characteristics of the benign and malignant tumour cells in micrographs (b) and (d) respectively and contrast them with the normal colonic epithelial cells present at the tumour margins in each case. The malignant cells are more pleomorphic and less differentiated than are the cells of the benign neoplasm.

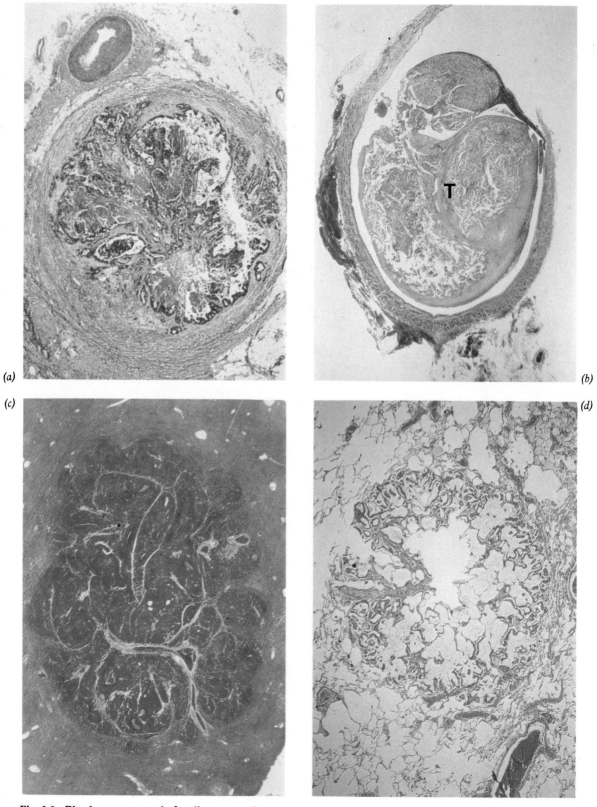

Fig. 6.6    Blood stream spread of malignant neoplasms

# Fig. 6.6 Blood stream spread of malignant neoplasms *(illustrations opposite)*
## (a) malignant colonic neoplasm (MP)    (b) malignant renal neoplasm (LP)
## (c) metastatic deposit in liver (LP)    (d) metastatic deposit in lung (LP)

The vascular system provides a ready means of spread for many types of malignant tumour (*haematogenous spread*). Malignant cells gain access to the bloodstream usually through the thin-walled vessels of the venous system; invasion of arterial vessels tends to result in severe haemorrhage or infarction rather than tumour spread. After infiltrating through the vessel walls, malignant cells may grow along veins in solid cores from which fragments may break off to form *tumour emboli*. Such emboli tend to lodge in the first capillary beds encountered; in the case of most malignancies these are the pulmonary capillaries but in the case of gut malignancies, the capillaries of the liver. The lungs and liver are therefore frequent sites of metastatic deposition. Small clumps of tumour cells may also pass through liver and lung capillaries and are then distributed by the arterial system throughout the entire body. Brain and bone marrow thus become common sites for metastatic deposition.

Micrograph (a) provides an example of venous invasion and is taken from the serosa of a colon in which there is an extensive malignant neoplasm. It shows a large serosal vein the lumen of which contains a solid mass of tumour which is growing along the vessel lumen; the site of invasion of the vessel wall was proximal to this section and therefore cannot be seen.

Venous invasion and permeation is particularly common in malignant neoplasms of the kidney, as in micrograph (b). In this case vessel invasion begins at the thin walled venous tributaries within the renal parenchyma, but the tumour then rapidly grows as a solid core along the lumina of increasingly large renal vein tributaries until, as shown here, the main renal vein itself becomes filled with tumour **T**; from the renal vein, the tumour may even extend into the inferior vena cava.

Micrographs (c) and (d) show examples of hepatic and pulmonary blood-borne metastases respectively. Hepatic metastases often arise from organs drained by the portal system; the lesion in micrograph (c) is from a poorly differentiated primary neoplasm in the stomach. Lung metastases on the other hand arise from tumour emboli from the systemic circulation and micrograph (d) is an example of secondary spread from an ovarian primary lesion.

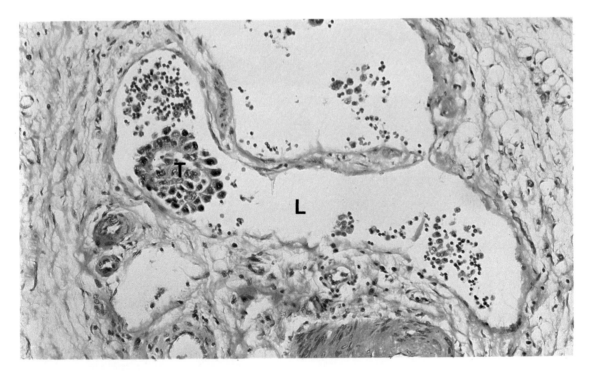

# Fig. 6.7 Lymphatic spread of malignant neoplasms (HP)

Malignant tumours may also invade through the walls of lymphatics, and tumour may then spread along lymphatic channels either by permeation of solid cores along the lymphatic lumina, or by fragments breaking off the intralymphatic tumour mass to form emboli which pass in the lymph drainage to regional lymph nodes. This micrograph illustrates a large, valved lymphatic **L** containing an embolic clump of malignant tumour cells **T** en route to a lymph node. Tumour embolization along lymphatics to regional lymph nodes is a very common mode of spread in malignant tumours of epithelial origin.

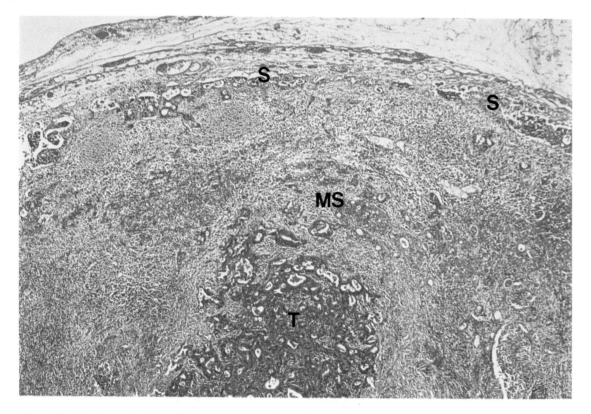

**Fig. 6.8  Metastasis of malignant tumour in a lymph node** (MP)

Embolization of clumps of malignant cells within lymphatic vessels leads to the formation of metastatic tumour deposits (*secondaries*) in the lymph nodes draining the primary site. This micrograph shows a lymph node draining a primary malignant tumour of the colon. Having arrived via afferent tributaries, the tumour cells have impacted in the subcapsular sinus **S** where they have proliferated to some extent. From here malignant cells have passed down a medullary sinus **MS** in one area and a small deposit of metastatic tumour **T** is beginning to grow in a new location deep within the node.

## Tumour nomenclature

The classification and nomenclature of neoplasia has developed from gross morphological, histological, and behavioural observation. Ideally the name given to a tumour should convey information about the cell of origin and the likely behaviour (either benign or malignant). While this is so for the majority of tumours of epithelial and connective tissues, there are a large number which are given eponymous or semidescriptive names out of either poor understanding of pathogenesis or long established tradition. Some tumours have several different names which are synonymous but derive from different classifications.

Benign neoplasms of surface epithelia, e.g. skin, are termed *papillomata* (singular *papilloma*). This term is prefixed by the cell of origin e.g. *squamous* for skin, *transitional* for bladder. Benign neoplasms of both solid and surface glandular epithelium are termed *adenomata* (singular *adenoma*). This is prefixed by the tissue of origin e.g. thyroid adenoma, salivary gland adenoma. Frequently benign tumours of surface glandular epithelium (almost always in the large bowel) assume a papillary growth pattern when they are termed *villous adenomata*.

A malignant tumour of any epithelial origin is termed a *carcinoma*. Tumours of glandular epithelium (including that lining the gut) are termed *adenocarcinoma*. Tumours of other epithelia are prefixed by the cell type of origin e.g. squamous cell carcinoma of skin, transitional cell carcinoma of bladder. To classify an adenocarcinoma, the tissue of origin is added, e.g. adenocarcinoma of prostate, adenocarcinoma of colon, adenocarcinoma of breast. A more detailed summary is given in Fig. 6.9 below.

In connective tissues there is a simpler and more descriptive classification of neoplasia. Firstly the tissue of origin is designated, with the addition of the suffix *-oma* for a benign tumour, or *-sarcoma* for a malignant tumour. As an example, a benign tumour of adipose tissue is termed a lipoma whilst a malignant tumour of the same origin is termed a liposarcoma. A detailed summary of other connective tissue tumours is shown in Fig. 6.10.

There are a variety of other neoplasms which do not fit into either epithelial or connective tissue category described above and these are grouped according to their tissue of origin. The main categories are as follows:

*Lymphomas* — tumours of the lymphoid system (see Chapter 15).

*Embryonal tumours* — tumours of childhood which are believed to derive from primitive embryonal "blastic" tissue; the most common are nephroblastoma of the kidney (Fig. 14.13), and neuroblastoma of the adrenal medulla (Fig. 19.10).

*Gliomas* — tumours derived from the non-neural support tissues of the brain (see Chapter 22).

*Germ cell tumours* — tumours derived from germ cells in the gonads (see Chapters 16 and 18).

*Teratomas* — tumours which contain elements of all three embryological germ cell layers, ectoderm, endoderm, and mesoderm; these are most commonly found in the testis and ovary. They vary in malignancy from benign to extremely malignant and are commonest in young people. Teratomas represent complex forms of germ cell tumours.

*APUD tumours* — tumours derived from cells of the APUD system, and which secrete polypeptide hormones or active amines. Examples include phaeochromocytoma of the adrenal medulla (Fig. 19.8), carcinoid tumour of the appendix (Fig. 12.10) and medullary carcinoma of the thyroid (Fig. 4.6).

In addition to the system described above, individual tumours may also be known by other names according to function e.g. insulinoma, appearance e.g. oat cell carcinoma, or by an eponym e.g. Hodgkin's disease.

Finally there is a group of tumour-like lesions known as *hamartomas* which represent non-neoplastic overgrowths of tissues indigenous to the site of their occurrence. These are thought to be developmental abnormalities. A common example is the 'port wine stain' of the skin composed of blood vessels and known as a *haemangioma*; note that the suffix -oma erroneously implies that this is a benign neoplasm. An example of a haemangioma in the liver is shown in Fig. 10.9.

The cytological appearances of a representative selection of different tumours from each group are illustrated in Figs 6.11 to 6.19.

**Fig. 6.9  Nomenclature of epithelial tumours**

| Tissue of origin | Benign | Malignant |
| --- | --- | --- |
| Surface epithelium | Papilloma | Carcinoma |
| Squamous | Squamous cell papilloma | Squamous cell carcinoma |
| Glandular (columnar) | Adenoma (villous or tubular) | Adenocarcinoma |
| Transitional | Transitional cell papilloma | Transitional cell carcinoma |
| Solid glandular epithelium | Adenoma | Adenocarcinoma |
| *Examples* | | |
| Thyroid | Thyroid adenoma | Thyroid adenocarcinoma |
| Kidney | Renal adenoma | Renal adenocarcinoma |
| Liver | Hepatic adenoma | Hepatic adenocarcinoma |

**Fig. 6.10  Nomenclature of connective tissue tumours**

| Tissue | Benign | Malignant |
| --- | --- | --- |
| Fibrous | Fibroma | Fibrosarcoma |
| Bone | Osteoma | Osteosarcoma |
| Cartilage | Chondroma | Chondrosarcoma |
| Adipose | Lipoma | Liposarcoma |
| Smooth muscle | Leiomyoma | Leiomyosarcoma |
| Skeletal muscle | Rhabdomyoma | Rhabdomyosarcoma |

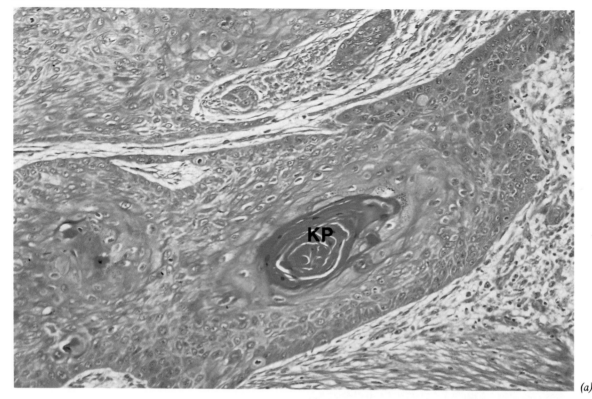

*(a)*

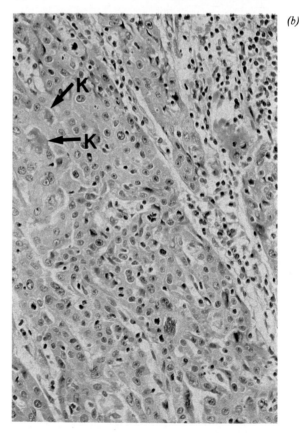

*(b)*

## Fig. 6.11   Squamous cell carcinoma
## (a) well differentiated (HP)
## (b) poorly differentiated (HP)

Squamous cell carcinomas may arise in any site of native
stratified squamous epithelium e.g. skin, oesophagus, tongue,
penis. They may also arise in stratified squamous epithelium
which has formed by the process of metaplasia e.g. bronchus,
urinary bladder.

The degree of differentiation varies widely. Well
differentiated tumours as seen in micrograph (a) have
cytological features similar to the prickle cell layer of normal
stratified squamous epithelium; the cells are large, eosinophilic
and slightly fusiform in shape. The nuclei exhibit a moderate
degree of pleomorphism and mitotic figures are not very
abundant. The cells are commonly arranged in broad sheets
and large clumps and at very high magnification intercellular
bridges (typical of normal prickle cells) may be visible. The
most characteristic feature of well differentiated squamous
carcinomas is the formation of keratin which may be seen
within individual cells but more often forms lamellated pink
stained masses known as *keratin pearls* **KP**.

In contrast, poorly differentiated squamous carcinomas as in
micrograph (b) lose most of their resemblance to normal
prickle cells and have a high nucleus-cytoplasmic ratio. Keratin
pearl formation is not seen although individual cell
keratinization **K** may be present. In the most anaplastic
squamous carcinomas the only evidence of cell of origin may
be intercellular bridges only visible at high magnification after
careful search.

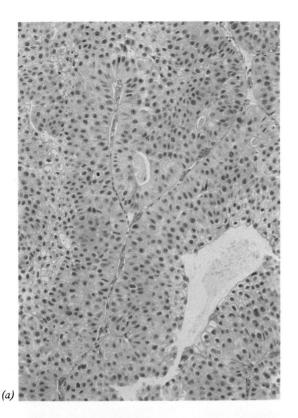

*(a)*

### Fig. 6.12  Transitional cell carcinoma
### (a) well differentiated (papillary) (HP)
### (b) poorly differentiated (HP)

These tumours arise almost exclusively from native transitional epithelium in the urinary tract. The well differentiated lesions usually adopt a papillary growth pattern and the cytological features are almost indistinguishable from that of normal transitional epithelium. Micrograph (a) shows a papillary tumour closely resembling normal urothelium but with slight nuclear pleomorphism and minimal evidence of mitotic activity. As the tumours become less differentiated, the growth pattern becomes more solid and nuclear pleomorphism becomes more marked. In anaplastic tumours it may not be possible to determine the tissue of origin except by knowing that the tumour has arisen in the urinary tract. Micrograph (b) shows a poorly differentiated solid tumour from the bladder wall; note the nests of highly pleomorphic tumour cells **T** invading between bundles of smooth muscle **M**.

*(b)*

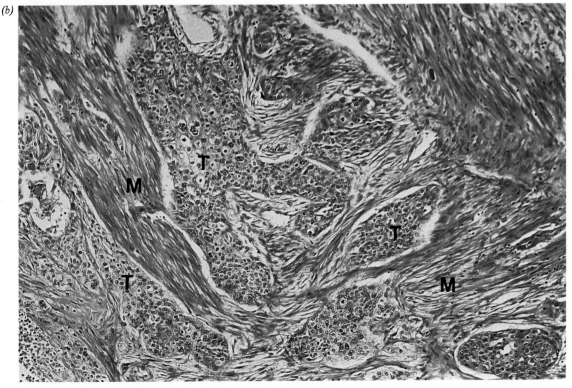

## Fig. 6.13   Adenocarcinoma
## (a) well differentiated colonic (HP)
## (b) poorly differentiated colonic (HP)

Carcinomas which derive from surface glandular epithelium such as large bowel and stomach tend to exhibit a glandular pattern of growth which is characteristic of well differentiated tumours but which may be lost as tumours become less differentiated. Such tumours are known as *adenocarcinomas* whatever their state of differentiation. The same is true of carcinomas arising in solid glandular tissues such as kidney, breast and prostate, and of tumours of the liver (which in embryological terms develops as an outgrowth of primitive gut epithelium).

Micrograph (a) illustrates a typical well differentiated adenocarcinoma from the colon. It exhibits a well formed glandular pattern **G**; the cells are hyperchromatic, have high nuclear-cytoplasmic ratio and numerous mitoses **M** are seen. Unlike the normal colon, the glandular pattern is irregular and there is little evidence of mucin secretion.

In contrast, the poorly differentiated colonic adenocarcinoma shown in micrograph (b) shows no tendency to form a glandular pattern and the cells are extremely pleomorphic. The only evidence of its glandular origin is the presence of occasional cells with a large secretory vacuole **V** which could be shown with special staining techniques to contain mucin. In these cells, the nucleus is displaced to one side giving rise to the term *signet cells* from their supposed resemblance to signet rings. Signet cells stained by the P.A.S. method are illustrated in Fig. 12.8 (d).

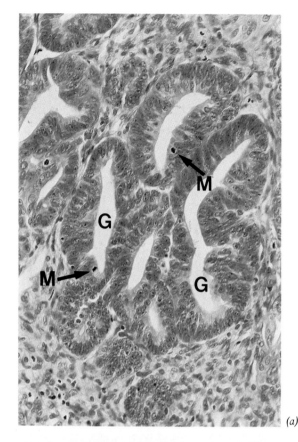

*(a)*

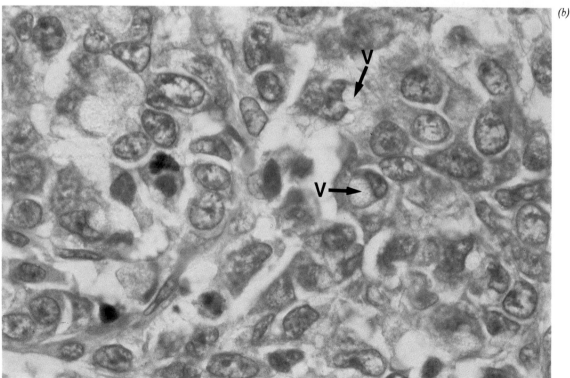

*(b)*

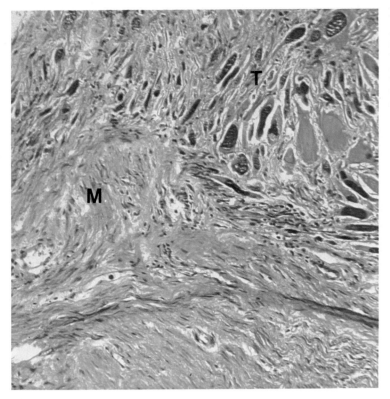

## Fig. 6.14 Sarcoma (HP)

Sarcomas are malignant tumours derived from connective tissues including adipose tissue, bone, cartilage and smooth muscle. Many sarcomas resemble the tissue of origin either cytologically, structurally or by producing characteristic extracellular materials such as collagen and ground substance. For example fibrosarcomas produce collagen, liposarcomas have intracellular lipid vacuoles and chondrosarcomas produce cartilagenous ground substance.

Poorly differentiated sarcomas may not show any evidence of tissue of origin and consist of pleomorphic spindle shaped cells with numerous mitotic figures. Such tumours are termed *spindle cell sarcomas* or *undifferentiated sarcomas*.

This micrograph shows a sarcoma derived from uterine smooth muscle. Normal myometrium **M** is being invaded by large spindle shaped tumour cells **T** with huge nuclei and abundant pink cytoplasm similar to that of smooth muscle cells; this is thus a *leiomyosarcoma*. This degree of pleomorphism is unusual in a leiomyosarcoma; in these tumours the degree of malignancy is usually determined by the invasiveness of the tumour and the number of mitotic figures rather than on cytological criteria.

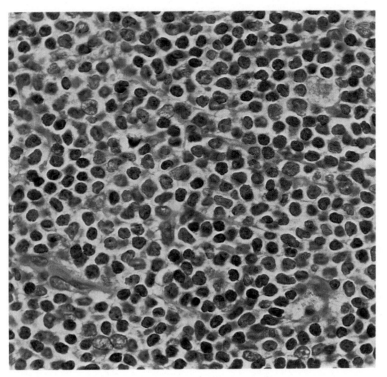

## Fig. 6.15 Lymphoma (HP)

Lymphomas are a group of solid tumours derived from cells of the lymphoreticular system. They tend to be confined to lymphoid organs such as lymph nodes, spleen, bone marrow and liver but many spread to other tissues particularly the skin and CNS; occasionally primary lymphomas occur in the gastrointestinal tract especially the small bowel.

Histologically, lymphomas consist of sheets of lymphoid cells arranged either diffusely or in a follicular pattern. The latter arrangement is usually a good prognostic indicator. Lymphomas are discussed in detail in Chapter 15.

This micrograph illustrates a highly malignant lymphoma composed of diffuse sheets of large lymphoid cells with no evidence of follicular formation. Such tumours may have a rapidly progressive clinical course and respond poorly to treatment.

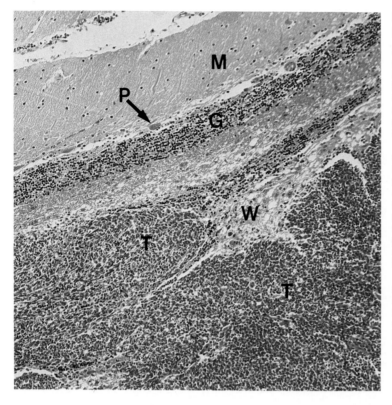

## Fig. 6.16   Embryonal tumour (HP)

Embryonal tumours are derived from cells similar to those of various primitive embryonal tissues. They usually present in childhood, are rapidly growing and many are highly malignant. The tumour cells are small with dark staining nuclei and very little cytoplasm whatever the organ of origin.

This micrograph shows a tumour occurring in the cerebellar region and thought to be derived from primitive neural cells; it is known as a *medulloblastoma*. The tumour **T** is composed of sheets of very small cells and appears to have arisen in the cerebellar white matter **W**; note the inner granular **G** and outer molecular layers **M** of the cerebellum with intervening Purkinje cells **P**.

Other types of embryonal tumours may show some features of maturation or organoid structure suggestive of their tissue of origin. Examples are the nephroblastoma (Wilms' tumour) of the kidney (see Fig. 14.13) and neuroblastoma of the adrenal gland (see Fig. 19.10).

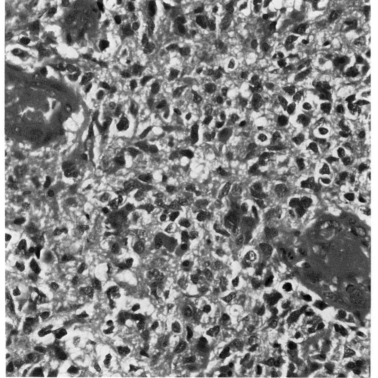

## Fig. 6.17   Glioma (HP)

Tumours derived from CNS support cells are known as *gliomas* and are classified according to the cell of origin eg. astrocytes, oligodendrocytes. Like tumours elsewhere, gliomas exhibit varying degrees of differentiation which correspond to prognosis.

The cells of well differentiated gliomas are usually cytologically indistinguishable from normal cells however the tumour cells are extremely prolific and spread diffusely through the otherwise normal brain structure. The cells of poorly differentiated gliomas on the other hand may be extremely pleomorphic.

This micrograph shows a poorly differentiated astrocytoma composed of homogeneous sheets of tumour cells with large, moderately pleomorphic nuclei. The tumour has completely replaced the normal brain tissue. Other examples of gliomas are shown in Figs 22.6 to 22.8.

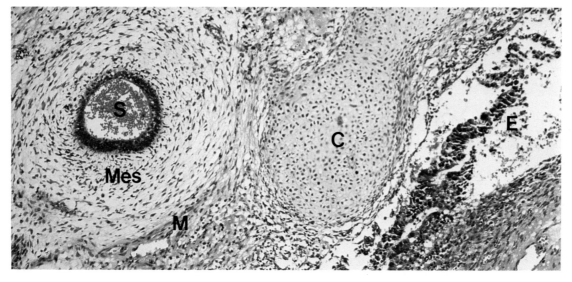

## Fig. 6.18  Teratoma (HP)

Teratomas are tumours derived from germ cells and most commonly arise in the testis or ovary. The tumours contain neoplastic tissues derived from any of the three germ cell layers, endoderm, mesoderm and ectoderm (including neurectoderm) and thus may contain tissues as diverse as teeth, thyroid, brain and muscle. The tumours range from benign to highly malignant.

A malignant teratoma of the testis is shown in this micrograph. Respiratory type epithelium has formed a cystic space **S** into which haemorrhage has occurred. This is surrounded by pale mesenchyme-like tissue **Mes**. There is also immature cartilage **C** and bands of smooth muscle **M**. An area of desquamated epithelium **E** of indeterminate type is also seen. When a malignant teratoma metastasizes all these tissue elements may be present in the secondary deposits.

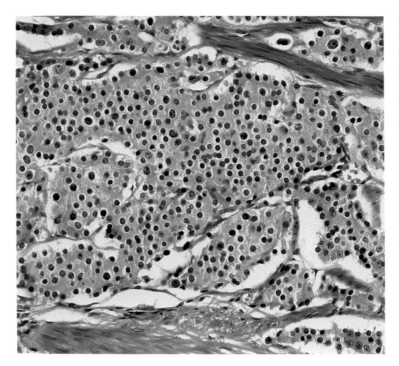

## Fig. 6.19  APUD tumour (HP)

The APUD cell system is composed of a diverse group of cells which synthesise and secrete peptide and amine hormones. Neoplasms in this group of tissues are known as APUD cell tumours. A functional classification is applied where the secretory product can be identified eg. insulinoma, gastrinoma, and glucagonoma. By long usage the APUD cell tumours which secrete 5 hydroxytryptamine are termed *carcinoid tumours*. Some APUD cell tumours have no identifiable secretory product. APUD tumours may be benign or malignant and mainly arise in the gastrointestinal tract, the pancreas and thyroid glands.

Tumours of APUD cells have certain common histological features. As shown in this micrograph, the cells are relatively small and uniform with prominent, round nuclei and characteristic granular cytoplasm due to the presence of secretory granules; these may be demonstrated using special stains as in Fig. 12.10 (b) or immunohistochemistry. Electron microscopy may also be used to identify cells according to the ultrastructural features of the secretory granules.

# 7. Atherosclerosis

## Introduction

Hardening and thickening of vessel walls in the arterial tree is a major cause of illness and death particularly in affluent societies, and the term *arteriosclerosis* is often used as a general descriptive term for such diseases.

The commonest type of arteriosclerosis is that in which the underlying histopathological lesion is *atheroma* which mainly affects large and medium sized arteries; this form of arteriosclerosis is thus known as *atherosclerosis*. Other forms of arteriosclerosis occur, such as that in which the walls of arterioles are thickened in association with hypertension (see Figs 10.1 and 10.2); from a histopathological and clinical point of view however, atherosclerosis is the condition of overwhelming importance.

Atherosclerosis occurs to some extent in almost everyone, but pathological consequences mainly occur in associaton with severe atherosclerosis only. The factors predisposing to severe lesions with a high incidence of complications are now well recognized, but the pathogenic mechanisms are still incompletely understood.

In outline, the atheromatous lesion first begins in the tunica intima by infiltration of lipids into certain intimal cells; this stage is probably represented macroscopically by the *fatty streak*. The lesion progressively enlarges by further accumulation of intracellular and extracellular lipids causing tissue degeneration and fibrosis which begins to involve the tunica media; this stage is represented by the raised *fibrous plaque*. Further development of the lesion is often complicated by internal haemorrhage, calcification, ulceration and thrombus formation resulting in the so-called *complicated lesions* which characterize the advanced form of atherosclerosis. The processes of atheroma formation are illustrated in Figs 7.1 and 7.2. Atherosclerosis may affect many vessels but the aorta, cerebral arteries, coronary arteries, carotid arteries and iliofemoral arteries are those which are most frequently severely affected and are those in which the various complications of atheroma have their major impact. The main histopathological complications are shown in Figs 7.3 to 7.6.

The most important pathological and clinical sequelae of atherosclerosis are: (a) narrowing of the vessel lumen producing partial or complete obstruction to blood flow leading to *ischaemia* and *infarction* of the target tissue (see Chapter 9); (b) formation of a clot or *thrombus* which, if it detaches, forms an *embolus* which blocks one or more smaller vessels distally (see Chapter 8); (c) weakening of the vessel wall, predisposing to dilatation; such a dilatation is known as an *aneurysm*. Rupture of the weakened and aneurysmally dilated artery wall is a further serious complication and is seen most commonly in the abdominal aorta.

**Fig. 7.1  Early atheromatous lesions** (*illustrations opposite*)
**(a) early atheromatous plaque** (LP)
**(b) foam cells and lipid** (HP)

The normal arterial tunica intima is a delicate layer of fibroelastic connective tissue lined on its luminal aspect by a layer of simple flat endothelial cells. In elastic arteries (such as the aorta, subclavian and carotid arteries), the intima is bounded externally by the interspersed layers of elastic tissue and smooth muscle which makes up the tunica media, whereas in muscular arteries (such as the coronary and femoral arteries), the intima is separated from the muscular tunica media by a discrete internal elastic lamina. The intima contains scattered cells which are responsible for collagen and elastin synthesis but which also have ultrastructural characteristics of smooth muscle cells and are thus often referred to as *myointimal cells*.

These two micrographs show the early changes of atheroma in the aorta. Micrograph (a) shows a pale staining area of thickening in the intima **I** representing an early atheromatous

lesion and consisting of aggregated myointimal cells containing lipid, and some intimal fibrous tissue. Because the lesions appear macroscopically as slightly raised flat areas they are termed *atheromatous plaques*. Note that the medial layer of the vessel **M** is uniform and appears normal at this stage; early atheroma is a disease confined to the intima.

At higher power, a detail of the intimal thickening is shown in micrograph (b). Myointimal cells full of lipid appear as large, pale staining cells **F** with very vacuolated cytoplasm giving rise to the term *foam cells*. As the lesion progresses, some of these foam cells break down and liberate lipid into the intima where it is represented by non-staining angular clefts **C**. The presence of free lipid appears to induce a fibrous reaction in the surrounding tissues which appear eosinophilic (pink staining) due to the presence of increased amounts of collagen.

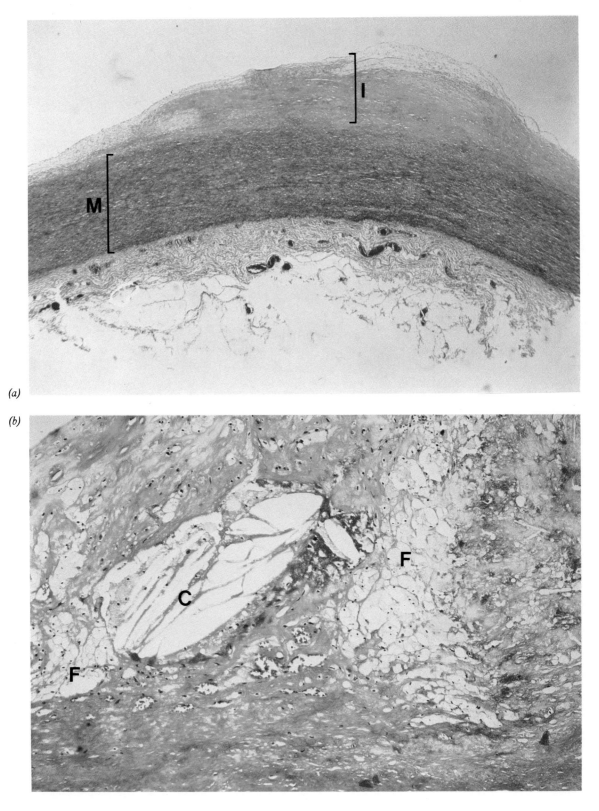

*(a)*

*(b)*

Fig. 7.1   **Early atheromatous lesions**

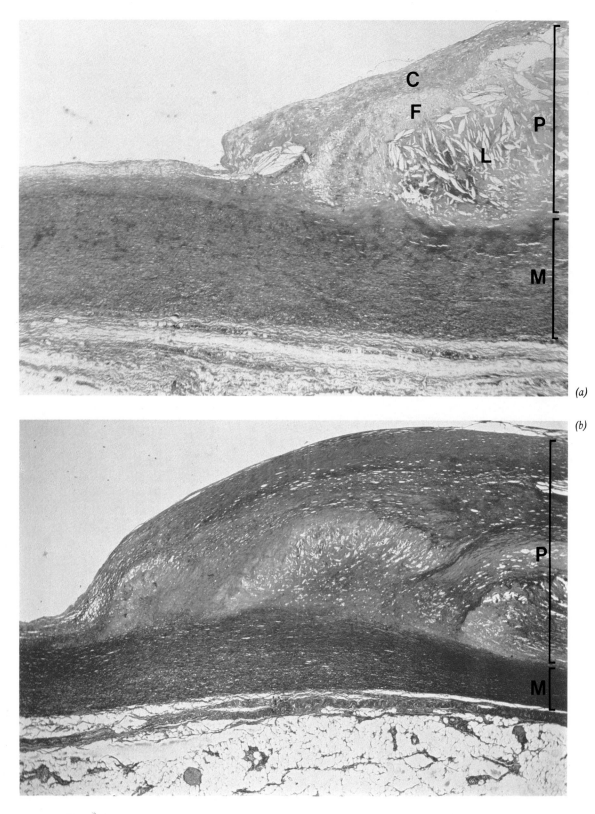

*(a)*

*(b)*

**Fig. 7.2    Fibrous atheromatous plaques**

### Fig. 7.2 Fibrous atheromatous plaques *(illustrations opposite)*
### (a) fibrolipid plaque (LP)
### (b) fibrous plaque (LP)

Early intimal atheromatous lesions enlarge by further accumulation of lipid in foam cells and also free within the extracellular intimal tissue. This is associated with a more marked fibrotic response in the intima leading to increased thickening of the plaque. Once a more significant degree of fibrous tissue develops in an atheromatous lesion, it is termed a *fibrolipid plaque*.

Micrograph (a) shows a section of aorta with part of a fibrolipid plaque **P**. Note the areas of nonstaining lipid **L** surrounded by pink staining fibrous tissue **F**, making up the thickened intima. A zone of denser, more intensely stained fibrous tissue, sometimes termed a fibrous cap **C**, runs

between the endothelial surface and the underlying fibrolipid aggregate. With progression of the lesion the fibrous cap thickens and the intimal lesion becomes larger and more raised. Micrograph (b) shows such a plaque, being composed mostly of fibrous tissue. Note in both micrographs that there is early thinning of the tunica media **M** beneath the plaque compared to the adjacent normal vessel wall. This is accompanied by loss of supporting elastic tissue, atrophy of smooth muscle cells and progressive medial fibrosis. With time, the medial fibrous tissue stretches due to loss of elastic recoil in the vessel wall, and the vessel dilates. This dilatation is the basis of the formation of an *atheromatous aneurysm*.

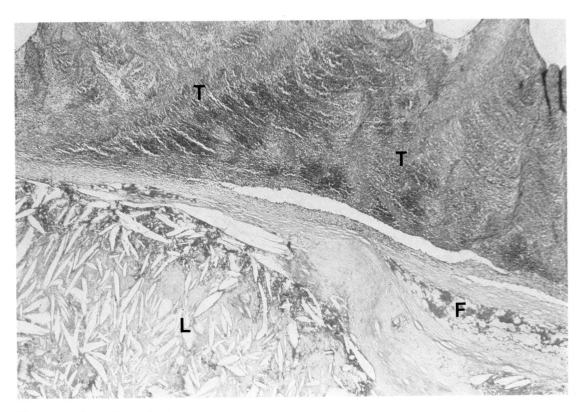

### Fig. 7.3 Complicated atheroma (MP)

As an atheromatous plaque enlarges it may become very thick relative to the normal thickness of the vessel wall and as well as lipid, foam cells and fibrous tissue, calcium may be deposited in the lesion. With thickening and fibrosis, the blood supply to the abnormal intima may become insufficient and the lesion may undergo necrosis and surface ulceration; this is then described as a *complicated atheromatous lesion*. The normal smooth endothelial lining having gone, the collagen and lipid

of the atheromatous lesion are exposed directly to the blood flow. The coagulation sequence is thus activated and thrombus is formed on the vessel wall at the site of ulcerated atheroma.

This micrograph shows the top of an atheromatous plaque with foam cells **F** and lipid **L**. The surface has ulcerated and is encrusted with thrombus **T** composed of fibrin, platelets and entrapped blood cells.

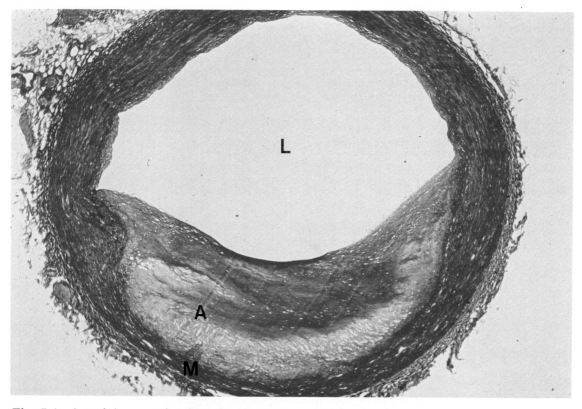

## Fig. 7.4  Arterial narrowing by atheroma (LP)

The formation of a large plaque of atheroma **A** in the intima of a small or medium sized artery, such as the coronary artery branch shown here, can greatly reduce the size of the lumen **L**. The consequent reduction in blood flow leads to ischaemia of the tissues supplied, in this case the myocardium. Note that the media **M** underlying the thickest mass of atheroma is markedly thinned. Such partly occlusive atheroma is very frequent in the coronary arteries of cigarette smoking males, particularly in the region of the bifurcation of the left coronary artery. A frequent symptom of this arterial narrowing is the condition known as *angina pectoris*, a gripping pain in the chest particularly experienced on exertion, disappearing with rest. This pain is a manifestation of ischaemia of the

myocardium, and patients with long standing angina often show replacement of small areas of myocardial muscle by fibrous scar tissue, the end result of anoxic necrosis of muscle fibres.

Luminal narrowing by atheroma occurs similarly in many other arteries. In the leg arteries, such changes can produce severe calf pain on walking (*intermittent claudication*) and may eventually lead to the development of gangrene of the lower leg. In the vertebrobasilar arterial system to the cerebellum and brain stem, severe atheroma can produce transient ischaemia manifest clinically as dizziness, loss of balance and occasional unconsciousness.

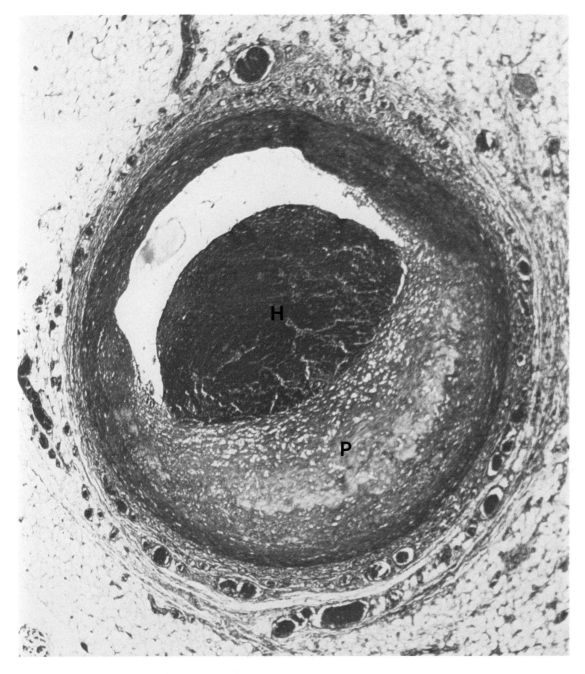

## Fig. 7.5  Haemorrhage into atheromatous plaque (LP)

Within an established fibrolipid atheromatous plaque of some duration, small thin walled capillaries are present, particularly in the loose fibrous tissue adjacent to the foam cells and free lipid. Occasionally, rupture of the wall of one of these vessels may produce a small localized haemorrhage. Because of the confined space in which this often apparently trivial bleed occurs, the consequences can be disproportionately devastating. In this micrograph, a small haemorrhage **H** has occurred in the superficial area of a fibrolipid atheromatous plaque **P**; the accumulated blood has tracked beneath the nonulcerated endothelium, causing it to bulge markedly into the arterial

lumen. This has led to even greater narrowing of a lumen already reduced to about half its normal size by the pre-existing atheromatous plaque. Such an abrupt reduction in arterial flow leads to acute ischaemia in the supplied tissues.

In this patient, the lesion was situated in the anterior descending branch of the left coronary artery and resulted in a substantial area of the anterior wall of the left ventricle and the anterior half of the interventricular septum becoming acutely ischaemic. Extensive myocardial necrosis ensued, a process known as myocardial infarction (see Fig. 9.3).

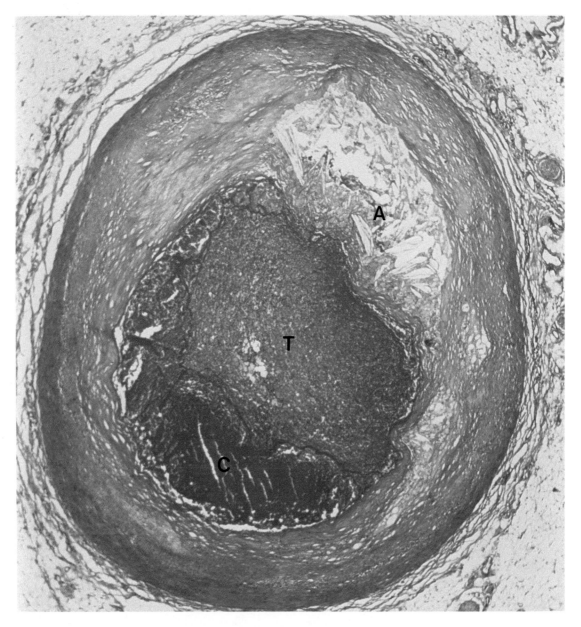

## Fig. 7.6   Thrombus formation on atheroma (LP)

The most important complication of atheroma in small and medium sized arteries is the development of a *thrombus* on the surface of an atheromatous plaque; the process of thrombus formation is discussed in detail in Chapter 8. Thrombus, which consists of a mass of platelets and insoluble fibrin, tends, in the arterial system, to form on any intimal surface which is damaged and roughened. Endothelial ulceration over an atheromatous plaque is the commonest cause of intimal roughening in the arterial system.

This micrograph of a coronary artery shows an ulcerated atheromatous plaque **A** which has already significantly constricted the arterial lumen. A thrombus **T** has then developed on the ulcerated surface, largely obliterating the remaining lumen. The thrombus is deep pink in colour, and is composed of fibrin and platelets. The residual lumen is

occupied by bright red postmortem blood coagulum **C** composed entirely of tightly packed red blood cells. The naked eye distinction between genuine antemortem thrombus and postmortem coagulum is important; thrombus is pinkish red, granular and firm, whereas coagulum is predominantly dark red, shiny and jelly-like.

When thrombus formation occurs on an atheromatous lesion in a large diameter artery, such as the aorta or carotid arteries, the thrombus may be small and cause little significant obstruction to blood flow at the site. Fragments of thrombus may however become detached and pass into the peripheral circulation to block a smaller vessel and cause ischaemia or infarction in its area of distribution. This phenomenon is known as *thrombo-embolism* and is described more fully in Chapter 8.

# 8. Thrombosis and embolism

## Introduction

In health, a variety of factors override the latent haemostatic processes of platelet aggregation and blood clotting to ensure free circulation of blood. Under certain pathological circumstances, these dynamics may be disrupted leading to the formation of a solid mass of blood products in a vessel lumen; this process is known as *thrombosis* and the mass of blood products is referred to as a *thrombus*.

*Embolism* is the process in which any abnormal mass forming in, or entering, the bloodstream passes with the circulation to lodge in an organ with resulting pathological consequences; the abnormal mass is known as an *embolus*. Emboli are most commonly caused by detachment of all or part of a thrombus from its site of formation and this form of embolism, often called *thrombo-embolism*, is of the greatest clinical importance; nevertheless emboli may arise from other sources. Atheromatous debris, clumps of tumour cells, bacterial vegetations from heart valves, fat, bone marrow and air may also form emboli with important clinical sequelae. The most dramatic outcome of embolism is the blockage of a major blood vessel resulting in necrosis of the tissue supplied; this phenomenon, known as *infarction*, is described in detail in the next chapter. Embolism may also be the means of spread of tumour or infection.

Thrombus consists of aggregations of platelets bound together by fibrin strands with variable numbers of erythrocytes and leucocytes trapped in the tangled mass and contributing to the bulk of the thrombus. Thrombosis may occur in any part of the circulation but most particularly in large veins, large arteries, in the heart chambers, and on heart valves. Three major conditions, alone or in combination, predispose to thrombosis:

(a) damage to the vessel wall, such as atheroma in arteries, inflammation involving veins (phlebitis), or myocardial death and resultant endocarditis as in myocardial infarction

(b) disordered blood flow such as stasis or undue turbulence

(c) abnormally enhanced haemostatic properties of the blood such as increased platelet concentration or stickiness, or factors promoting blood clotting or diminished fibrinolysis; subtle physiological changes such as occur in dehydration, major illness and the postoperative state are included in this category.

Unlike a blood clot formed *in vitro* or *postmortem*, a thrombus has a defined architecture and consistency which reflects the manner and stages of its formation and the nature of blood flow in the vicinity. For example, thrombus formed in an artery is usually dense and composed mainly of aggregated platelets and fibrin, whereas thrombus formed in slowed or static blood more closely resembles clotted blood in that it contains masses of erythrocytes and leucocytes. The process of thrombus formation is shown in Fig. 8.1.

Thrombus may partially or completely occlude a vessel lumen, again according to the conditions predisposing to its formation. In the heart or major arteries, thrombus often covers only part of the vessel wall and in this case is known as *mural thrombus*; for example, mural thrombus may form on the ventricular endocardium following a myocardial infarct (see Fig. 8.2), in an aneurysmal dilatation or on an atheromatous lesion in the aorta (see Fig. 7.6). In other situations, thrombosis may completely occlude a vessel lumen; this is particularly common in the deep veins of the legs in immobilized, debilitated patients, and results in obstruction of venous return from the feet and lower legs. Stasis of blood resulting from occlusion or partial obstruction of blood flow by thrombus may lead to *propagation* of the thrombus in the static blood. As previously outlined, thrombus formed under such conditions contains many blood cells and relatively less fibrin and is thus much more prone to become detached to form a thrombo-embolus. For example, following deep venous thrombosis in the leg, the thrombus may propagate as far as the common iliac vein or even the inferior vena cava; such a huge thrombus may readily become detached and pass via the right side of the heart to the pulmonary arterial tree as a *pulmonary embolus* which is often fatal (see Fig. 8.3).

Finally, whatever the clinical consequences of thrombosis i.e. embolism, infarction etc., a thrombus may be dealt with in one of two ways: resolution or organization and repair. Resolution involves the normal physiological phenomenon of fibrinolysis as well as autolytic disintegration of the cellular elements of the clot. Alternatively, the thrombus may undergo organization by ingrowth of granulation tissue from the vessel wall and subsequent fibrous repair. By an extraordinary mechanism, the organised thrombus may undergo *recanalization*, with the formation of new vascular channels, the larger channels acquiring muscular walls (see Fig. 8.4).

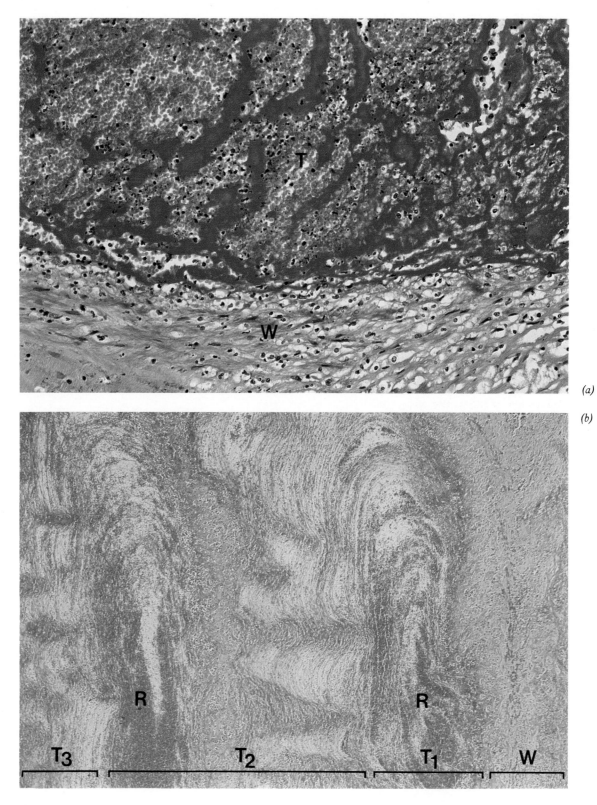

*(a)*

*(b)*

Fig. 8.1   Thrombus formation

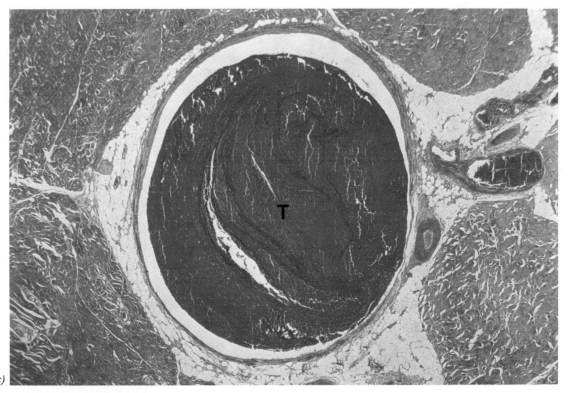

*(c)*

## Fig. 8.1  Thrombus formation *(illustrations (a) and (b) opposite)*
**(a) early thrombus** (HP)
**(b) enlargement of thrombus** (MP)
**(c) thrombosis in a vein** (LP)

Damage of a vessel wall usually involves damage to the endothelial lining and exposure of intimal collagen resulting in first adherence, and then aggregation of platelets at the site of damage. At the same time, tissue damage and collagen exposure activate the extrinsic and intrinsic blood clotting systems respectively, the latter system also depending on release of platelet factor 3 from aggregated platelets. The result is activation of prothrombin to thrombin which in turn catalyses the conversion of soluble plasma fibrinogen into insoluble fibrin. Thus the flimsy platelet aggregates become bound together into a solid resilient mass, the thrombus.

Micrograph (a) illustrates an arterial wall **W** damaged by atheroma. The endothelium has become ulcerated with the formation of thrombus **T** at the site of injury. This thrombus consists of platelet aggregates within a meshwork of eosinophilic (red staining) fibrin; entrapped erythrocytes and leucocytes are present, but are not themselves involved in the specific haemostatic processes.

Small areas of thrombus formed on vessel walls may be resolved completely by fibrinolytic mechanisms, however under appropriate conditions the thrombus continues to enlarge. Micrograph (b) illustrates this process. The abnormal vessel wall **W** has become coated by a thin layer of fibrin and platelet thrombus $T_1$ with entrapped red cells **R**. This has

formed the basis for the deposition of another layer of fibrin-platelet thrombus $T_2$, again with entrapped red cells. A third layer $T_3$ can be seen forming at the left of the picture. Thus thrombi enlarge by the successive deposition of a number of layers, a feature which is apparent to the naked eye in the laminated cut surface seen in an established thrombus (*lines of Zahn*).

In the arterial system, damage to the intimal layer is the most common predisposing factor in thrombus formation, but in the venous system the most important factor is the rate of blood flow; reduced flow rates increase susceptibility to thrombus formation.

Micrograph (c) shows venous thrombosis **T** completely occluding the lumen of a vein in a neurovascular bundle from the muscle of the calf. This is known as deep vein thrombosis (DVT) and is frequently seen in postoperative patients who are confined to bed.

Propagation of thrombus along the veins and detachment of a fragment may lead to pulmonary embolism (Fig. 8.3) and infarction (Fig. 9.5). This sequence of events is the most important and serious sequel of venous thrombosis. It occurs because of low blood flow resulting from postoperative immobility and increased concentrations of coagulation factors in the blood after any forms of trauma, including surgery.

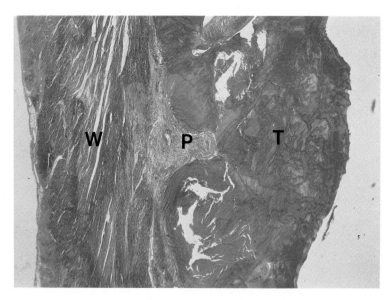

### Fig. 8.2 Left ventricular mural thrombus (LP)

Thrombosis within the heart chambers most commonly occurs upon endocardium damaged by myocardial infarction (see Fig. 9.3). This micrograph illustrates infarcted ventricular wall **W** with mural thrombus **T** laid down on the luminal surface; the thrombus surrounds a papillary muscle **P**.

The left ventricle is the most common site of mural thrombosis after myocardial infarction and is an important source of potentially disastrous systemic thrombo-emboli to such organs as the brain, kidneys, gut and spleen.

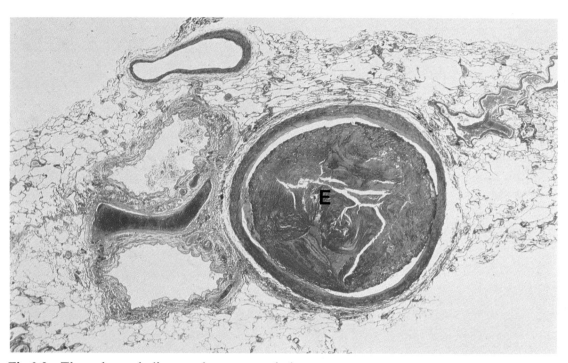

### Fig.8.3 Thrombo-embolism: pulmonary embolus (LP)

When fragments of thrombus become detached from their site of formation they travel in the circulation (venous or arterial, according to site of origin) as thrombo-emboli. On reaching vessels of small enough calibre to prevent further passage, the thrombo-emboli impact producing sudden vascular occlusion. Depending on the size of the thrombo-embolus, the tissue or organ involved, and the extent of alternative vascular supply, the result may be either inadequate blood flow for normal sustenance of the tissue (ischaemia) or frank tissue necrosis (infarction); these phenomena are described in the next chapter.

This micrograph illustrates lung tissue in which the pulmonary artery branch is occluded by an embolus **E** originating from thrombus in the deep veins of the leg.

This condition, known as *pulmonary embolism*, is an important cause of sudden death, especially in debilitated or immobilized patients predisposed to deep venous thrombosis.

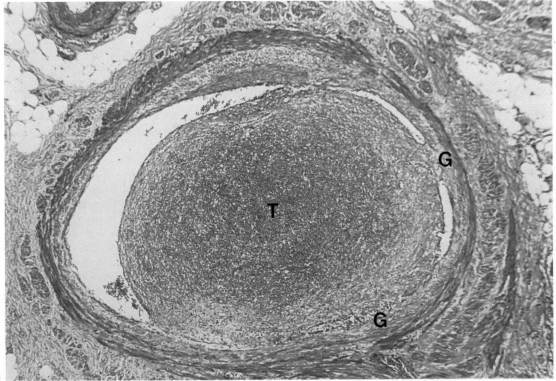

*(a)*

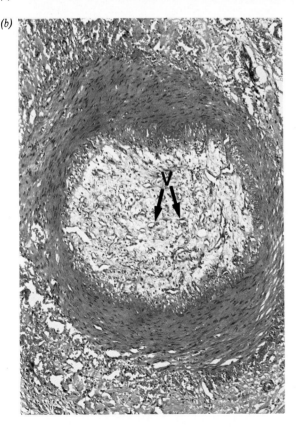

*(b)*

## Fig. 8.4 Fate of thrombi
### (a) organization (LP)
### (b) recanalization (MP)

Following occlusion of a vessel by thrombus, there is an initial inflammatory response in the vessel wall. Eventually the thrombus becomes organized by ingrowth of granulation tissue from the intima of the vessel wall. Micrograph (a) shows a vein occluded by thrombus **T**. At various points, granulation tissue **G** extends from the vessel wall into the thrombus. This eventually results in replacement of the thrombus by fibrovascular granulation tissue. In some cases, larger vessels develop within the fibrovascular granulation tissue of the organizing thrombus and may permit passage of blood through the damaged, previously occluded area. This occurs most commonly in arteries and is termed *recanalization*.

Micrograph (b) illustrates this process in an artery which has been occluded by thrombus and is at a later stage of organization than in micrograph (a). Note that the granulation tissue in the lumen contains numerous small blood vessels **V**. These vessels may conduct blood across the thrombosed area and some will enlarge with time and acquire smooth muscle walls.

# 9. Infarction

## Introduction

Infarction occurs in any tissue when there is interruption of blood supply sufficient to cause tissue necrosis; the area of tissue involved is described as an *infarct*. On the other hand, disturbance of blood supply may not be sufficient to cause frank tissue necrosis but may instead cause temporary or permanent damage to the tissue or some of its functional elements; this situation is known as *ischaemia* and may in due course, though not necessarily, lead to infarction.

Infarction may result either from obstruction of arterial supply or, much less commonly, from obstruction of venous drainage. Arterial occlusion is usually due to thrombosis or embolism (see Chapter 8); examples from the kidney and myocardium are shown in Figs 9.1 and 9.3 respectively. Alternatively, organs which receive their blood supply via a vascular pedicle may become infarcted if the pedicle becomes twisted e.g. torsion of the testis (see Fig. 18.4) or constricted by becoming entrapped in a narrow space e.g. bowel infarction due to hernial strangulation (Fig. 9.6). In such cases, complete arterial obstruction is often preceded by venous obstruction since extrinsic pressure affects the thin walled, low pressure veins before compromising the arteries; venous obstruction causes the tissue to become deeply congested and ischaemic, and subsequent arterial obstruction causes overt infarction.

When infarction is due to simple cessation of arterial supply, the shape of the infarct reflects the geographical distribution of the artery involved. In most organs (e.g. kidney, spleen, brain) the infarct appears wedge-shaped on section with the broad part of the wedge at the periphery. In contrast, infarcts in the heart are not wedge-shaped but rather involve part or full thickness of the myocardium and its overlying endocardium and/or visceral pericardium.

Like most forms of tissue damage, infarction excites an acute inflammatory response followed by replacement of necrotic tissue by granulation tissue which then undergoes fibrous repair and scarring (see Chapter 2). The naked eye and histological appearances of infarcts thus depend on how far this sequence has progressed. One important exception to this process is the brain which does not have the capacity for the usual processes of granulation tissue formation and fibrous repair. Cerebral infarcts undergo central liquefaction with reactive gliosis at the margins of the lesion and old infarcts are usually marked by a cystic area surrounded by a zone of gliosis; brain infarction is illustrated in Fig. 22.2.

Organs in which there are extensive capillary, sinusoidal or arteriovenous anastamoses often have infarcts which in their earliest stages are dark red in colour due to congestion with blood and haemorrhage (from the Latin, *infarcire* — to stuff); important examples are the lung (see Fig. 9.5) and spleen.

## Fig. 9.1  Renal infarction *(illustrations opposite)*
## (a) early infarct (LP)
## (b) margin of infarct (MP)

The general features of infarction induced by thrombo-embolism are well illustrated by renal infarcts which usually result from emboli originating from thrombus in the left ventricle (e.g. mural thrombus after myocardial infarction) or the left atrial appendage (e.g. in atrial fibrillation).

In the very early stages (i.e. within 12 hours of infarction), gross examination shows the infarcted area to be ill defined and dark, but progressively the lesion becomes paler until its wedge-shaped margins may be clearly distinguishable. Micrograph (a) shows the histological appearance of a typical early renal infarct. The recently infarcted necrotic area **Inf** stains less intensely than the normal cortex **N** but the general architecture of the infarct remains intact with still discernible 'ghosts' of glomeruli and renal tubules. The infarcted area has become demarcated from normal cortex by a narrow hyperaemic zone **H** representing the earliest stages of a typical acute inflammatory response. Between this hyperaemic zone and the necrotic tissue is a purple staining band containing the neutrophils of an early cellular acute inflammatory exudate.

Micrograph (b) shows, at higher magnification, the edge of the infarct in micrograph (a). Note that the normal cortical tissue **N** with its well defined glomeruli and tubules gives way to a zone of hyperaemia **H**; next to this is a purplish band of acute inflammation **In** at the margin of the infarcted area where marked necrotic changes are evident in both glomeruli and tubules (see Fig. 1.5a). The acute inflammatory zone exhibits typically dilated and congested capillaries and an influx of small, dark staining neutrophil polymorphs.

The necrotic tissue is progressively removed by neutrophils and macrophages and replaced by granulation tissue which eventually undergoes fibrous repair to form a small fibrous scar (see Fig. 9.2).

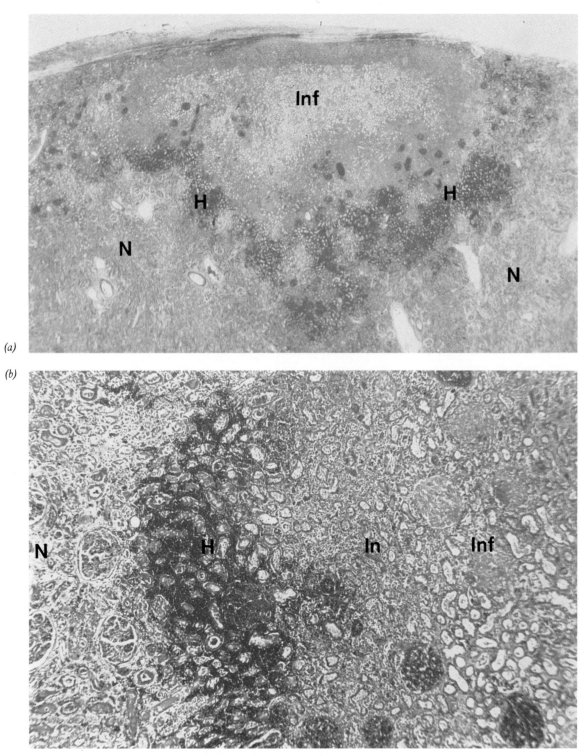

Fig. 9.1    Renal infarction

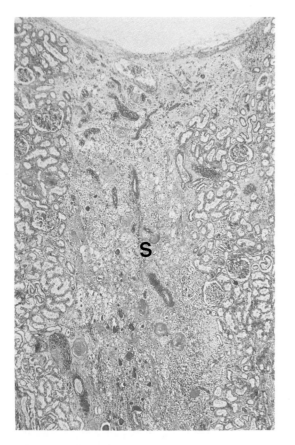

## Fig. 9.2  Old renal infarct (MP)

This micrograph illustrates the end result of a renal infarct occurring two months previously; the infarct was of similar size to that shown in Fig. 9.1. All that now remains is a small, narrow, pink staining, wedge-shaped scar **S** with its broad aspect at the capsular surface. Note that the capsular surface at the site of the scar is depressed as a result of contraction of the collagen fibres within the scar (cicatrization; see Fig. 2.10).

## Fig. 9.3  Myocardial infarction (illustrations opposite)
**(a) 24 hour infarct** (HP)
**(b) 3 day infarct** (HP)
**(c) 10 day infarct** (HP)
**(d) 14 day infarct** (HP)

The most common clinical example of infarction is that of the myocardium following occlusion of a coronary artery.

Using routine staining methods, the earliest histological evidence of infarction is visible some 12 to 24 hours after the onset of acute ischaemia, as illustrated in micrograph (a). The infarcted cardiac muscle fibres **In** exhibit patchy loss or blurring of cross striations and tend to become more intensely stained by eosin when compared to normal myocardial fibres **My**; there may also at this stage be some degree of early capillary engorgement and interstitial oedema, representing an incipient acute inflammatory response.

By about 2 to 3 days, as shown in micrograph (b), the infarcted fibres are intensely eosinophilic and most have lost their nuclei; there is marked infiltration by neutrophils **N** into the oedematous interstitium. The acute inflammatory process evolves during the succeeding days during which time the necrotic myocardium undergoes autolysis and fragmentation, and the neutrophil infiltration becomes more intense.

By about the tenth day, as illustrated in micrograph (c), most of the necrotic muscle has disappeared as a result of the combined phagocytic activity of neutrophils and macrophages (see Fig. 2.6). The infarcted area is now largely occupied by residual macrophages, some lymphocytes and plasma cells, in a loose oedematous mesh in which a few capillaries and fibroblasts herald the earliest signs of granulation tissue formation.

By about the fourteenth day, the infarct is almost wholly replaced by fibrovascular granulation tissue **G**, as illustrated in micrograph (d), and the necrotic myocardium has been almost completely removed by the phagocytic activity of macrophages and neutrophils.

Over succeeding weeks, the fibrovascular granulation tissue becomes progressively more fibrous and less vascular, leading to the formation of a highly collagenous and relatively acellular scar by about the end of the second month following infarction; examples of myocardial scars are shown in Fig. 9.4.

The infarcted myocardium offers the least resistance to pressure around about the tenth day and at this time the patient is most vulnerable to myocardial rupture. This not uncommon complication is almost invariably fatal when a ventricle wall ruptures, spilling blood into the pericardial cavity (haemopericardium). If the interventricular septum is involved in the infarct, there may be rupture of the septum with the sudden appearance of a systolic murmur. Similarly, rupture of an infarcted papillary muscle may lead to mitral valve incompetence with the sudden appearance of a characteristic systolic murmur.

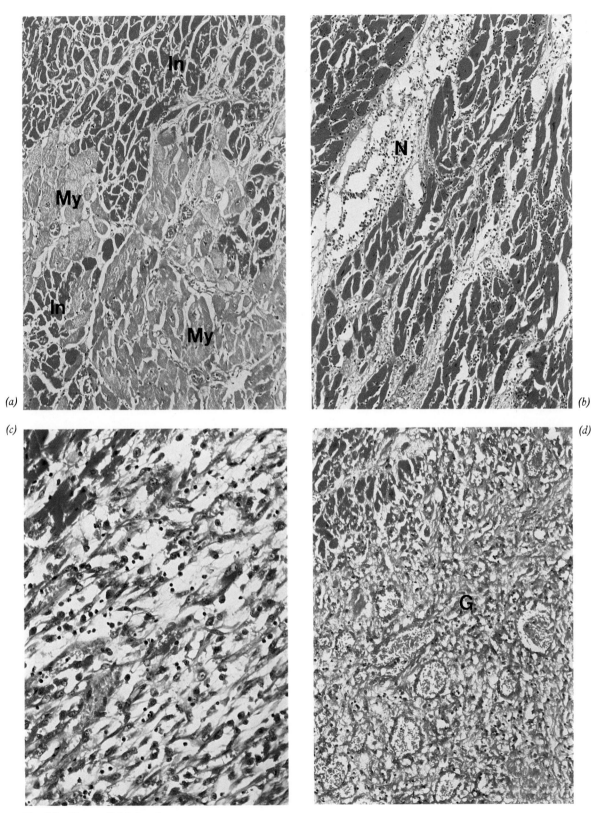

Fig. 9.3  Myocardial infarction

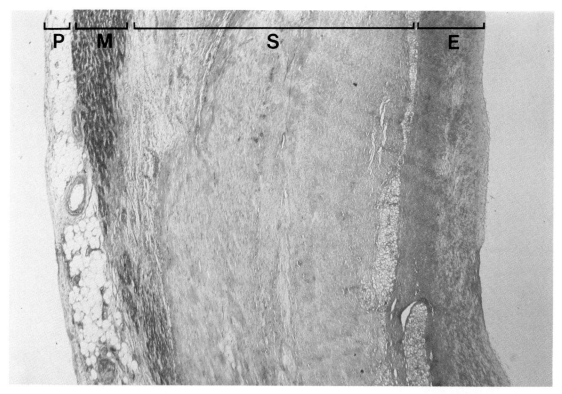

*(a)*

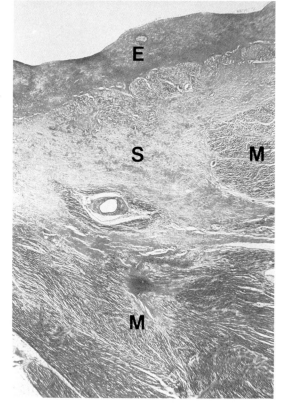

*(b)*

## Fig. 9.4   Old myocardial infarcts
**(a) full thickness scar** (LP)
**(b) partial thickness scar** (LP)

These two micrographs show examples of myocardial scars
several months after infarction. The sites of infarction are
marked by densely collagenous pale pink staining scar **S**,
contrasting with the more heavily staining surviving
myocardial muscle **M**. Continuing contraction (cicatrization) of
the fibrous scar over succeeding months leads to thinning of
the infarcted area of the ventricular wall. If the scar is
inadequate to withstand ventricular pressures (most likely after
a full thickness infarct), a ventricular aneurysm may develop
by ballooning of the ventricular wall. With or without
aneurysm formation, stasis in the region of the non-contractile
scar predisposes to formation of a ventricular mural thrombus
(see Fig. 8.2).

If the original infarct involves the endocardium **E** or visceral
pericardium **P**, or both as in some full thickness infarcts, these
normally delicate layers become markedly thickened as a result
of their involvement in the inflammatory process and
subsequent organization and repair.

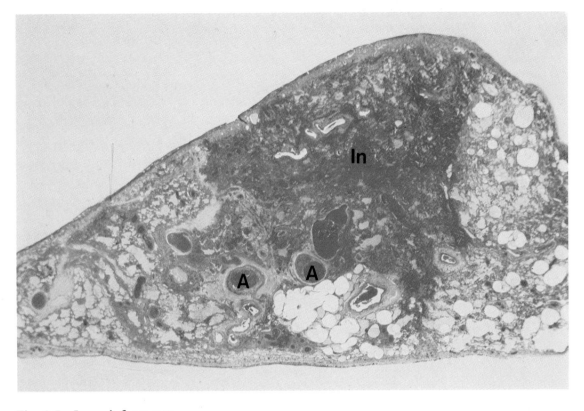

## Fig. 9.5  Lung infarct (LP)

Infarcts of the lung usually result from small pulmonary emboli arising from fragments of thrombus within the veins of the legs (see Fig. 8.1c). In their early stages, lung infarcts are firm, dark red, wedge-shaped areas at the lung periphery; their firmness and colour derive from the fact that the alveolar spaces are filled with erythrocytes, partly due to leakage from damaged capillary walls and partly from blood carried by the unobstructed bronchial arterial circulation. The pleura becomes involved in the resulting acute inflammatory response; in this case the fibrinous pleurisy results in characteristic sharp pleuritic pain and a pleural friction rub.

This micrograph illustrates the edge of a lung with a small congested infarct **In**. Note the obstructed branches of the pulmonary artery **A** and the clearly defined margins of the infarct demarcating the area supplied by this vessel.

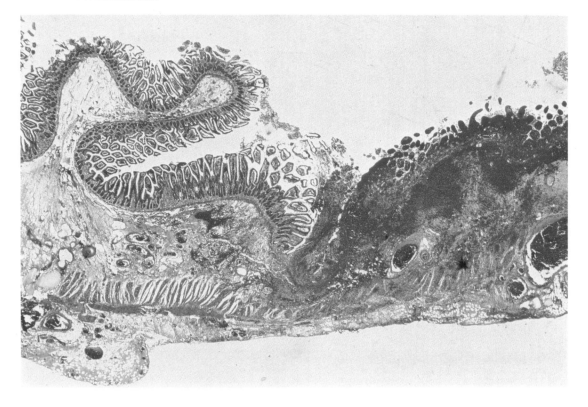

**Fig. 9.6   Bowel infarction following volvulus** (LP)

Bowel infarction may occur either as a result of arterial occlusion e.g. mesenteric thrombosis or embolism, or, more commonly, as a result of venous obstruction. Venous obstruction may occur either through torsion (twisting) of a free loop of bowel around its vascular pedicle (*volvulus*), entrapment in a tight hernial orifice (e.g. indirect inguinal hernia) or obstruction by fibrous peritoneal adhesions (e.g. following previous surgery).

Venous obstruction initially causes the bowel to become intensely congested with blood, giving it a plum coloured appearance on gross examination; as the dammed-back blood prevents arterial inflow, the bowel becomes progressively anoxic. Frank necrosis follows unless the venous obstruction is relieved.

In this micrograph of a small bowel volvulus, the necrotic bowel at the right hand end of the picture is stained bright red due to massive suffusion with blood; the outline of the necrotic mucosal villi is still apparent. Note the sharp demarcation between normal and necrotic bowel, and the marked engorgement of all vessels.

# PART 2

# Basic Systems Pathology

# 10. Cardiovascular system

## Introduction

Diseases of the cardiovascular system are the commonest cause of death and serious illness in developed countries. Pre-eminent is atherosclerosis which, because of its numerous associated disorders and complications, is the exclusive topic of one chapter (Ch. 7). Of similar order of importance are the phenomena of thrombosis and embolism, which are the subject of Chapter 8, and their frequent sequel, infarction, which is described in Chapter 9.

## The heart

Of the diseases involving the heart, ischaemic heart disease, is of paramount importance. In the vast majority of cases, the cause of ischaemic heart disease is atherosclerosis of the coronary arteries with or without accompanying thrombosis; coronary artery atheroma and thrombosis are illustrated in Figs 7.4 and 7.6, and the stages of myocardial infarction are shown in Figs 9.3 and 9.4.

Functional and structural abnormalities of the heart may develop as a result of hypertension due to increased peripheral resistance in the systemic circulation (hypertensive heart disease) or pulmonary circulation (cor pulmonale). In both cases the ventricle exposed to hypertension undergoes hypertrophic thickening of its muscular wall; ventricular failure often ensues.

*Rheumatic fever,* a systemic connective tissue disorder with an immunological basis, often affects the heart with important immediate and long term clinical consequences; rheumatic heart lesions are illustrated in Fig. 10.3. Viral, bacterial and parasitic infections of the heart may involve pericardium, myocardium, and the endocardium and heart valves; those of greatest clinical and histological importance are shown in Fig. 10.4. Inflammation of the pericardium is now rarely caused by microbial agents but more often occurs in response to myocardial infarction, tumour invasion or uraemia; an example of acute pericarditis is provided in Fig. 2.3.

## The arterial and venous systems

The most common pathological abnormality of the arterial tree is thickening and hardening of the walls, a condition known as *arteriosclerosis*. Atheroma (atherosclerosis) is the most frequent cause of arteriosclerosis and is discussed in Chapter 7. The other important causes of artery and arteriole wall thickening and hardening are those associated with hypertension and diabetes mellitus; in both cases however, the specific vascular changes are often superimposed upon features of the ubiquitous atherosclerosis. Some of the important arterial wall changes associated with hypertension are illustrated in this chapter in Figs 10.1 and 10.2 and in Fig. 14.8. Diabetic vascular changes are illustrated in relation to their important impact on the kidney in Fig. 14.7.

Abnormal dilatations of arterial vessels, known as *aneurysms,* may be divided into five different types. First, those arising as a complication of atherosclerosis (e.g. in abdominal aorta). Second, *syphilitic aneurysms,* usually involving the ascending aorta, result from damage inflicted upon the aortic media by the chronic inflammatory lesions of syphilitic aortitis (Fig. 3.19). A third type of aneurysm is that resulting from idiopathic degeneration of the tunica media and usually involving the thoracic aorta; these *dissecting aneurysms* are discussed in Fig. 10.5. Fourth, areas of developmental weakness in the walls of the cerebral arteries may undergo aneurysmal dilatation under the stress of transient or persistent high blood pressure; such aneurysms are known as *berry aneurysms* (Fig. 10.6). Finally, hypertensive and diabetic vascular disease predispose to aneurysm formation in small vessels of the brain and retina respectively; rupture of these *microaneurysms* may lead to brain haemorrhage and blindness.

Arterial walls become the specific target of inflammation in a group of diseases of probable autoimmune aetiology. The most common of these *arteritides* are *polyarteritis nodosa* and *giant cell arteritis* illustrated in Figs 10.7 and 10.8 respectively. Arteritis is also an important histological feature of organs affected by some systemic autoimmune diseases such as systemic lupus erythematosis.

The venous system is relatively free of diseases of any great clinical importance although veins are an important site of thrombus formation as discussed in Chapter 8.

Benign and malignant tumours, known as angiomas and angiosarcomas respectively, may arise from the blood or lymph vascular tissues. Most common among these are *haemangiomas* illustrated in Fig. 10.9, many of which are regarded as hamartomas rathre than neoplasms.

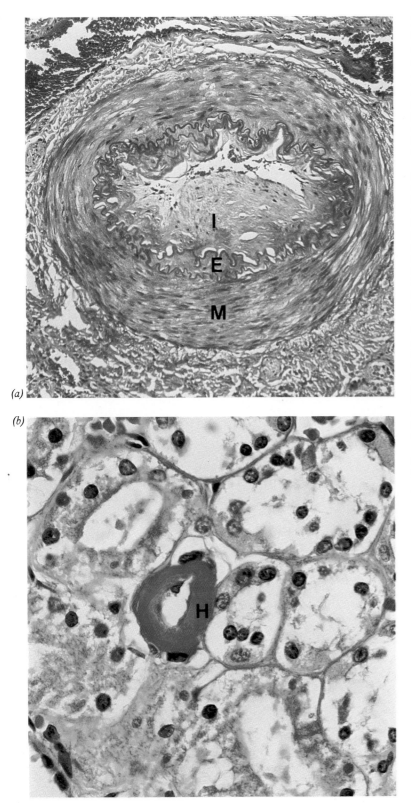

(a)

(b)

## Fig. 10.1 Arterial changes in essential hypertension (a) medium sized artery (MP) (b) arteriole (HP)

Hypertension, whether idiopathic or secondary to known pathology, is known to be associated with concurrent changes in peripheral arterial vessels; whether such changes are part of the primary causative process, secondary, or contributory remains unresolved.

When the increase in blood pressure is moderate and gradual in onset (*essential* or *benign hypertension*), muscular arteries exposed to the persistently raised diastolic pressure undergo progressive thickening of their walls. Three features are prominent and are shown in micrograph (a): symmetrical hypertrophy of the muscular media **M,** extensive reduplication of the internal elastic lamina **E** and regular fibrotic thickening of the intima **I**. All these changes lead to reduction of luminal diameter.

Arterioles show a different type of wall thickening sometimes referred to as *hyaline arteriolosclerosis* and shown in micrograph (b). The normal layers of the wall become ill defined and replaced by homogeneous eosinophilic (pink stained) material called *hyaline* **H** now thought to be of basement membrane-like composition. This results in reduction in size of arteriolar lumina and may contribute to further hypertension.

Similar arteriolar changes occur in diabetes mellitus and are illustrated with respect to the kidneys in Fig. 14.7.

### Fig. 10.2 Arterial changes in accelerated hypertension (a) medium sized artery (HP) (b) arteriole (HP)

When the increase in blood pressure is of marked degree and rapid onset (*accelerated* or *malignant hypertension*), muscular arteries develop extensive thickening of the tunica intima **I** by proliferation of intimal cells; this gives the appearance of concentric lamellae which encroach upon the arterial lumen as seen in micrograph (a). In contrast to the findings in moderate hypertension, the tunica media **M** and internal elastic lamina **E** remain largely unchanged.

The impact of sudden and severe hypertension on arterioles is even more dramatic as shown in micrograph (b). The intimal cells undergo rapid proliferation (as in the muscular arteries) which is often complicated by disruption of the vessel wall with leakage of plasma proteins including fibrinogen into and beyond the arteriolar wall. This change, known inaccurately as *fibrinoid necrosis*, is characterized by obliteration of the wall by intensely eosinophilic amorphous proteinaceous material **P**; the lumen is often completely occluded.

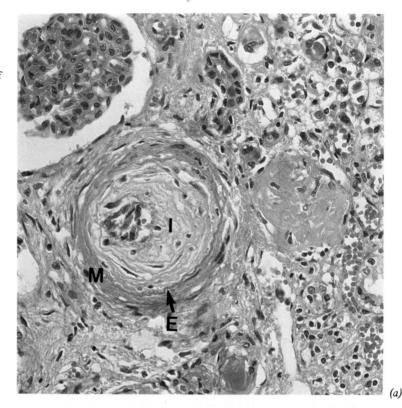

*(a)*

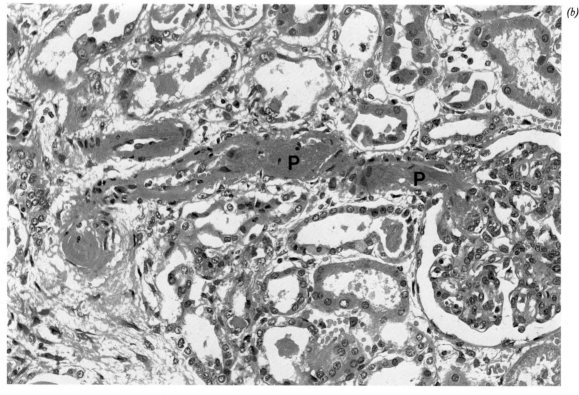

*(b)*

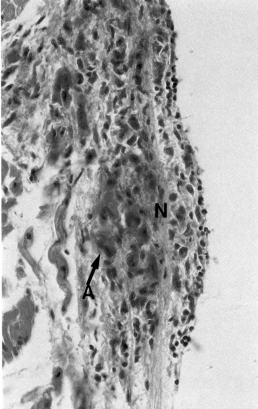

*(a)*

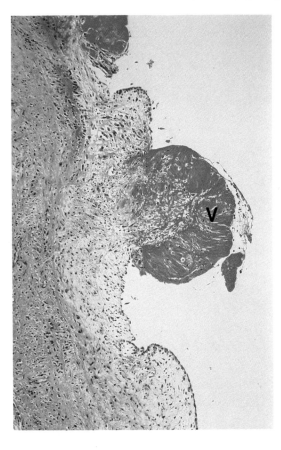

*(b)*

## Fig. 10.3   Rheumatic heart disease
## (a) Aschoff body (HP)
## (b) acute rheumatic endocarditis (MP)

*Rheumatic fever* is a systemic inflammatory disease which, in susceptible individuals, appears to follow infection by *group A β haemolytic streptococci;* such infections commonly occur in the throat and are themselves relatively innocuous.

The systemic manifestations are thought to represent a disordered immunological response resulting in inflammation of connective tissues. Connective tissues in all parts of the body may be involved e.g. the joints and skin, with painful short term consequences, but involvement of the heart is the most important clinically because of its potentially fatal acute course and long term consequences.

In its acute phase, rheumatic fever may produce a *pancarditis* affecting concurrently pericardium, myocardium and endocardium. The characteristic rheumatic lesion is the *Aschoff body* one of which is shown in micrograph (a). The fully developed  Aschoff body has a central ill-defined area of degenerate or necrotic material **N** surrounded by a mixture of inflammatory leucocytes and an occasional multinucleate giant cell. Amongst these cells can often be seen a so-called *Anitschow myocyte* **A** recognized by its peculiar, irregular, ribbon-like nucleus and extensive eosinophilic cytoplasm. Despite their name, these cells are considered to represent large modified fibroblasts. Aschoff bodies are found in the interstitial connective tissue of the myocardium particularly near vessels, in the subepicardial fibrous tissue, and (as in this micrograph) in the subendocardial connective tissue.

Involvement of the pericardium and myocardium in the acute phase leads to pericarditis and myocarditis respectively, each with possibly life-threatening consequences. The importance of endocardial involvement lies in its effects upon the heart valves. Valvular lesions result in endocardial roughening which in turn induces formation of fibrin and platelet thrombi along the free margins of the valve leaflets. Organization and progressive fibrous scarring of the inflamed and thrombus-bearing valves continues over many years with eventual fibrous thickening and distortion of the valve leaflet or cusp. Contraction of the fibrous scar tissue causes shrinkage of the valve, whilst the fibrosis and occasional calcification may lead to great rigidity and immobility. Fibrous thickening and fusion of chordae tendinae also occurs in affected atrioventricular valves further reducing valve mobility. Such destructive changes may render the valve stenotic or incompetent.

Micrograph (b) illustrates part of a mitral valve leaflet affected by acute rheumatic endocarditis. A small thrombotic vegetation **V** has formed on the upper (atrial) surface of the valve leaflet at the site of the remnants of a large Aschoff body. The edge of a similar thrombotic vegetation, now becoming covered with endocardial cells as a first step in its organization and fibrosis, can be seen at the top of the picture.

Apart from the destructive long term consequences of rheumatic endocarditis itself, such damaged valves are thereafter susceptible to infection causing the condition commonly called *subacute bacterial endocarditis* (see Fig. 10.4).

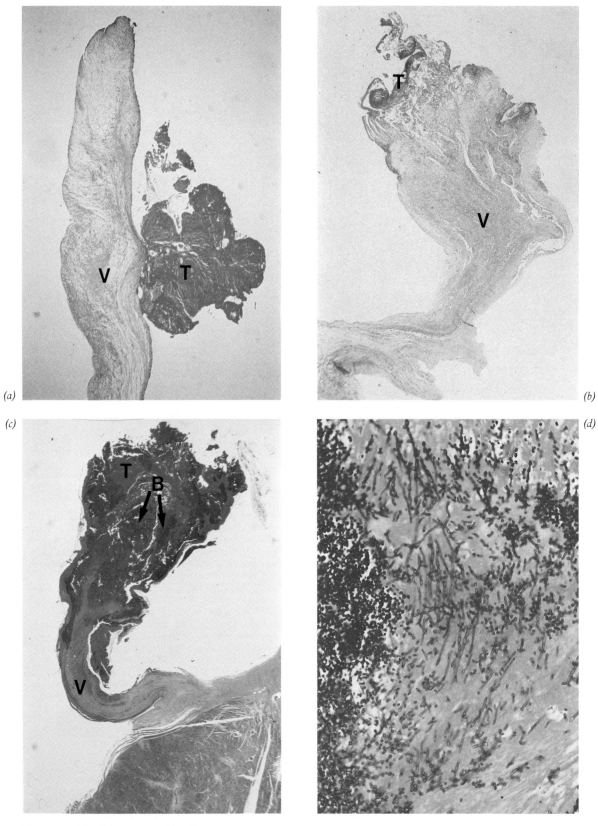

*(a)*

*(b)*

*(c)*

*(d)*

**Fig. 10.4   Valvulitis (endocarditis of valves)**

# Fig. 10.4   Valvulitis (endocarditis of valves) *(illustrations opposite)*
## (a) marantic (thrombotic, nonbacterial) endocarditis (LP)
## (b) bacterial endocarditis (subacute) (LP)
## (c) bacterial endocarditis (acute) (LP)
## (d) fungal (Candidal) endocarditis (P.A.S. stain; HP)

The heart valves may under certain conditions become subject to a variety of vegetative lesions which have traditionally been described as various forms of *endocarditis*. The primary phenomenon underlying all these conditions is the formation of thrombus on the valve leaflets or cusps. As in the arterial system, roughening of the endocardial surface predisposes to thrombus formation (see Chapter 8); this may occur when valve leaflets or cusps have been previously damaged by rheumatic fever or ischaemic heart disease, but may also follow autoimmune valve damage in systemic lupus erythematosis (*Libman-Sachs endocarditis*) and in the acute phase of rheumatic fever (acute rheumatic carditis, see Fig. 10.3). The most frequent type of valve thrombi, however, occur in so-called *marantic endocarditis* in which warty thrombotic vegetations develop on mitral and aortic valves. This phenomenon occurs in seriously ill patients, often those with widely disseminated malignancy, and is usually associated with a state of hypercoagulability of the blood. Despite use of the term endocarditis in these conditions, inflammation itself is usually not a feature of the valve at the time of thrombus formation.

True valvular inflammation may arise however if these thrombotic vegetations on the valves then become infected with bacteria, fungi or other organisms, conditions collectively referred to as *infective endocarditis*. Bacterial endocarditis tends to be divided into two clinicopathological patterns. In the first, traditionally known as *subacute bacterial endocarditis,* the thrombotic vegetations develop on previously damaged valves (usually scarred rheumatic mitral or aortic valves) which then become colonized by bacteria of low virulence such as *Streptococcus viridans;* such organisms tend to reach the valves via a transient bacteraemia e.g. following dental extraction. The major clinical consequences are those resulting from detachment of small thrombotic emboli, often infected, into the systemic circulation.

In the second type of bacterial endocarditis, known traditionally as *acute bacterial endocarditis,* thrombi form on previously normal valves and become infected by virulent organisms such as *Staphylococcus aureus*. In this case, the patient is usually already severely debilitated and septicaemic, such as from an infected venous or urinary catheter, and the infecting organism is that which is responsible for the septicaemia. In contrast with the subacute pattern, in the acute form the fulminating infection extends into the substance of the valve causing tissue necrosis. Rapid destruction of the valve leaflet leads to valvular incompetence and acute cardiac failure is the usual clinical outcome.

*Fungal endocarditis,* formerly rare, is now appearing more commonly, sometimes as a complication of immunosuppressive therapy or heroin addiction; *Candida albicans* is the most common culprit and the clinical course of the disease tends to be rather acute.

The incidence of these types of endocarditis has changed over the past few decades for many reasons including the widespread use of broad spectrum antibiotics and decreasing incidence of rheumatic fever. Furthermore, understanding of the nature of these conditions has changed markedly in recent years leaving behind a somewhat inappropriate terminology.

Micrograph (a) illustrates a mitral valve lesion of marantic (thrombotic, nonbacterial) endocarditis; masses of thrombus **T** have developed on the superior surface of the valve leaflet **V.** Such thrombotic masses are only loosely attached to the underlying, normal noninflamed valve, and therefore are readily detached, whole or in part, leading to major embolic episodes such as cerebral, renal and splenic infarction (see Chapter 9). In practice, this type of endocarditis is rarely diagnosed in life but is a common necropsy finding.

The subacute form of bacterial endocarditis affecting a mitral valve is demonstrated in micrograph (b). The valve leaflet **V** is covered at its tip by pink staining thrombus **T** containing small colonies of blue-purple staining bacteria. Note that the underlying valve, though thickened due to previous rheumatic fever, shows no evidence of bacterial destruction and that the organisms are present in relatively small numbers (compare with micrograph c). Fragments of such vegetations frequently become detached giving rise to multiple small embolic episodes.

An example of the acute form of bacterial endocarditis involving an aortic valve is shown in micrograph (c). In this case, highly virulent bacteria **B** causing septicaemia have settled on heart valves probably colonizing small pre-existing thrombi; bacterial proliferation then stimulates further formation of thrombus **T** forming large vegetations which, in contrast to the subacute situation, erode and destroy the previously normal valve **V.** Compare the huge mass of bacteria and thrombus in this case with that of the subacute form shown in (b). Since destruction is so rapid, the clinical picture is usually of rapidly developing cardiac failure rather than thrombotic episodes.

Micrograph (d) shows a vegetation on an aortic valve from a patient with fungal endocarditis. The section is stained by the P.A.S. method to demonstrate the yeasts and pseudohyphae of *Candida albicans* (stained magenta) which populate the thrombotic mass. Candida usually gains access to the bloodstream from the skin (where it is an abundant commensal) as a result of nonsterile intravenous injection procedures (e.g. in heroin addicts as in this case) or from infected surgical wounds.

## Fig. 10.5 **Dissecting aneurysms of the aorta** (LP)

*Dissecting aneurysms* most commonly affect the thoracic aorta. A laceration of the tunica intima **I** leads to tracking of blood into the tunica media **M,** the plane of cleavage (dissection) usually being between the middle and outer thirds of the media, as in this example; note that the site of intimal laceration is not included in this photographic field. The medial haematoma **H** then frequently bursts through the tunica adventitia **A** with rapidly fatal consequences.

The pathogenesis of dissecting aneurysms is poorly understood but almost all cases exhibit a peculiar type of non-inflammatory degeneration of the smooth muscle and elastic tissue of tunica media. In this condition, known as *medial mucoid degeneration* or *cystic medionecrosis,* areas of the tunica media become replaced by irregular masses of acellular polysaccharide material. Dissecting aneurysms may occur in adults at any age though they are most common in middle age, with males outnumbering females.

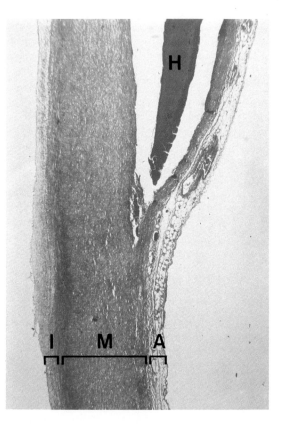

## Fig. 10.6 **Berry aneurysm** (Elastic van Gieson stain; LP)

*Berry aneurysms* are a characteristic type of aneurysm found in the cerebral circulation particularly at junctions in the circle of Willis or at bifurcations of the major cerebral arteries (especially the middle cerebral). Berry aneurysms most often become manifest in middle age by rupturing to cause *subarachnoid haemorrhage.* These aneurysms are, however, an occasional incidental finding at all ages and are often multiple.

This micrograph illustrates a berry aneurysm **B** arising from the anterior cerebral artery **A** just proximal to the point where it gives rise to its anterior communicating branch **C.** The vessel has a normal tunica media **M,** adventitia **Ad** and internal elastic lamina **E** (elastin stains black with this staining method). Note that at the point of origin of the aneurysm, the tunica media is deficient (arrow). The wall of the aneurysm **W** is composed of loose fibrous intimal tissue and the lumen contains blood. There is no medial muscle or elastin in the aneurysm wall.

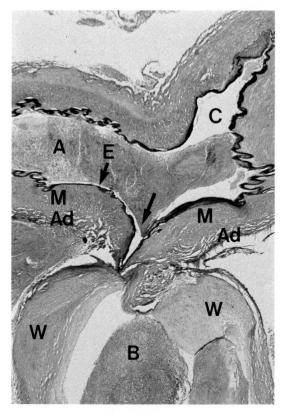

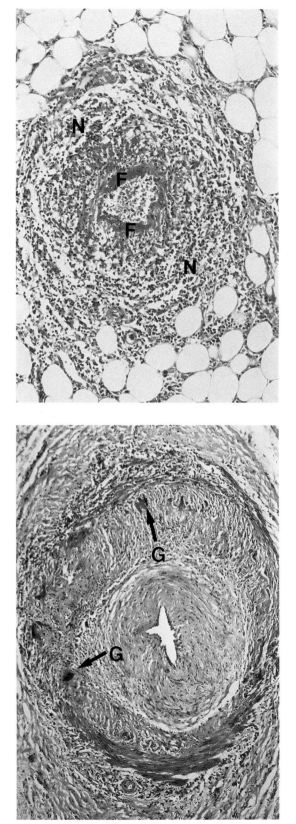

## Fig. 10.7 Polyarteritis nodosa (MP)

*Polyarteritis nodosa* is a rare, systemic immunological disease characterized by acute inflammation of the walls of medium and small sized muscular arteries; the lesions are discrete and scattered and may be found in all organs but in particular the kidneys, heart, liver and gastrointestinal tract, lungs, peripheral nerves and skin.

Histologically, the appearance is of an acute necrotizing inflammation of the arterial wall with heavy infiltration of neutrophils **N** accompanied by a variable, sometimes large, number of eosinophils. The vessel wall almost invariably exhibits the features of so called *fibrinoid necrosis* **F** (see Fig. 10.2) and the lumen may become occluded by thrombus. Subsequent fibrous healing leaves the vessel wall thickened and nodular with a defective internal elastic lamina. Apart from generalized symptoms such as fever, malaise, weakness and weight loss, the clinical presentation of this disease is extremely variable depending on which tissues become ischaemic or infarcted as a result of the arterial lesions. For example, kidney involvement may be manifest by pain, haematuria or proteinuria, heart involvement by angina, myocardial infarction or pericarditis, and skin involvement by tender subcutaneous nodules. Clinical diagnosis must usually be substantiated by tissue biopsy.

## Fig. 10.8 Giant cell (cranial or temporal) arteritis (MP)

Giant cell arteritis is another systemic immunological disease of blood vessels particularly medium sized arteries of the head, thereby resulting in the synonyms of *cranial* and *temporal arteritis.*

Histologically, the walls of involved vessels exhibit features more reminiscent of granulomatous than acute neutrophilic inflammation. Multinucleate giant cells **G** are the most characteristic finding and these tend to be arranged circumferentially, apparently in relation to degenerate fragments of the internal elastic lamina. Marked fibrous thickening of the intimal layer may be complicated by thrombosis, which may produce acute blindness if the ophthalmic artery is affected.

In addition to vague constitutional symptoms, the condition often presents as localized throbbing pain or tenderness e.g. over the temporal artery, or alternatively, as more generalized muscle pain in the condition known as *polymyalgia rheumatica.* Diagnosis is confirmed by temporal artery or muscle biopsy according to the clinical presentation although results will be negative unless a discrete inflammatory lesion is included in the biopsy specimen.

This photomicrograph shows a temporal artery biopsy from a 76 year old man who presented with sudden onset of impaired vision in one eye.

In contrast to polyarteritis nodosa which mainly afflicts men aged from 20 to 50 years, giant cell arteritis is unusual before the age of 50 and is predominantly a disease of the elderly with females being slightly more susceptible than men.

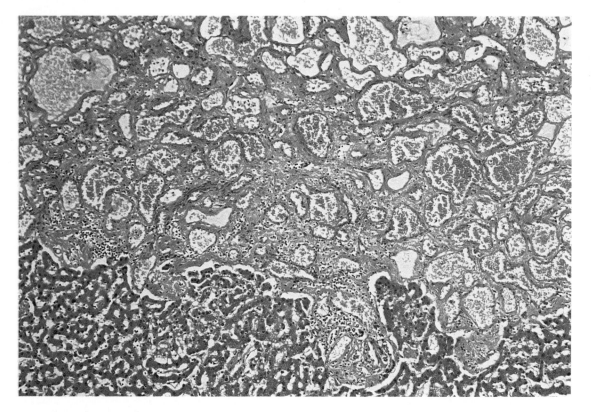

## Fig. 10.9   Haemangioma (MP)

Benign tumours of vascular tissues most commonly occur in
the skin and liver. The most frequent type is the simple
*haemangioma* composed of blood-filled vascular spaces lined by
endothelium. When large vascular spaces predominate the
lesion is called a *cavernous haemangioma*, but alternatively the
spaces may be small and of capillary dimensions, when the
lesion is known as a *capillary haemangioma;* frequently, both
forms are present in the same lesion. This angioma was an

incidental finding in the liver at necropsy.

Tumour-like masses of vascular tissue are found in the brain
and other sites and are often regarded as *hamartomas* (see
Chapter 6). Benign tumours or hamartomas of lymphatic
vessels (*lymphangiomas*) also occur but are rare. Malignant
tumours of vasoformative tissue, *angiosarcomas,* are extremely
rare.

# 11. Respiratory system

## Upper respiratory tract

There are only a few conditions of general histopathological interest in the upper respiratory tract. *Nasal polyps* (Fig. 11.1) are a common sequel of prolonged or recurrent inflammation. Malignant tumours of the nasal passages and sinuses are rare but *nasopharyngeal carcinoma* (Fig. 11.2) is of special interest because it may have a viral aetiology. The stratified squamous epithelium of the larynx may undergo hyperplastic or dysplastic change to form benign squamous papillomata or invasive squamous carcinoma (Fig. 11.3).

## Lower respiratory tract

The trachea and bronchi may become acutely inflamed as a result of infections by viruses or pyogenic bacteria to cause *acute tracheobronchitis* (Fig. 11.4). This latter infection is frequently complicated by extension of the infection and inflammation into the surrounding lung parenchyma to cause a pattern of lung infection known as *bronchopneumonia* (Fig. 11.5), a common cause of illness and death in the debilitated and elderly. Another common pattern of bacterial lung infection is *lobar pneumonia* which involves a whole segment or lobe; usually a more virulent bacterium such as the pneumococcus is involved and fit young people may be almost as susceptible as the elderly and debilitated. Lobar pneumonia illustrates many important principles of acute inflammation and the phenomenon of resolution, and is discussed in Chapter 2 (Figs 2.5 and 2.12). In contrast, tuberculosis and sarcoidosis are classical examples of specific chronic inflammations and are discussed fully in Chapter 3.

Recurrent episodes of acute bronchitis or persistent noninfective irritation of bronchial mucosa (e.g. due to cigarette smoking) may produce *chronic bronchitis* (Fig. 11.6) which is frequently associated with persistent alveolar dilatation and alveolar wall destruction, a condition known as *emphysema* (Fig. 11.7). Recurrent or persistent suppurative bacterial infections of bronchi and bronchioles may lead to irreversible dilatation of these airways with marked thickening and chronic inflammation of the walls, a condition known as *bronchiectasis* (see Fig. 3.3). *Abscess* formation in the lungs (Fig. 2.13) is a serious complication of certain pneumonias, particularly Staphylococcal Klebsiella pneumonias. Lung abscesses may also result from septic emboli or infarction of the lung, bronchiectasis (particularly where bronchi are obstructed by tumour) or as a complication of pulmonary tuberculosis.

*Asthma* (Fig. 11.8) is a disorder of the airways often provoked by certain organic allergens in susceptible individuals. A histologically important group of parenchymal lung diseases follows the inhalation of certain inorganic particulate substances, usually as a result of industrial exposure; these disorders, which include *silicosis* (Fig. 11.9) and *asbestosis* (Fig. 11.10), are collectively known as *pneumoconioses* and exhibit the common feature of progressive pulmonary fibrosis.

The massive capillary bed of the lungs makes them vulnerable to a variety of haemodynamic and other vascular disorders. Left ventricular failure results in engorgement of pulmonary capillaries and fluid transudation into the alveolar spaces causing *pulmonary congestion* and *oedema* (Fig. 11.11). Chronic pulmonary congestion e.g. due to mitral stenosis may result in numerous small intra-alveolar haemorrhages followed by red cell lysis; phagocytosis of released iron pigments, mainly haemosiderin, leads to the gross appearance known as *brown induration.*

Two other common vascular disorders of great clinical importance are *pulmonary embolism* and *pulmonary infarction* illustrated in Figs 8.3 and 9.5 respectively. The lung vasculature may also be affected by the relatively uncommon primary arteritis known as Wegener's granulomatosis.

The airways are a common site of primary malignant tumours which are of three main types: *squamous cell carcinoma* (Fig. 11.12) and *oat cell carcinoma* (Fig. 11.13), which occur most frequently in the main bronchi and their major branches, and *adenocarcinoma* (Fig. 11.14) which tends to arise more peripherally. In contrast, benign tumours of the lung and bronchi are rare. In addition, the lung is an extremely common site of metastatic tumour deposits, usually blood-borne from distant organs (see Fig. 6.6d).

Finally, the pleura is the site of several important pathological processes. Acute inflammation of the pleura (*pleurisy*) is a frequent accompaniment of lung infections and infarcts, and is characterized by a marked fibrinous exudate typical of serosal surfaces (Fig. 2.3). Rarely, a primary malignant tumour arises in the pleural serosa; this tumour, known as a *mesothelioma* (Fig. 11.15), is almost exclusively confined to people with a history of exposure to certain forms of asbestos.

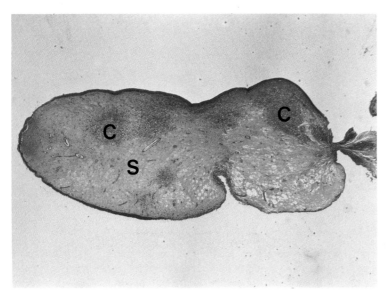

### Fig. 11.1   Nasal polyp (LP)

Chronic inflammation of the nasal mucosa, whether infective or allergic in nature, results in marked oedema and engorgement of the supporting connective tissue and infiltration by chronic inflammatory cells; eosinophils are prominent in allergic rhinitis. Nasal polyps merely represent focal areas in which this response has been exaggerated resulting in the development of polypoid masses.

In this example, note the grossly oedematous stroma **S** and stretched but otherwise relatively normal covering epithelium. The predominant inflammatory cells present in this polyp are plasma cells and eosinophils, mainly in clumps **C** at the periphery of the polyp.

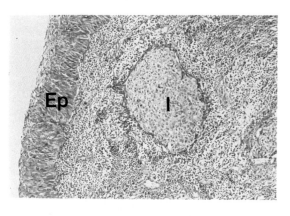

### Fig. 11.2   Nasopharyngeal carcinoma (MP)

In the nasal cavities and nasopharynx, malignant tumours may be either transitional, squamous or adenocarcinomas although anaplastic carcinomas also occur, particularly in the nasopharynx. In this micrograph, an invasive transitional cell carcinoma of the nasal cavity is shown. The stroma is very heavily infiltrated by lymphocytes, a common feature of tumours in this site, particularly transitional cell tumours; this gave rise to the inaccurate term 'lymphoepithelioma' formerly used to describe such tumours. A possible viral aetiology (EB virus) has been postulated for some nasopharyngeal carcinomas. Note the islands **I** of invasive carcinoma beneath the dysplastic surface transitional epithelium **Ep.**

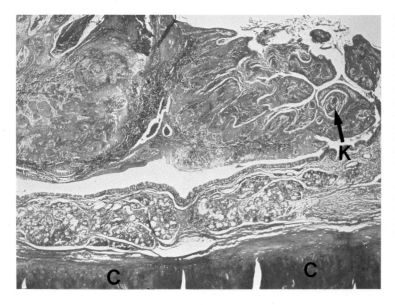

### Fig. 11.3   Carcinoma of the larynx (LP)

Squamous cell carcinomas form the vast majority of malignant tumours of the larynx, most commonly originating in the vocal cords (intrinsic), but also occasionally arising in epiglottis, aryepiglottic folds and pyriform fossae (extrinsic carcinoma of larynx). Squamous carcinomas of the larynx are usually well differentiated and exhibit keratin pearl formation.

This micrograph shows a squamous carcinoma arising from vocal cord; note the presence of keratin pearls **K.** The section also includes part of the normal laryngeal wall including laryngeal cartilage **C.**

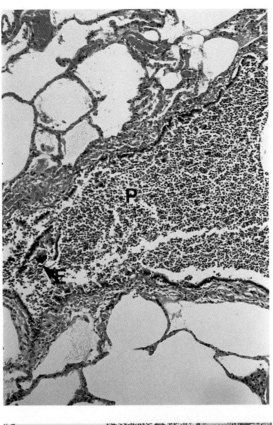

### Fig. 11.4  Acute purulent bronchitis (MP)

Bacterial infections of the upper respiratory tract (often following a transient viral infection) tend to spread down the respiratory tract where they may produce an acute purulent *tracheobronchitis* and *bronchiolitis*. The mucosa of the airways becomes acutely inflamed and congested, and the smaller lobular bronchi and bronchioles become filled with purulent exudate **P** composed of fluid and numerous neutrophils; strips of necrotic epithelium **E** are often shed into the pus. The inflammatory process inhibits ciliary activity but promotes secretion of mucus which, with the dead and dying pus cells, pools in the airways and is coughed up as yellow-green sputum. In the early stages, the lung parenchyma is usually unaffected but the alveolar spaces adjacent to the affected bronchioles often become filled with oedema fluid. In susceptible patients, this may then proceed to the development of bronchopneumonia as shown in Fig. 11.5.

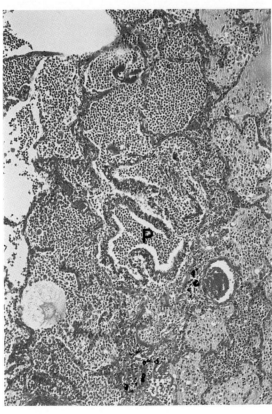

### Fig. 11.5  Bronchopneumonia (MP)

Extension of bacterial infection from bronchioles into the surrounding lung parenchyma leads to a patchy pattern of purulent pneumonic consolidation known as *bronchopneumonia*; this is in marked contrast to the involvement from the outset of a whole lobe or lobule as occurs in *lobar pneumonia* (see Fig. 2.5).

Each peribronchial focus of pneumonic consolidation has within it a small bronchus or bronchiole exhibiting the features of acute purulent bronchitis **P** as demonstrated in Fig. 11.4. As each focus of bronchopneumonia expands, it tends to merge with adjacent foci until the consolidation becomes confluent.

Bronchopneumonia is a threat to the very young, elderly or those debilitated by pre-existing illness such as congestive cardiac failure or carcinomatosis, and is a very common terminal event. No specific organism is responsible, but *Streptococcus pneumoniae* and *Haemophilus influenzae* are the most frequent in Britain.

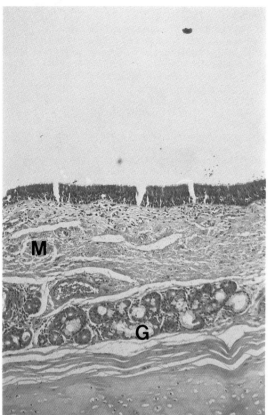

(a)

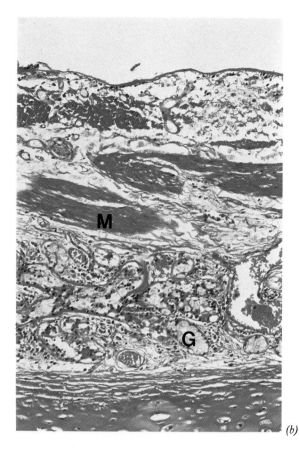

(b)

## Fig. 11.6 Chronic bronchitis
## (a) normal bronchial wall (MP)
## (b) bronchial wall in chronic bronchitis (MP)

Chronic irritation of the bronchial mucosa, either by tobacco smoke, atmospheric pollution or by repeated episodes of infection, induces chronic inflammatory and hyperplastic changes resulting in marked thickening of the bronchial wall. This feature is well illustrated in micrograph (b) when compared to the normal bronchial wall shown in micrograph (a) at the same magnification.

Three factors contribute to the increased thickness of the bronchial wall: infiltration of the submucosa by chronic inflammatory cells, marked hypertrophy of mucosal smooth muscle **M** and marked hyperplasia of the mucous glands **G** with the production of copious mucus. In addition, the surface epithelium undergoes hyperplasia or even squamous metaplasia (see Fig. 5.5) and the consequent loss of ciliary activity then compounds the problem of excessive mucus production and provides an ideal environment for superimposed bacterial infection.

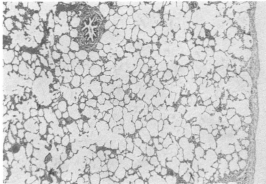

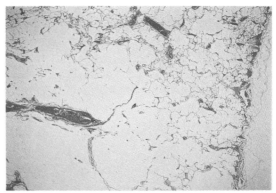

(a)

(b)

## Fig. 11.7   Pulmonary emphysema
## (a) normal lung (LP)
## (b) emphysematous lung (LP)

*Emphysema* is a condition characterized by permanent enlargement of the alveolar spaces almost invariably accompanied by some destruction of alveolar septal tissue, yet in the apparent absence of inflammation. Comparison of emphysematous and normal lungs (shown here at the same magnification) demonstrates the marked increase in alveolar volume and consequent  marked reduction in area of alveolar

wall available for gaseous exchange in emphysema. This problem is compounded by the loss of elastic 'guy rope' support which alveolar walls normally provide to the airways; thus in emphysema, the airways tend to collapse during expiration, a factor which, combined with commonly coexisting chronic bronchitis, greatly inhibits alveolar ventilation.

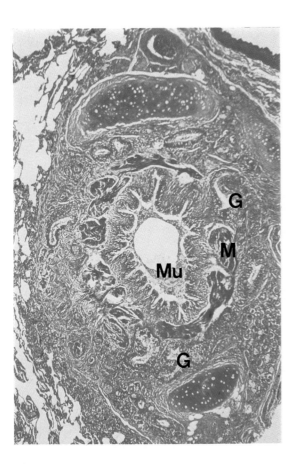

## Fig. 11.8   Chronic asthma (MP)

*Asthma* is an allergic phenomenon which results in marked diminution of functional airway diameter thereby causing severe shortness of breath (dyspnoea); clinically this is manifest by expiratory difficulty and wheezing. The reduction in luminal diameter has three components: bronchospasm, mucosal oedema and luminal occlusion by excessive mucus production.

Single acute asthmatic attacks resolve spontaneously or with therapy leaving no apparent structural disorder; however in chronic asthmatics as in this example, the bronchial walls become thickened due to hypertrophy of smooth muscle **M,** hyperplasia of submucosal mucous glands **G,** protracted oedema of supporting connective tissues and marked infiltration by eosinophils. Eosinophils characteristically accumulate in a variety of allergic states and may be involved in deactivation of some of the chemical mediators of the allergic inflammatory response. The bronchial lumen becomes obstructed by mucus **Mu** containing inflammatory cells, predominantly eosinophils.

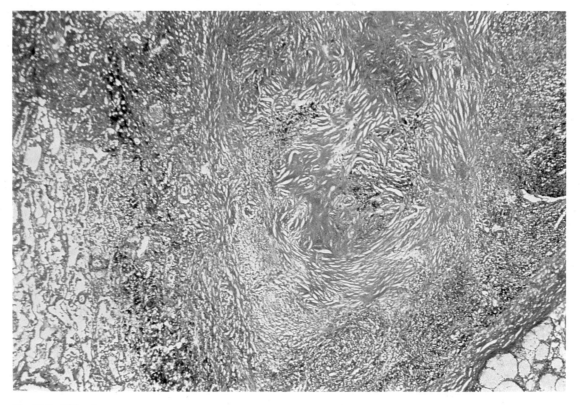

Fig. 11.9   **Silicosis**

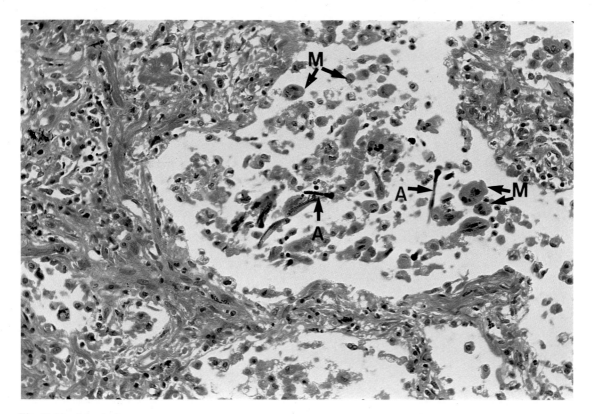

Fig. 11.10   **Asbestosis**

### Fig. 11.9  Silicosis (MP; *illustration opposite above*)

*Silicosis* is the form of pneumoconiosis which tends to occur in miners and others with industrial exposure to silica dusts. Initially, the inhaled silica particles are phagocytosed by macrophages which accumulate in clumps, very occasionally forming granuloma-like masses. The presence of silica-laden macrophages excites a vigorous focal fibrotic reaction resulting in the formation of nodules of collagenous tissue. The centre of each focus becomes progressively hyaline and acellular, and is surrounded by a variable zone of more cellular fibrous tissue exhibiting a relatively sparse chronic inflammatory cell infiltrate in which black carbon-laden macrophages abound. Usual histological methods do not reveal the presence of silica which can however be demonstrated as refractile particles by

polarised light microscopy.

As the process continues, the fibrotic nodules may coalesce, resulting in widespread pulmonary fibrosis.

Silicosis is the most common of the pneumoconioses; other examples are asbestosis (see Fig. 11.10), and berylliosis, in which the inhaled particles excite a giant cell granulomatous reaction similar to that seen in sarcoidosis (see Fig. 3.18). All the clinically significant inorganic dust diseases of the lung lead to progressive fibrosis, with ventilatory failure and diminished gaseous exchange. Disruption of the pulmonary microvasculature may lead to pulmonary hypertension and right heart failure (cor pulmonale).

### Fig. 11.10  Asbestosis (HP; *illustration opposite below*)

*Asbestos,* a complex silicate, occurs in the form of long needle-like fibres which when inhaled into the lung parenchyma become coated with proteinaceous material to form segmented *asbestos bodies.* The presence of asbestos fibres excites a macrophage and giant cell response which ultimately leads to fibrosis in a similar manner to that of silicosis described in Fig. 11.9. The major fibrotic lesions occur initially in the subpleural zone of the lower lobes.

This micrograph shows an alveolar space containing alveolar macrophages **M** and typical asbestos bodies **A**; the brownish

colour of the asbestos bodies derives from the incorporation of haemosiderin in the proteinaceous coat.

Apart from its deleterious effect on pulmonary function, exposure to asbestos predisposes to neoplastic change. Mesotheliomas of the pleura and less often the peritoneum (see Fig. 11.15) may follow exposure to an uncommon form of asbestos known as 'blue asbestos' whilst common asbestos exposure greatly increases the risk of bronchogenic carcinomas especially in cigarette smokers.

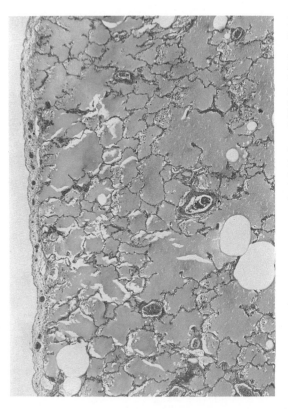

### Fig. 11.11  Pulmonary congestion and oedema (LP)

Any condition in which the left ventricle or atrium fails to empty adequately increases pressure in the affected chamber which is transmitted back to the pulmonary venous system and pulmonary capillaries. The pulmonary capillaries become *congested* and dilated with erythrocytes and the increased hydrostatic pressure results in *transudation* of plasma fluid into the alveolar spaces causing *pulmonary oedema.*

As progressive cardiac failure is a terminal event in many diseases, pulmonary congestion and oedema is a common postmortem finding. This condition also provides an ideal environment for the growth of pathogens of relatively low virulence, so superimposed bronchopneumonia is a common sequel (see Fig. 11.5).

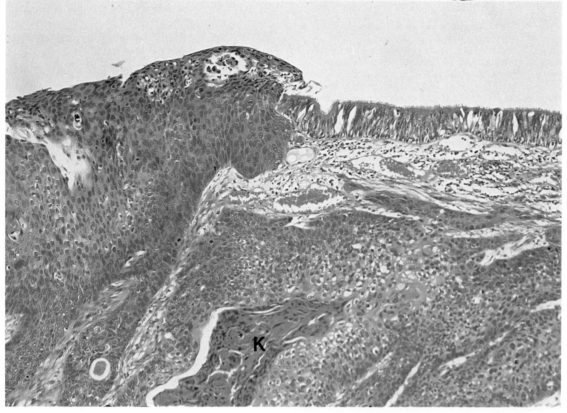

*(a)*

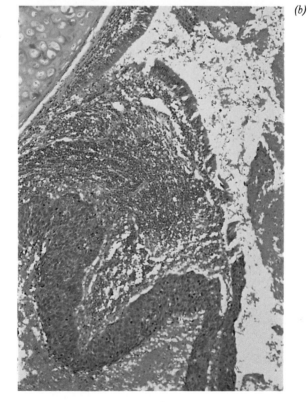

*(b)*

## Fig. 11.12   Squamous cell carcinoma of bronchus
### (a) well differentiated (HP)
### (b) poorly differentiated (HP)

Squamous cell carcinoma, the commonest primary malignancy of the lung, usually arises in the main bronchi or their larger branches close to the lung hilum and often in an area of epithelium which has previously undergone focal squamous metaplasia. Such tumours invade the local parenchyma and tend to obstruct the involved airway as well as spreading via local lymphatics to regional lymph nodes. These tumours have the typical features of squamous cell carcinoma but tend to vary widely in degree of differentiation. At one extreme is the well differentiated  keratinizing type as in micrograph (a) where a basic stratified squamous pattern is evident and there is formation of keratin **K** in some areas. Towards the other end of the spectrum are tumours such as that shown in micrograph (b) in which squamous characteristics such as intercellular bridges are only visible at high magnification (see Fig. 6.11). Some tumours are so poorly differentiated that their squamous features can only be ascertained by electron microscopy; with light microscopy therefore such tumours are often merely classified as *large cell undifferentiated carcinoma.*

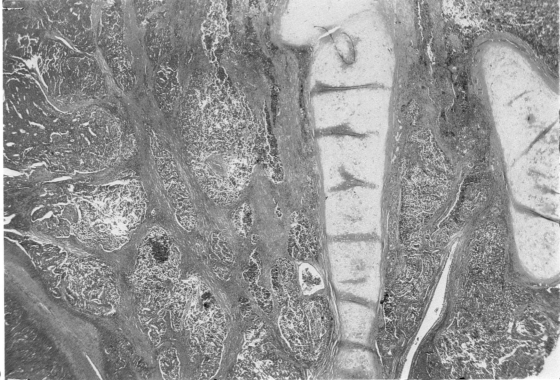

*(a)*

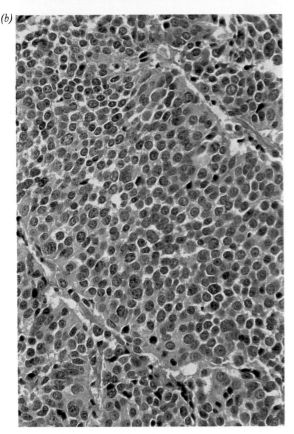

*(b)*

### Fig. 11.13 Oat cell carcinoma
**(a)** LP
**(b)** HP

In addition to squamous carcinoma, the proximal bronchi may also give rise to another important carcinoma known as *oat cell carcinoma*. As seen at high magnification in micrograph (b), the name derives from the supposed resemblance of the small, tightly packed, darkly stained, ovoid tumour cells to oat grains; from these histological features and rampant clinical course, some authorities prefer to apply the term *small cell undifferentiated carcinoma*. These tumours rapidly and extensively invade the bronchial wall and surrounding parenchyma as seen in micrograph (a), and may compress and invade nearby pulmonary veins. Lymphatic and blood-borne spread is an early feature of these tumours, and oat cell tumours have the worst prognosis.

The origin of oat cell tumours is a mystery but there is some evidence that they are derived from cells of the APUD system scattered within the bronchial mucosa. Apart from their local and metastatic effects, these tumours may also secrete peptide hormones such as ACTH giving rise to various tumour-related endocrine syndromes.

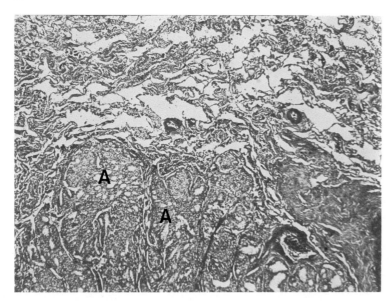

## Fig. 11.14   Adenocarcinoma of the lung (LP)

Adenocarcinomas are the third and least common type of primary lung tumour and tend to arise more peripherally in small bronchi and bronchioles; they have a particular predilection for old areas of scar tissue e.g. healed tuberculosis. The main histological feature of this type of tumour is the formation of the tumour cells into a glandular acinar pattern **A**, the acini often being filled with mucus. Very poorly differentiated variants of adenocarcinoma constitute another type of *large cell undifferentiated carcinoma* (see also Fig. 11.12); here also, only electron microscopy can demonstrate the glandular origin of such tumours. The cytological features of adenocarcinomas are shown in Fig. 6.13.

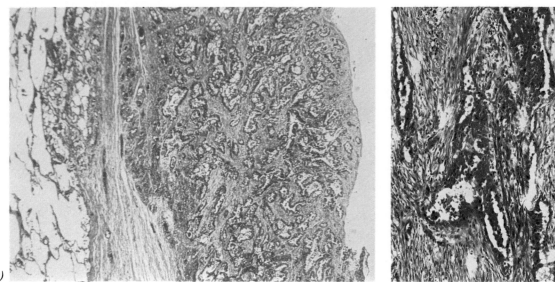

*(a)*   *(b)*

## Fig. 11.15   Mesothelioma of pleura
**(a)** LP
**(b)** HP

The pleura is frequently involved in secondary spread of bronchial and breast carcinoma but primary tumours of the pleura are rare. Nevertheless, these tumours, known as *mesotheliomas* because of their origin from mesothelial cells, are of great interest since they are related to exposure to asbestos dust, although often exposure is trivial and in the distant past. Even more rarely, mesotheliomas of the peritoneum occur also with a history of exposure to asbestos.

Pleural mesotheliomas present as a dense sheet of tumour extending over the pleural surface as in micrograph (a), often encasing the lung in a hard white shell; the tumour extends only a little distance into the lung parenchyma and metastatic spread is rare.

At low magnification, the tumour can be seen to have both a glandular epithelial component and a fibrous stromal component. At high magnification as in (b), both epithelial and spindle-celled stromal components exhibit the pleomorphism characteristic of malignancy; most mesotheliomas contain both components, but occasionally one pattern predominates.

# 12. Alimentary system

## Oral tissues

The mouth and associated structures may be involved in a wide variety of disease states which may be loosely divided into three categories. First, many systemic diseases, particularly dermatological conditions, exhibit oral manifestations (e.g. lichen planus, syphilis) and in most cases the histological features are merely variants of the equivalent skin lesions. Second, all oral tissues may be subject to acute or chronic inflammatory states, the most common being *dental caries* and its sequelae (e.g. *periapical abscess formation*) and *periodontal disease* (i.e. inflammation of the gums); such topics are dealt with in specialist dental texts. Of more general histopathological interest is inflammation of the salivary glands, commonly due to obstruction of ducts by calculi, leading to *chronic sialadenitis* (Fig. 12.2). Third, many benign and malignant tumours may arise in the oral tissues, the most common being squamous cell carcinomas of the lips, oral mucosa and tongue (see Fig. 12.1). Salivary tumours, both benign (see Figs 12.3 and 12.4) and malignant (see Fig. 12.5), are relatively common.

## Oesophagus

The lower oesophagus frequently becomes inflamed as a result of gastric acid reflux, producing either oesophagitis or sometimes chronic peptic ulceration identical to that seen in stomach and duodenum (see Figs 3.1 and 12.7). The most common oesophageal neoplasm is squamous cell carcinoma (Fig. 12.6) although adenocarcinomas may arise in ectopic gastric mucosa at the lower end of the oesophagus; the lower oesophagus may also be involved by local spread from a primary adenocarcinoma of the upper end of the stomach.

## Stomach

Inflammation of the stomach is a frequent transient response to viral and bacterial infections and ingested toxins, both bacterial and chemical (e.g. alcohol). More permanent and clinically significant inflammation may occur in response to excessive gastric acid production resulting in chronic ulceration of either stomach or first part of the duodenum. Peptic ulceration exhibits characteristic features of chronic inflammation and is thus discussed in detail in Chapter 3, (Fig. 3.1). Malignant tumours of the stomach are common and are almost invariably adenocarcinomas; examples are shown in Fig. 12.8. Benign tumours of the stomach are less common.

## Small intestine and appendix

Primary disorders of the small intestine are relatively uncommon with the exception of *coeliac disease* (see Fig. 12.9), in which sensitivity to gluten causes mucosal atrophy and malabsorption, and *Crohn's disease* (see Fig. 12.12), a chronic inflammatory disease which may also effect all other parts of the alimentary tract especially the colon. Primary tumours of the small intestine and appendix are very rare with the exception of *carcinoid tumours* (see Fig. 12.10). *Appendicitis* (see Fig. 12.11) is an extremely common disorder and is a classical example of acute inflammation.

## Large intestine

The colon and rectum are subject to various viral, bacterial and parasitic infections which are short lived and readily diagnosed by microbiological methods; an important exception is *amoebic colitis* (Fig. 12.14) which is often diagnosed only after histological examination of biopsy specimens. Of great importance is the chronic relapsing inflammatory disease of the large intestine known as *ulcerative colitis* (see Fig. 12.13); this condition must be distinguished from Crohn's colitis, not least because ulcerative colitis involving the whole large bowel eventually leads to malignant change in a significant proportion of cases. Raised intraluminal pressure in the colon, probably due to low residue diet, commonly leads to saccular herniation of mucosa through the muscle layers of the bowel wall; the diverticula so formed may become infected giving rise to *diverticulitis* (see Fig. 12.17) which may have serious sequelae such as abscess formation, ulceration and bleeding, perforation, fistula formation (e.g. with other segments of bowel, urinary bladder etc) and widespread peritoneal inflammation and fibrosis. The large intestine may undergo infarction either as a result of mesenteric artery occlusion by thrombus or embolus, or more commonly by venous infarction following hernial strangulation or volvulus; an example is shown in Fig. 9.6.

Benign tumours of the large bowel are of two main types. The most common is the *tubular adenoma* (*adenomatous polyp*) which has the appearance of a relatively smooth-surfaced ovoid polyp arising from a short stalk; it is this type of polyp which also occurs in large numbers throughout the large bowel in the hereditary condition, familial polyposis coli. The other type of benign tumour is the *villous adenoma* (*villous papilloma*) which is composed of narrow frond-like outgrowths of epithelium arising from a broad base giving it a papillary appearance naked eye. Many benign colonic adenomas exhibit histological features of both types within the same lesion although one pattern usually predominates; such tumours are described as *tubulovillous adenomas*. Benign colonic adenomas of all types usually present with rectal bleeding, and all have the potential for malignant transformation. The three types are illustrated in Fig. 12.15.

Malignant tumours of the colon and rectum are very common, and almost all are adenocarcinomas (see Fig. 12.16); most appear histologically moderately differentiated with a clearly defined glandular pattern. The anal canal, being lined by squamous epithelium, is occasionally the site of a squamous carcinoma (see Fig. 6.11) although local invasion of the anal canal by an adenocarcinoma of the lower rectum also occurs.

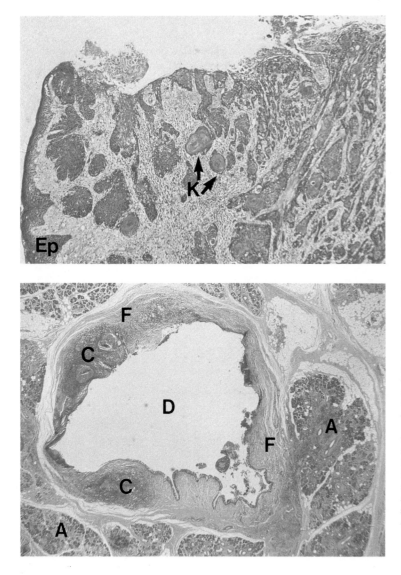

### Fig. 12.1  Carcinoma of the tongue (LP)

Malignant tumours of the mucosa of the lips, tongue, cheeks and gums are almost invariably squamous cell carcinomas and are all histologically very similar; they tend to be well differentiated and, although locally invasive, rarely metastasize beyond regional lymph nodes.

This micrograph illustrates a typical oral squamous carcinoma involving the tongue. Note the adjacent normal stratified squamous epithelium **Ep** from which the tumour has arisen. The tumour has deeply infiltrated the tongue and exhibits characteristic keratin pearl formation **K**. Cytological details are shown in Fig. 6.11(a).

### Fig. 12.2  Chronic sialadenitis (LP)

Prolonged obstruction of a large salivary gland duct by a calculus (*sialolith*) results in chronic inflammation and acinar atrophy in the gland drained by the obstructed duct; these features are collectively known as *chronic sialadenitis* and are shown in this micrograph of submandibular gland, the gland most commonly involved.

The large salivary duct **D,** a major tributary of Wharton's duct, is dilated, and the periductal tissue exhibits fibrosis **F** and infiltration by masses of chronic inflammatory cells **C.** The surrounding secretory acini **A** have undergone marked atrophy and the expanded interstitial spaces have become filled by fibrous and adipose tissue.

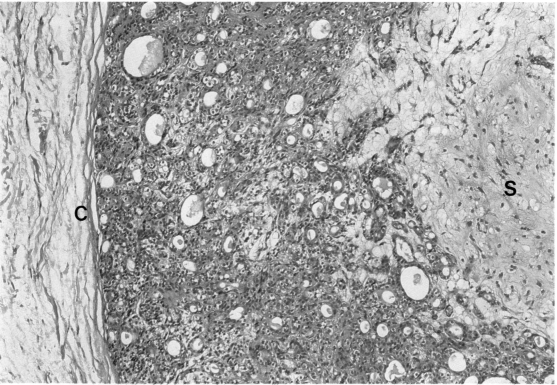

*(a)*

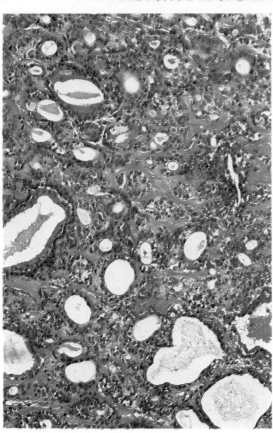

*(b)*

## Fig. 12.3   Benign pleomorphic salivary adenoma
### (a) typical pleomorphic form (MP)
### (b) monomorphic variant (HP)

The most common salivary gland tumour is the *pleomorphic adenoma*, formerly known as *mixed salivary tumour*; the latter term was acquired from the histological appearance of columns and islands of benign epithelial tumour tissue separated by loose myxomatous connective tissue stroma in which areas resembling immature cartilage may be found.

Pleomorphic adenomas occur most commonly in the parotid gland and are often irregular in shape and poorly circumscribed; in the parotid gland this leads to difficulty in achieving total excision (bearing in mind the facial nerve) and local recurrence is common.

Micrograph (a) demonstrates the typical features of benign pleomorphic adenomas namely a strongly staining neoplastic glandular element and a pale blue stained, loose connective tissue stroma **S** somewhat resembling cartilage. Note that the tumour is circumscribed by a thin fibrous capsule **C.**

Much less commonly, salivary adenomas are entirely composed of the glandular epithelial component and contain none of the myxomatous stromal component which often dominates the picture in the typical pleomorphic salivary adenoma; this variant is described as a *monomorphic salivary adenoma* and an example is shown in micrograph (b).

## Fig. 12.4 Adenolymphoma (MP)

This unusual benign tumour occurs almost exclusively in and around the parotid gland; it commonly arises in middle aged and older men. It is composed of large glandular acini **A** embedded in dense lymphoid tissue **L** in which typical lymphoid follicles **F** are sometimes seen. The glandular element consists of tall columnar epithelium rather resembling that of large salivary ducts.

The histogenesis of this tumour is not understood but the glandular element may represent hamartomatous salivary duct tissue within lymph nodes in and around the parotid gland. Adenolymphomas are also known by the eponymous name, *Warthin's tumour.*

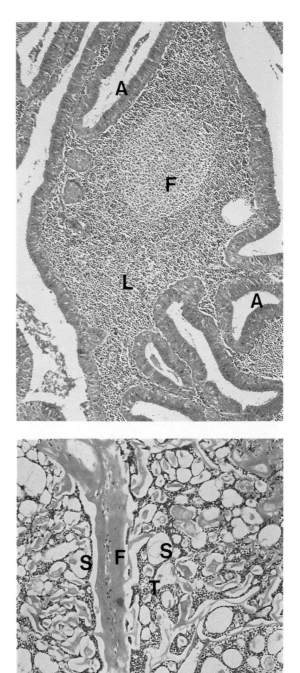

## Fig. 12.5 Adenocystic carcinoma (MP)

The most common malignant tumour of salivary tissue is the *adenocystic carcinoma* formerly known by the unsatisfactory and inaccurate term *cylindroma.* Histologically, it has a characteristic cribriform (seive-like) appearance due to the presence of small spaces **S** in an otherwise solid mass of tightly packed tumour cells **T.** The tumour cells are arranged in clumps and cords separated by a fibrous stroma **F** which may exhibit a marked degree of hyalinization.

As well as occurring in the major salivary glands, adenocystic carcinomas commonly arise in the minor or accessory salivary glands of the palate. These tumours are locally invasive and prone to recurrence following surgical excision. Spread to regional lymph nodes is frequent and wide systemic spread is common.

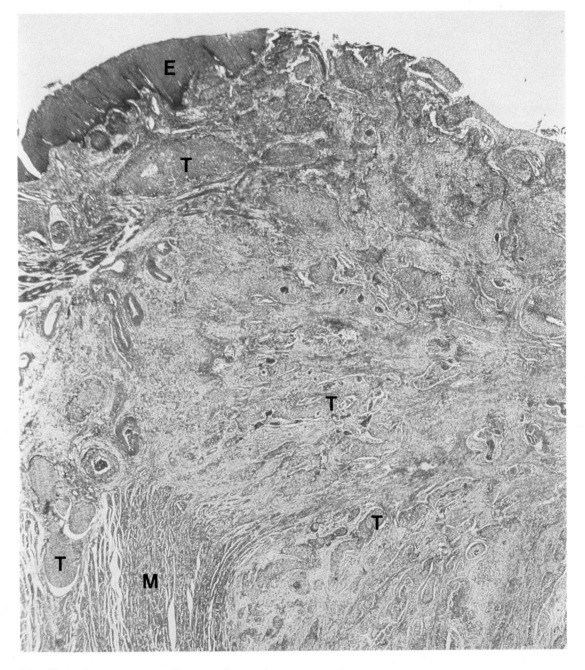

**Fig. 12.6   Squamous carcinoma of oesophagus** (LP)

The oesophagus is lined by stratified squamous epithelium and, the majority of malignant oesophageal tumours are typical squamous carcinomas with occasional keratin pearl formation see Fig. 6.11; most are only moderately well differentiated.

Obstructive symptoms do not usually occur until the lesions are well advanced with extensive local invasion of surrounding mediastinal tissues, and metastases particularly to regional lymph nodes and the liver. In this example, note the origin of the tumour from normal stratified squamous epithelium **E** and full thickness infiltration of the muscular wall **M** by blue-staining islands of tumour **T** .

Adenocarcinomas (see Fig. 6.13) form a small proportion of oesophageal malignancies and usually arise from ectopic gastric mucosa; their clinical course is similar to that of squamous carcinomas.

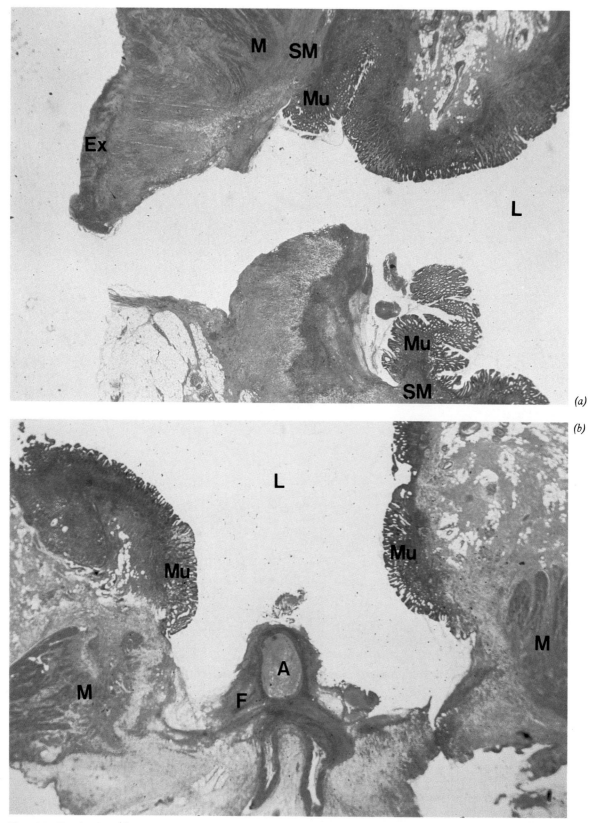

*(a)*

*(b)*

Fig. 12.7   Peptic ulceration

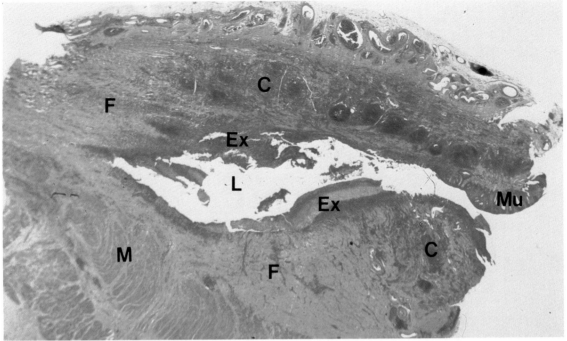

(c)

## Fig. 12.7    Peptic ulceration *(illustrations (a) and (b) opposite)*
## (a) perforated gastric ulcer (LP)
## (b) bleeding gastric ulcer (LP)
## (c) peptic stricture of oesophagus (LP)

The histological details of chronic peptic ulceration in the stomach have already been described in Chapter 3 (Fig. 3.1) as an example of nonspecific chronic inflammation. Acid-induced necrosis of the gastric wall, the acute inflammatory response to that necrosis, organization of the acute inflammatory exudate to form granulation tissue, and fibrous repair of the granulation tissue to form a fibrous scar, all occur concurrently. The outcome of this dynamic process depends on which is the dominant element, the damaging stimulus (in this case, gastric acid) on the one hand or the attempts of the body to heal the damage (organization and fibrous repair) on the other. These three illustrations further demonstrate the manner in which the process may affect the oesophagus, stomach and duodenum.

If tissue destruction proceeds at a pace which outstrips the attempts to confine or repair it, the process may extend rapidly through the full thickness of the wall of the bowel, leading to *perforation*. In the perforated gastric ulcer shown in micrograph (a), note that tissue necrosis has extended through the full thickness of the wall, with complete destruction of the mucosa **Mu,** submucosa **SM** and muscle layers **M.** Discharge of gastric contents into the peritoneal cavity has excited an acute inflammatory exudate **Ex** on the serosal surface of the stomach. The margins of the perforated ulcer are lined by necrotic tissue, beneath which is a zone of acute inflammation similar to that found in the floor of a more chronic ulcer (see Fig. 3.1b), but there is no evidence of fibrous granulation tissue or fibrous scar since the destructive process has been too acute. Perforations such as this occur most commonly in peptic ulcers in the first part of the duodenum, but also occur in the stomach as in this example.

Under other circumstances, the tissue necrosis, although not involving the full thickness of the intestine wall, extends

deeply enough to involve the wall of a large artery. This is most common in long standing chronic gastric ulcers situated on the posterior wall in the region of the left gastro-epiploic artery. This vessel tends to become incorporated in the fibrous scar on the serosal aspect of a chronic gastric ulcer, and its wall may then be eroded in a subsequent episode of tissue necrosis during an acute exacerbation of the ulceration. This may produce torrential haemorrhage leading to haematemesis, melaena and death. Micrograph (b) illustrates such a chronic gastric ulcer; note the eroded artery **A** trapped in the fibrous scar tissue **F** forming the floor of the ulcer. Part of the wall of the artery is undergoing necrosis as a result of the acid attack and massive haemorrhage will follow.

Another important sequel of the chronic inflammatory process results from persistent attempts at fibrous repair; this leads to progressive formation of dense fibrous scar tissue which after the process of shrinkage (cicatrization) may grossly distort the wall of the viscus. At the lower end of the oesophagus or in the pyloric region, the narrowing may be so great as to cause stricture formation with partial or even complete obstruction of the lumen. When the ulcerative process is still active, this obstruction may be compounded by the inflammatory oedema of the mucosa surrounding the ulcer. Micrograph (c) shows a longitudinal section of a long standing peptic ulcer of the lower oesophagus demonstrating many of these features. Note how the lumen **L** is narrowed by fibrous scarring **F**; the mucosa is extensively ulcerated and replaced by inflammatory exudate **Ex** and there is considerable chronic inflammation **C** in the wall.

In endoscopic biopsies of such lesions, peptic ulceration can be diagnosed by the presence of fragments of necrotic ulcer slough, acute inflammatory exudate, and swollen and inflamed mucosa.

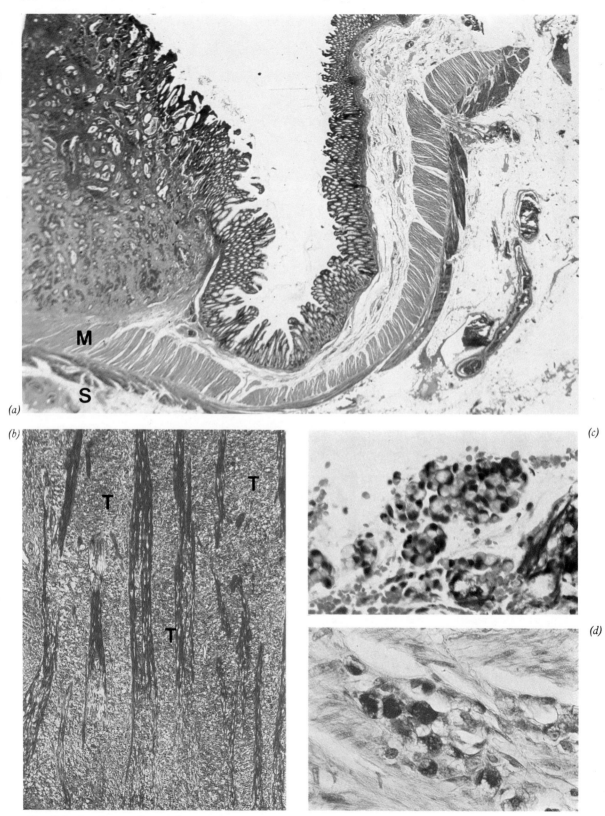

Fig. 12.8   Carcinoma of stomach

**Fig. 12.8    Carcinoma of stomach** *(illustrations opposite)*
**(a) well differentiated, polypoid adenocarcinoma** (LP)
**(b) poorly differentiated adenocarcinoma in linitis plastica** (MP)
**(c) signet ring cells** (HP)
**(d) signet ring cells** (P. A. S. staining method; HP)

Gastric carcinoma may assume a wide variety of gross morphological forms such as malignant ulcer, fungating polypoid tumour and diffuse infiltration of the wall (*linitis plastica*). Nevertheless, the histological form is invariably that of adenocarcinoma (Fig. 6.13).

Gastric adenocarcinoma is only moderately well differentiated in the majority of cases although the whole spectrum of differentiation through to marked anaplasia is encountered. In general, the tumours which take the form of a fungating polypoid tumour are relatively well differentiated; in the example shown in micrograph (a), note the well formed glandular pattern of the tumour which is sill confined to the submucosa, the muscular layer **M** and serosal layer **S** being not yet involved.

In contrast, in linitis plastica as illustrated in micrograph (b),

sheets of pale blue stained cells **T** infiltrate in narrow cords and strands between the red stained bundles of muscle fibres towards the serosa. Glandular spaces cannot be seen within the tumour since this type is almost invariably very poorly differentiated.

Micrograph (c) shows some of the cells from this tumour at high magnification. The cells are ovoid in shape with the darkly staining nucleus pushed to one pole of the cell by a large nonstaining vacuole which occupies most of the cytoplasm; they have the typical appearance of signet ring cells (see also Fig. 6.13). The vacuoles are full of mucin which can be demonstrated by special staining methods such as P.A.S. illustrated in micrograph (d), in which mucin droplets (mucopolysaccharide) stain magenta.

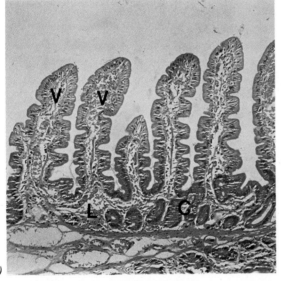

(a)

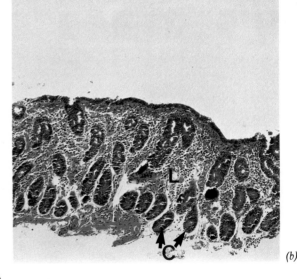

(b)

**Fig. 12.9    Coeliac disease (gluten enteropathy)**
**(a) normal jejunal mucosa** (MP)
**(b) atrophic jejunal mucosa** (MP)

Atrophy of the small intestinal mucosa is a feature of several diseases, the most common and important being hypersensitivity to gluten (a constituent of wheat, oats and rye flour) giving rise to the condition known as *coeliac disease* or *gluten enteropathy*. In this disease, the villi of the duodenal and jejunal mucosa undergo complete or almost complete atrophy leaving a featureless mucosal surface with greatly diminished absorptive capacity. Clinically this results in a malabsorption syndrome characterized by marked weight loss and *steatorrhoea* (diarrhoea containing much unabsorbed lipid).

Diagnosis is usually confirmed by jejunal biopsy either using a Crosby capsule or by endoscopy. The typical histological features are shown in micrograph (b) compared with that of normal jejunal mucosa in (a). The normal villi **V** have undergone complete atrophy, however the crypts **C** between the villi increase in length and the lamina propria **L** becomes heavily infiltrated by chronic inflammatory cells predominantly lymphocytes and plasma cells. Change to a gluten-free diet results in restoration of the normal villous pattern after several weeks.

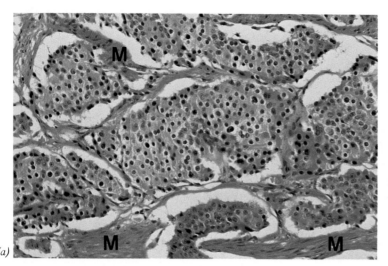
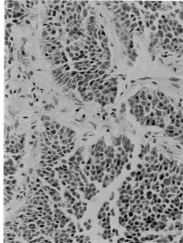

(a)                                                                                          (b)

### Fig. 12.10   Carcinoid tumour of appendix
(a) H & E; (HP)
(b) alkaline diazo staining method; (HP)

The most common abnormality of the appendix is acute
appendicitis which is illustrated and discussed in Fig. 12.11.
Another important lesion in the appendix is the carcinoid
tumour which is often discovered incidentally in appendices
removed for real or suspected appendicitis; this tumour also
occurs in the small intestine and represents the only relatively
common primary tumour in this site. Carcinoid tumours arise
from APUD cells of the appendiceal and small intestinal
mucosa.

As seen in micrograph (a), the tumour cells are small,
polygonal or cuboidal in shape with regular rounded nuclei
and the tumour cells are arranged in cords and clumps which
sometimes exhibit a tendency towards glandular formation.
Carcinoid tumours spread readily through the submucosa and

muscle layers of the intestinal wall and beyond into the
mesentery; this micrograph shows clumps of tumour cells
infiltrating between bundles of smooth muscle cells **M** deep in
the bowel wall.

Special stains such as the alkaline diazo method shown in
micrograph (b) demonstrate prominent cytoplasmic granules
(brick-red by this technique) in the cytoplasm of carcinoid
cells; this characteristic is common to many cells with neuro-
endocrine function (APUD cells). In carcinoid tumours, the
most important secretory product is serotonin
(5-hydroxytryptamine). Other examples of APUD cell tumours
are medullary carcinoma of the thyroid (see Fig. 4.6) which
secretes calcitonin, and phaeochromocytoma (Fig. 19.9) which
secretes adrenaline and noradrenaline.

### Fig. 12.11   Acute appendicitis *(illustrations opposite)*
**(a) early acute appendicitis** (MP)
**(b) later acute appendicitis** (MP)
**(c) late appendicitis with peritonitis** (LP)
**(d) gangrenous appendicitis** (MP)

Acute inflammation of the appendix is one of the most
common surgical emergencies in children and young people.
The earliest change, shown in micrograph (a), is ulceration of
the mucosa **U** with purulent exudate **P** entering the lumen and
a fibrinopurulent acute inflammatory exudate **Ex** replacing the
lost mucosa. At this stage, the patient may experience vague
central abdominal pain.

As the condition progresses, the inflammation spreads
throughout all layers of the wall of the appendix and the
mucosal ulceration becomes more extensive as illustrated in
micrograph (b); few of the original mucosal glands **G** now
remain intact and large numbers of neutrophils have infiltrated
through the submucosa **SM** and muscle layer **M** to the serosa
**S**, where at one point a fibrinous exudate **F** is beginning to
form on the peritoneal surface. Acute inflammation of the
visceral peritoneum soon involves the nearby parietal
peritoneum and it is this peritonitis, usually localized to the
right iliac fossa, which is responsible for the classical clinical
features of acute appendicitis.

The peritoneal exudate often spreads to cover most of the
serosal surface of the appendix and the mesoappendix even
though the point at which the inflammation spreads through
the appendix wall may remain well localized. This stage has
been reached in micrograph (c); the peritoneal surface is
covered by a thick fibrinopurulent exudate **Ex** extending onto
the fatty mesoappendix, even though the appendix wall is not
markedly inflamed at the level at which the histological section
was taken. Note however, that there is some purple staining
pus in the lumen of the appendix.

Severe continuing inflammation of the appendix wall often
leads to extensive necrosis of the muscle layer (*gangrenous
appendicitis*) which predisposes to perforation of the appendix
with more widespread peritonitis. This feature can be seen in
micrograph (d); the red staining muscle layer **M** is identifiable
up to a point where it has undergone necrosis **N**. Perforation
of the appendix is imminent and will almost certainly take
place at this point; the pus **P** which fills the lumen will then
be discharged into the peritoneal cavity.

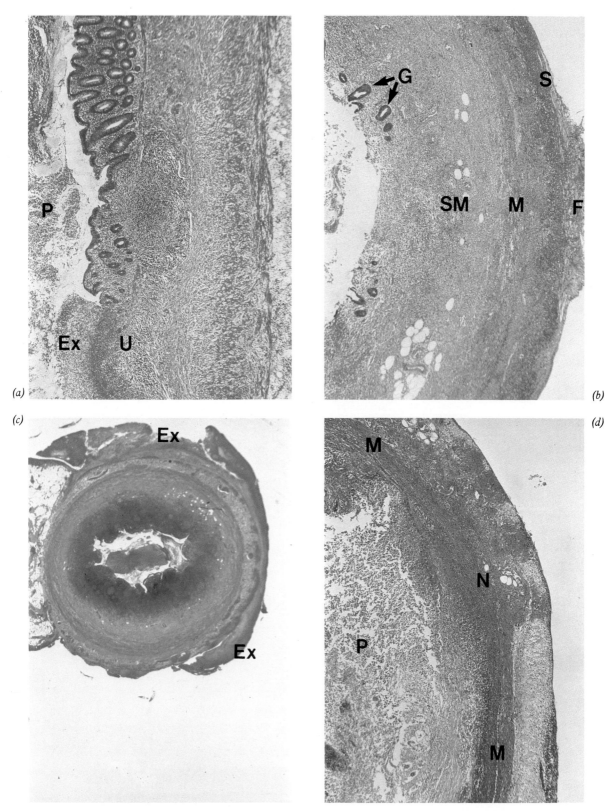

*(a)*

*(b)*

*(c)*

*(d)*

Fig. 12.11   **Acute appendicitis**

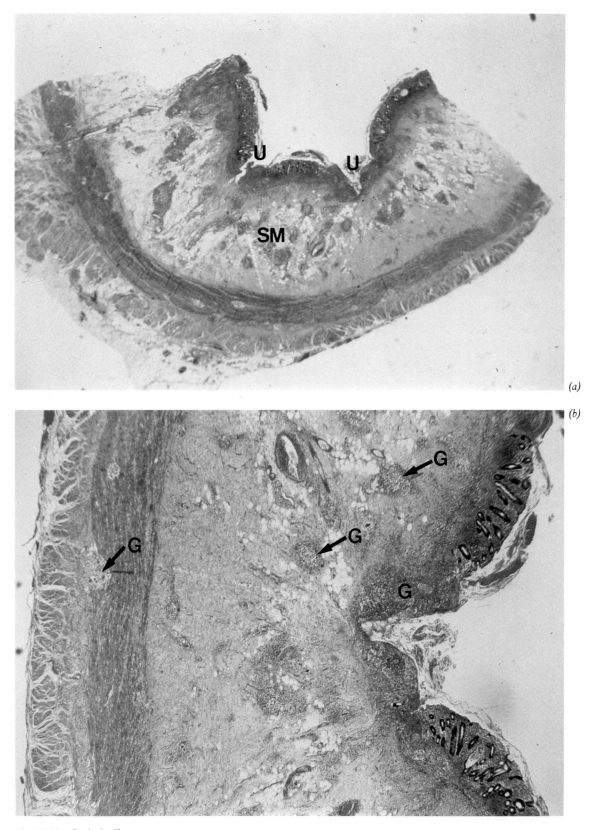

*(a)*

*(b)*

**Fig. 12.12   Crohn's disease**

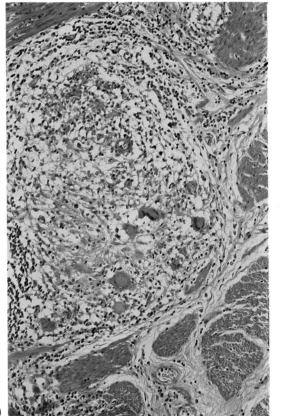

(c)

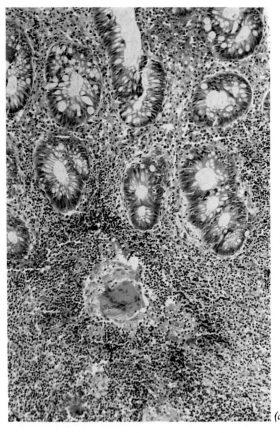

(d)

**Fig. 12.12   Crohn's disease** *(illustrations (a) and (b) opposite)*
**(a) ileal lesion** (LP)
**(b) fissured ulcer** (MP)
**(c) Crohn's granuloma** (HP)
**(d) rectal biopsy** (HP)

*Crohn's disease* is a chronic inflammatory disease of unknown
aetiology which mainly involves the small intestine, especially
the terminal ileum, but may also often affect the large bowel
and anus. In the latter sites it may be confused clinically with
ulcerative colitis and anal fissures and fistulae respectively. In
the small intestine it is characteristically patchy in distribution,
affecting short segments with lengths of normal bowel in
between (*skip lesions*). As shown in micrograph (a) the affected
segments of small intestine show gross thickening of the wall
mainly due to marked oedema and inflammation of the
submucosa **SM**. This oedema produces the typical
'cobblestone' macroscopic appearance of the mucosa in which
domed areas of swollen mucosa and submucosa are criss-
crossed by linear depressions caused by narrow fissured ulcers
**U**. A typical fissured ulcer can be seen more clearly in
micrograph (b) which also demonstrates two other features of
Crohn's disease, namely, that the chronic inflammatory

changes are transmural (i.e. affect all layers from mucosa to
serosa), and that chronic inflammatory granulomas **G**, often
containing giant cells, may be found in all layers. The giant
cell granuloma between the muscle layers is illustrated at
higher magnification in micrograph (c); the well circumscribed
granuloma contains macrophages and multinucleate giant cells,
as well as lymphocytes. Giant cell granulomata such as these
may also be found in lymph nodes draining the affected
segment of bowel. Micrograph (d) shows a similar, but smaller,
giant cell granuloma in the chronically inflamed mucosa
obtained by rectal biopsy in a case of suspected chronic
ulcerative colitis; its presence resulted in Crohn's disease being
diagnosed.

The result of this long standing chronic inflammation is
widespread fibrosis which may cause bowel obstruction; the
deep fissured ulceration predisposes to the formation of
fistulae, a common complication of Crohn's disease.

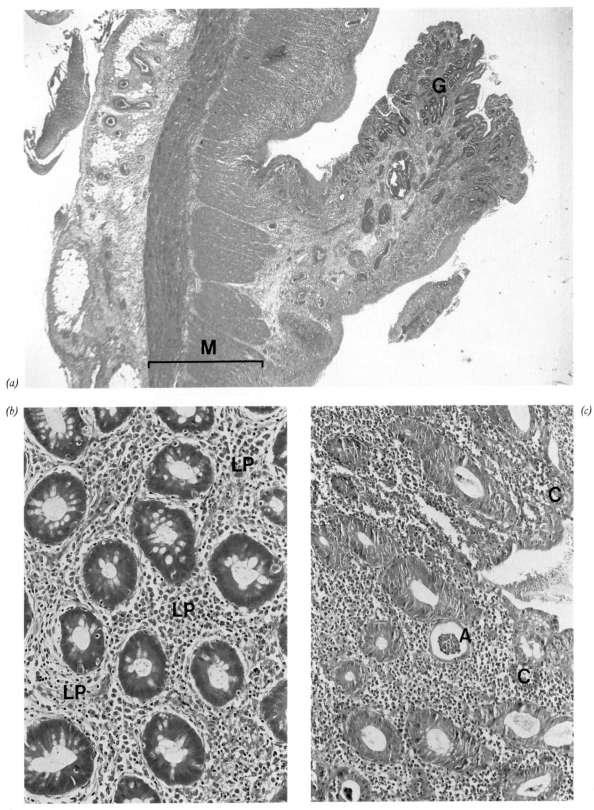

Fig. 12.13   Ulcerative colitis

## Fig. 12.13   Ulcerative colitis *(illustrations opposite)*
### (a) active disease with pseudopolyp formation (LP)
### (b) quiescent phase (HP)
### (c) reactivated chronic disease (HP)

*Ulcerative colitis* is a chronic relapsing inflammatory disease of the large bowel, sometimes accompanied by systemic features such as anaemia, arthritis and uveitis. In many clinical respects, ulcerative colitis may be difficult to distinguish from Crohn's disease affecting the colon, and large bowel biopsy may be a crucial element in the diagnosis (see Fig. 12.12d). The disease always involves the rectosigmoid region but often extends to involve the whole colon.

In the earliest acute lesions, there is acute inflammation of the mucosa with neutrophils accumulating in the lamina propria and in the lumina of the colonic glands to form *crypt abscesses;* ulceration of the mucosa occurs, but the ulcers are superficial rather than fissured as in Crohn's disease (see Fig. 12.12a & b).

If the inflammation persists, the area of ulceration may spread extensively throughout the length of the colonic mucosa; an example is shown in micrograph (a). Note that the ulcerative process has destroyed much of the mucosa and submucosa in this field, leaving an isolated island of nonulcerated mucosa which is swollen by acute and chronic inflammatory changes in the submucosa and lamina propria; some of the colonic glands **G** remain. Non-ulcerated areas such as this project above the surrounding ulcerated areas to produce so-called *inflammatory pseudopolyps*. Despite the severity and extent of the inflammation and ulceration, the changes are mainly confined to the submucosa and mucosa, and the muscularis **M** is not involved; inflammatory changes

are rarely transmural, a useful distinguishing feature from Crohn's disease (c.f. Figs 12.12a & b). In micrograph (a), a peritoneal exudate is present but this resulted from peritonitis due to surgical instrumentation causing perforation; this does not represent transmural inflammation.

During quiescent periods between acute exacerbations, the mucosa damaged by earlier severe inflammation or ulceration shows mixed features of chronic inflammation and attempts at restitution. Micrograph (b) shows a typical mucosal fragment obtained by endoscopic biopsy during a quiescent phase. The lamina propria **LP** is expanded by a heavy infiltrate of chronic inflammatory cells, mainly lymphocytes and plasma cells; the colonic glands show marked reduction in the numbers of mucin-secreting goblet cells and there are mild dysplastic changes with some cellular pleomorphism and increase in nuclear-cytoplasmic ratio.

Micrograph (c) illustrates the features indicative of residual or renewed acute inflammatory activity namely the presence of crypt abscesses **A** in the glands, dilation of superficial capillaries **C** in the lamina propria often with polymorph margination, and neutrophilic infiltration amongst the chronic inflammatory cells.

Repeated episodes of inflammation, ulceration and epithelial regeneration leads to dysplastic change in the constantly irritated surface and glandular epithelium; this factor may contribute to the high incidence of colonic adenocarcinoma arising in patients with a long history of ulcerative colitis.

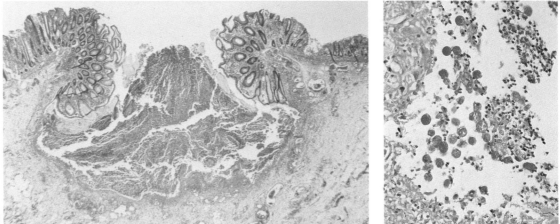

*(a)*  *(b)*

## Fig. 12.14   Amoebic colitis
### (a) amoebic ulcer (LP)
### (b) amoebae (P.A.S. staining method; HP)

This condition, caused by the parasite *Entamoeba histolytica*, is occurring with increasing frequency in developed countries particularly in people returning from less developed countries where sanitation is inadequate. It is a form of infective colitis producing severe diarrhoea containing blood and mucus; it may exhibit clinical features indistinguishable from Crohn's disease and ulcerative colitis.

Histologically, amoebic colitis is characterized by flask-shaped ulcers as seen in micrograph (a), with a typically broad base and narrow surface opening caused by invasion of colonic

crypts by amoebae which then spread laterally undermining the adjacent mucosa; the ulcers do not tend to coalesce however but remain isolated and do not extend beyond the submucosa. Amoebae may be recognisable in the ulcer margins in standard H & E stained sections but with the P.A.S. staining method, as shown in micrograph (b), they are stained a strong magenta colour. An unusual feature of amoebic colitis is the relatively meagre inflammatory response in the tissues surrounding the ulcers.

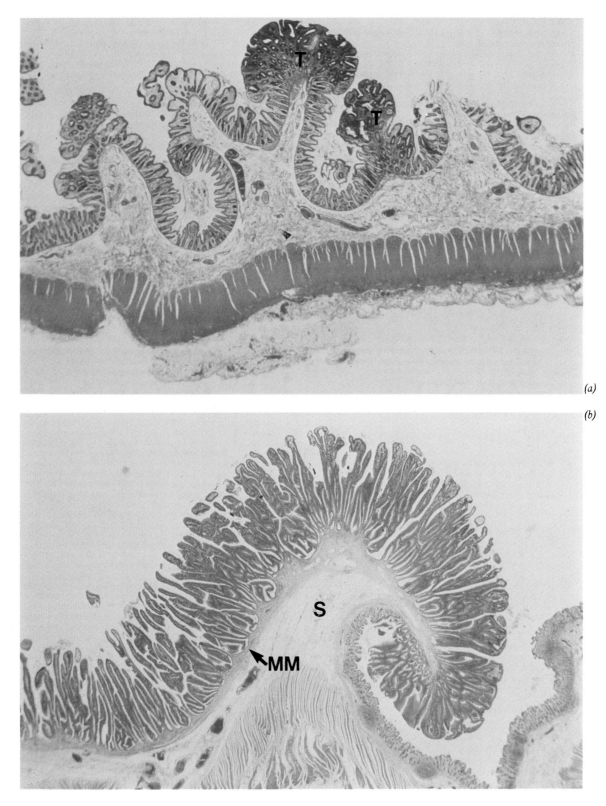

**Fig. 12.15   Colonic polyps**

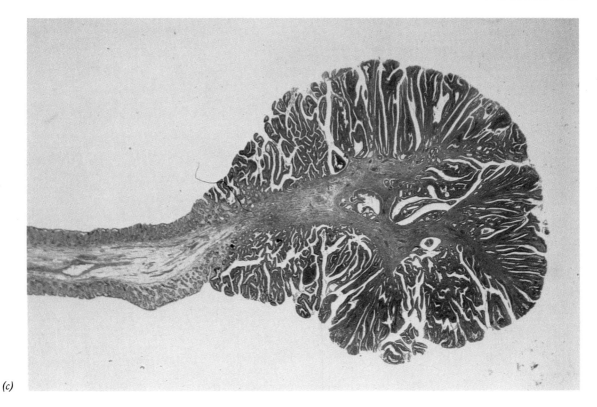

*(c)*

Fig. 12.15    Colonic polyps *(illustrations (a) and (b) opposite)*
**(a) tubular adenomas: polyposis coli** (LP)
**(b) villous adenoma** (LP)
**(c) tubulovillous adenoma** (LP)

*Colonic polyps* are usually benign adenomas of the epithelium
of the colonic mucosa. There are three main histological
patterns, *tubular adenoma, villous adenoma (papilloma)* and
*tubulovillous adenoma.*

Tubular adenomas are almost always pedunculated polypoid
lesions, the adenoma proper being connected to the mucosa by
a narrow stalk containing submucosal connective tissue and
muscularis mucosae and covered by normal non-neoplastic
colonic mucosa. The adenoma consists of dysplastic colonic
epithelium arranged in straight tubular glands, the cells being
dark staining because they lack the usually abundant
cytoplasmic mucin and have an increased nucleus/cytoplasm
ratio. When seen with the naked eye, these tumours have a
velvety smooth or slightly bosselated appearance. Tubular
adenomas may be either solitary or multiple. In one heritable
condition, known as *familial polyposis coli,* numerous small and
large tubular adenomas are scattered throughout the colon; the
importance of this condition is that there is a strong
predisposition to the transformation of the original benign
lesions into malignant colonic adenocarcinoma. Micrograph (a)
shows two tubular adenomas **T** in a segment of colon from a
patient with polyposis coli. Note the darkly stained
adenomatous masses connected to the underlying mucosa by
stalks which merely represent extensions of the normal mucosa

and submucosa. The cytological detail is shown in Fig. 6.2 (b).

*Villous adenoma (or papilloma)* is a sessile, rather than
pedunculated lesion, arising from a broad base; it is composed
of narrow frond-like outgrowths of epithelial cells arranged on
a delicate connective tissue stroma, giving a papillary
appearance both histologically and with the naked eye. A
typical sessile villous adenoma is illustrated in micrograph (b);
the lesion in this case is completely benign, showing no
evidence of invasion across muscularis mucosae **MM** into
submucosa **S**. Further cytological detail of this tumour is
shown in Fig. 6.5 (a) and (b).

Many long standing tubular adenomas acquire a partially
villous histological pattern, particularly at the surface, although
the general configuration of the lesion (pedunculated,
nonsessile) remains that of a pure tubular adenoma. Such
adenomas are called *tubulovillous adenomas*; in the example
shown in micrograph (c), note that the stalk is covered by
normal colonic-type mucosa which contrasts markedly with the
densely staining dysplastic epithelium of the adenoma.

All the above types of colonic polyps have the potential for
malignant change, the villous adenoma more frequently than
the other types. Early malignant transformation is first
manifest by invasion of tumour cells through the muscularis
mucosae into the underlying connective tissue stroma.

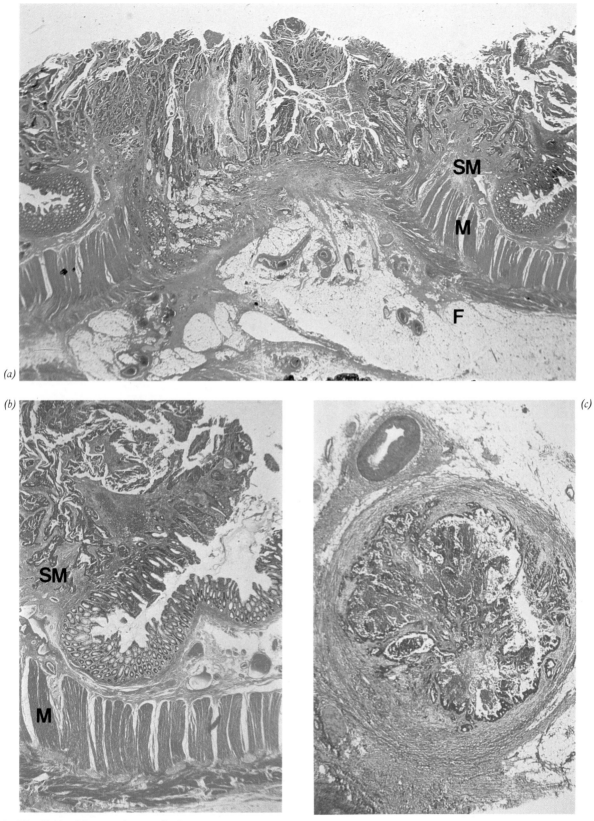

*(a)*

*(b)*

*(c)*

**Fig. 12.16　Adenocarcinoma of colon**

**Fig. 12.16    Adenocarcinoma of colon** *(illustrations opposite)*
**(a) invasive tumour** (LP)
**(b) edge of lesion in (a)** (MP)
**(c) invasion of vein** (MP)

Adenocarcinoma is the most common and important malignant tumour of the large bowel and arises most frequently in the descending and sigmoid colon and rectum. The tumours are usually raised with central ulceration and elevated margins but more extensive lesions may involve the whole circumference of the bowel forming an annular stricture; another growth pattern produces a protruberant cauliflower-like mass most commonly seen in the caecum and proximal colon.

Micrograph (a) shows an ulcerated adenocarcinoma of the rectum; the tumour has infiltrated deeply through the submucosa **SM**, muscularis **M**, and out into the paracolic fat **F.** Note that this tumour is moderately well differentiated as

evidenced by the well defined glandular pattern.

Micrograph (b) shows the raised everted edge of this tumour at higher magnification; note the abrupt transition between normal rectal mucosa and the abnormal malignant epithelium. In this area, the tumour has infiltrated into the submucosa **SM,** but not into the muscularis **M.**

The prognosis of colonic and rectal carcinomas depends on a number of factors, the most important being the depth of invasion of the bowel wall, the presence of distant metastases, and evidence of tumour invasion into veins. Micrograph (c) shows a vein in the serosa of the colon; it is filled with colonic adenocarcinoma which is growing along it as a solid cord.

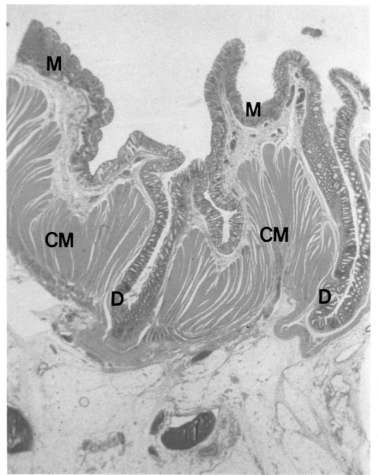

**Fig. 12.17    Diverticular disease** (LP)

Diverticular disease is a common condition in the elderly; it may involve any part of the colon, although the sigmoid colon is the most frequently and most severely affected part.

The normal muscular wall of the colon consists of an inner circular layer of smooth muscle and an outer longitudinal layer. However, the longitudinal layer does not completely surround the lumen but rather forms three distinct longitudinal bands known as taeniae coli. Possibly as a result of abnormally high intraluminal pressure associated with low residue diets, diverticula are formed by herniation of pouches of colonic mucosa **M** through weak areas of the circular muscle layer lacking support from the discontinuous outer longitudinal layer.

The characteristic histological feature is marked hypertrophy of the circular muscle layer **CM**; the longitudinal taeniae coli may also be hypertrophied. The diverticula **D** bulge towards the outer surface and often contain faecal material. The luminal openings of the diverticula are narrow and acute purulent inflammation readily develops in and around the diverticula; this condition, known as *diverticulitis*, may lead to torrential rectal haemorrhage, perforation, pericolic abscess formation, peritonitis, and fistula formation with other viscera such as bladder and vagina.

# 13. Hepatobiliary system and pancreas

## Acute inflammation of the liver

Hepatocytes, with their high degree of metabolic activity, are readily disturbed by toxins, especially drugs or alcohol, and demonstrate the classical histological cellular responses known as cloudy swelling, fatty change and necrosis as described in Chapter 1. Since the connective tissue component of liver is normally inconspicuous apart from in the portal tracts, acute inflammation of the liver is mainly evidenced by subcellular changes and inflammatory cell infiltrate of parenchyma rather than by the more typical vascular and exudative changes seen in other tissues where connective tissue is a more significant constituent..

*Hepatitis* is a general term for inflammation of the liver parenchyma which can then be further classified according to probable aetiology, e.g. viral hepatitis. Toxins are an important cause of hepatitic reactions; alcohol is probably the most common hepatic toxin, and liver biopsy is often employed to confirm a diagnosis of alcoholic hepatitis or establish its severity, especially where a reliable history cannot be obtained (see Fig. 13.2). A similar pattern of toxic hepatitis may result from overdosage with drugs such as paracetamol, exposure to carbon tetrachloride, and as an idiosyncratic response to drugs such as the anaesthetic gas halothane.

Hepatitis may also result from invasion of hepatocytes by viruses, most notably hepatitis A virus (*infectious hepatitis*), and hepatitis B virus (*serum hepatitis*), giving the histological appearance shown in Fig. 13.3. Rarely, agents such as *Leptospira* or *Toxoplasma* are the causative agent in hepatitis. Other infective agents usually involve the liver secondarily as part of disseminated disease, and may cause multiple minute infective lesions as in bacterial septicaemia and miliary tuberculosis, or large abscesses as in amoebiasis. Other parasites give rise to specific liver lesions such as cysts in hydatid disease, and granulomata in schistosomiasis. Chronic granulomatous lesions (gummata) also occur in tertiary syphilis (see Fig. 3.19b).

## Chronic inflammation of the liver

Apart from the forms of acute hepatitis described above, some patients develop clinical and biochemical manifestations of chronic inflammation of the liver. When this situation continues without improvement for 6 months or more, the condition is described as *chronic hepatitis*; this term however, excludes chronic inflammation of the liver caused by alcohol, bacterial agents and biliary obstruction. The commonest causes of chronic hepatitis are persistent viral infection and certain drugs, but there is a large group where there is no obvious causative agent and in which abnormal immunological phenomena may play an important role.

In clinical terms, chronic hepatitis exhibits a spectrum of activity from self limiting and relatively transient to severe and progressive. At one end of the spectrum is *chronic persistent hepatitis* (see Fig. 13.4), a prolonged relapsing but self-limiting form of hepatitis characterized histologically by inflammation confined to the connective tissue of the portal tracts and with no evidence of active destruction of liver cells. At the opposite end of the spectrum is an insidiously progressive form of hepatitis known clinically as *chronic active hepatitis* which if untreated culminates in cirrhosis and liver failure. Histologically, there is evidence of liver cell destruction and the inflammation extends from the portal tracts into the liver parenchyma; this histological appearance is described as *chronic aggressive hepatitis* (see Fig. 13.5).

In the management of chronic hepatitis, the diagnosis is made initially by correlating clinical appearances, biochemical results and histological appearances from biopsy specimens. The prognosis can then be established and treatment instituted in the non self-limiting cases. The clinical response to treatment is unfortunately not matched by consistent changes in the various biochemical disease markers. Histological examination of biopsy specimens taken at intervals in the progress of the disease provides a more reliable method of monitoring disease activity.

*Primary biliary cirrhosis* is another chronic inflammatory disease of the liver also with a probable immunological basis. In this condition, shown in Fig. 13.6, the intrahepatic bile ducts appear to be the focus of destruction with concurrent inflammation of the surrounding portal tract connective tissues.

## Other important liver disorders

Certain inborn errors of metabolism, in most cases probably reflecting single gene defects, result in the abnormal accummulation of various metabolites within hepatocytes. These are known as *storage diseases* and include glycogen storage diseases, mucopolysaccharidoses, lipidoses, haemochromatosis, and Wilson's disease. Liver biopsy may be useful in the diagnosis of such disorders and, as an example, haemochromatosis is illustrated in Fig. 13.7. In contrast, amyloidosis (see Fig. 4.4) is a condition involving extracellular accummulation of abnormal substances.

*Cirrhosis* is a general term applied to the end result of a variety of chronic liver disorders having the common feature of diffuse persistent destruction of hepatocytes accompanied by a concurrent reparative response which involves fibrosis in the connective tissue elements and focal, nodular regeneration of hepatocytes. The end result is impairment of liver function and gross distortion of liver architecture leading to portal hypertension. Various different types of cirrhosis are illustrated in Fig. 13.8.

Malignant disease frequently involves the liver, most commonly as secondary spread, especially from primary lesions in gut, breast and lung (see Fig. 6.6c); less frequently the liver becomes diffusely infiltrated in lymphoreticular malignancies such as Hodgkin's disease and other lymphomas (see Chapter 15). Primary malignancies of the liver, *hepatomas* (see Fig. 13.9), are uncommon and most often arise in pre-existing cirrhosis.

## Disorders of the biliary system

Gallbladder disease is a common surgical problem in developed countries and is often associated with stone formation and chronic obstruction of the cystic duct leading to *chronic cholecystitis* (see Fig. 13.11). Tumours of the biliary system are relatively rare and usually take the form of highly malignant adenocarcinomas (see Fig. 13.10).

## Pancreatic disorders

Inflammation of the pancreas is a relatively uncommon condition which may present in chronic or acute form; the latter carries a high mortality partly due to the release of pancreatic enzymes into surrounding tissues causing severe local tissue destruction (see Fig. 13.12). Malignant disease of the pancreas is now appearing with increasing frequency; these adenocarcinomas (see Fig. 13.13) are highly malignant and metastases are almost always present by the time of diagnosis.

## Fig. 13.1  Clinical features of hepatobiliary disease and their pathophysiology

| Sign/symptom | Clinical features | Mechanism |
|---|---|---|
| Jaundice | Yellow colouration of tissues due to bile. | Failure of metabolism or excretion of bile pigments. |
| Bleeding | Easy bruising and prolonged clotting time of blood. | Failure of protein synthesis i.e. clotting factors. |
| Oedema Ascites | Swelling of dependent parts due to extracellular accumulation of fluid. Fluid in the peritoneum | Failure of protein synthesis i.e. albumen thereby causing reduced oncotic pressure of plasma. |
| Gynaecomastia | Enlargement of male breast. | Failure to detoxify oestrogenic hormones. |
| Pruritis | Itching | Failure to excrete bile acids. |
| Encephalopathy | Altered consciousness and lack of co-ordination; may lead to coma. | Failure to detoxify ammonia and related substances from protein breakdown. |
| Haematemesis and melaena | Vomiting blood and passing altered blood per rectum. | Oesophageal varices due to portal hypertension. |

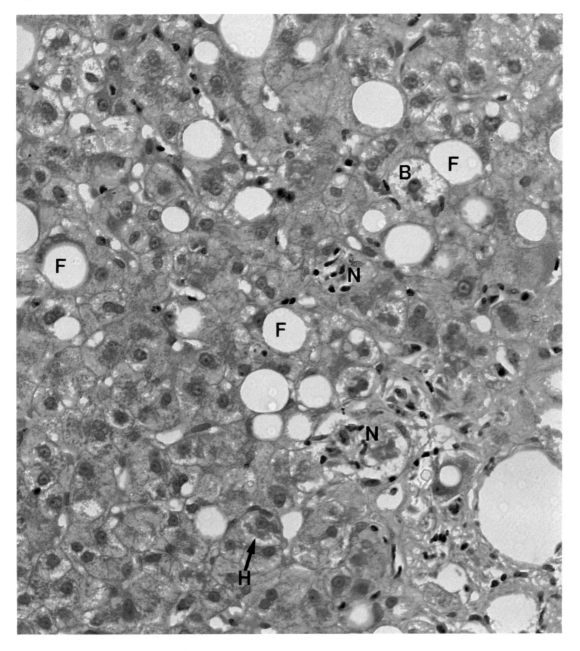

## Fig. 13.2  Alcoholic hepatitis (HP)

Alcohol is a potent hepatotoxin when taken in large quantities and liver changes occur even after isolated bouts of heavy drinking.

Early evidence of metabolic injury to the hepatocytes is the appearance of fatty change **F** manifest by the accumulation of lipid in the form of large cytoplasmic vacuoles within some hepatocytes usually displacing the nucleus to one side (see also Fig. 1.3). With more severe metabolic disruption, the hepatocytes undergo hydropic degeneration (see Fig. 1.2) and become swollen and vacuolated, an appearance described as *ballooning degeneration* **B**; in some cases, the metabolic disruption may be irrecoverable and some hepatocytes undergo necrosis. The location of necrotic hepatocytes **N** is marked by foci of neutrophils and lymphocytes. Some hepatocytes accumulate an eosinophilic material known as *Mallory's hyaline* **H** which is mainly seen in alcohol-induced cell damage; this material forms irregular cytoplasmic globules usually near the nucleus and stains a homogeneous pink colour slightly darker than normal cytoplasm. The hepatocytes around the centrilobular veins appear to be most vulnerable to alcohol toxicity and in some individuals delicate fibrosis may be seen around the central veins.

With prolonged alcohol abuse there is progressive fibrosis due to hepatocyte necrosis and regeneration of liver cells and this can progress further to alcoholic cirrhosis (see Fig. 13.17a).

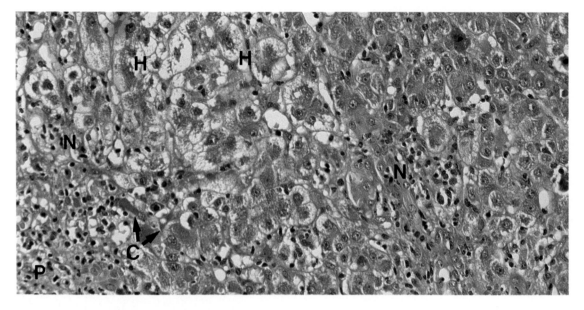

## Fig. 13.3    Acute viral hepatitis (HP)

The viral agents of acute hepatitis produce a similar picture whether due to virus type A or type B. There is widespread swelling and ballooning of hepatocytes due to hydropic degeneration **H** and this progresses to focal or spotty necrosis throughout the lobule; the areas of necrosis are identified by aggregates of neutrophils **N** or round eosinophilic (pink stained) bodies called *Councilman bodies* **C** representing the cytoplasm of necrotic liver cells. The Kuppfer cells are very active and within portal tracts **P** there are increased numbers of chronic inflammatory cells.

In time, regeneration of the dead hepatocytes occurs. In hepatitis A (infective type) the changes usually completely resolve but in hepatitis B (serum type) activity may persist or progress to chronic active hepatitis.

Rare cases of viral hepatitis occur in which there is massive liver necrosis instead of the focal type seen here. These fulminant cases are often fatal.

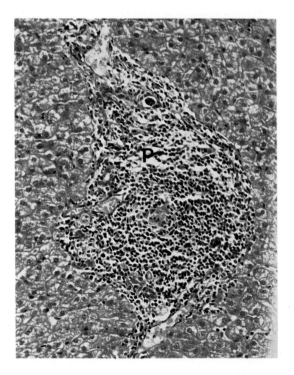

## Fig. 13.4    Chronic persistent hepatitis (HP)

This form of chronic hepatitis may be encountered after a previous episode of acute viral hepatitis. Clinically, it is noted that biochemical tests of liver function fail to return to normal and biopsy is performed to assess the degree of liver damage. Histologically, there is expansion of the portal tract **P** by mononuclear chronic inflammatory cells, mainly lymphocytes but with some plasma cells. Note that the inflammation is sharply limited to the connective tissue of the portal tract, in contrast to chronic aggressive hepatitis (see Fig. 13.4), where the inflammation spills out into the liver parenchyma. No necrosis of liver cells is seen in chronic persistent hepatitis. This form of chronic hepatitis carries a good prognosis and the histological changes remain stable or improve over a period of time. This biopsy was from a patient who had an episode of acute hepatitis due to hepatitis B virus, with mildly abnormal liver function tests 8 months after the illness.

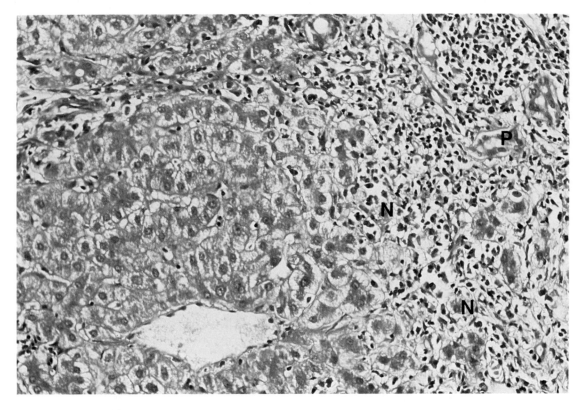

## Fig. 13.5   Chronic aggressive hepatitis (HP)

This disease is a form of chronic hepatitis characterized by continued active inflammation and hepatocyte damage commonly resulting in progressive fibrosis. The disease may progress to cirrhosis and liver failure if untreated. There are several causes of this histological picture including persistent hepatitis B infection; other patients have high titres of autoantibodies particularly against smooth muscle and an autoimmune aetiology has been postulated. Certain drugs may also cause this pattern of reaction.

Histologically, there are three main features. Firstly, there are marked chronic inflammatory changes in the portal tracts which become expanded by chronic inflammatory cells. Secondly, the layer of liver cells immediately adjacent to the portal tracts, known to pathologists as the *limiting plate*, undergoes necrosis **N** with lymphocytes and plasma cells spilling out of the portal tracts **P** into the liver parenchyma; this necrosis of cells in the limiting plate is patchy and is termed *piecemeal necrosis*.

Thirdly, the hepatocyte necrosis around the portal areas leads to fibrosis which may link the portal tracts with fibrous bridges. With further liver damage, the condition progresses to cirrhosis as shown in Fig. 13.8(c).

This histopathological appearance is known by the term *chronic aggressive hepatitis* and corresponds to the clinical condition described as *chronic active hepatitis*.

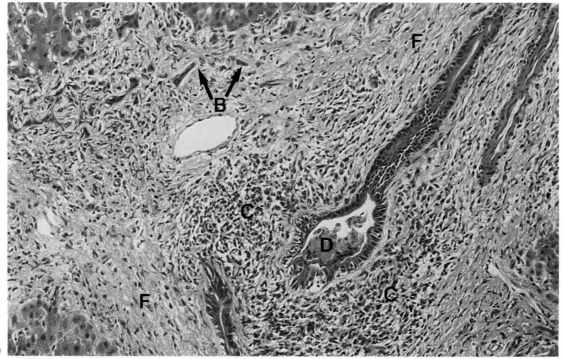

*(a)*

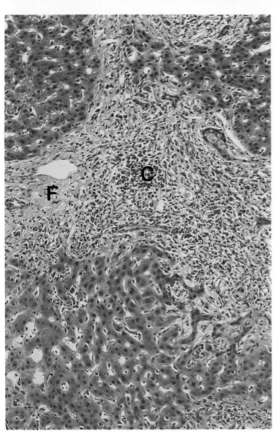

*(b)*

### Fig. 13.6   Primary biliary cirrhosis
### (a) early lesion (HP)
### (b) later lesion (HP)

Primary biliary cirrhosis is a chronic inflammatory disease of the liver in which destructive inflammatory changes are centred primarily on bile ducts but also affect hepatocytes.

The earliest changes are seen in the epithelium of the larger bile ducts **D** as shown in micrograph (a). There is vacuolation of the epithelial cells and infiltration of the wall and surrounding tissues by chronic inflammatory cells. A characteristic feature at this stage, though not shown here, is the formation of histiocytic granulomata in relation to damaged bile ducts.

Portal tracts then become progressively expanded by chronic inflammatory cells **C** and as the large bile ducts are destroyed they are no longer seen. As seen in micrograph (b), the inflammatory cells extend from the portal tracts into the liver parenchyma with piecemeal necrosis occurring along the limiting plate in a manner similar to chronic aggressive hepatitis (see Fig. 13.5). As liver cells are destroyed, the portal tracts also become expanded by fibrosis **F** .

At the periphery of the portal tracts there is proliferation of small bile ducts **B** which appear not to be canalised; this feature is best seen in micrograph (a).

If primary biliary cirrhosis proceeds unchecked, true cirrhosis develops (see Fig. 13.8); note that this disease is referred to as primary biliary cirrhosis even in the early stages when there is no evidence of cirrhotic changes.

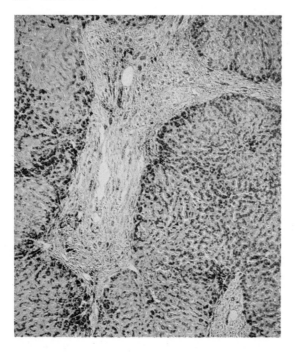

## Fig. 13.7 Haemochromatosis (Perls stain; MP)

*Haemochromatosis* is a condition characterized by excessive deposition of iron in the tissues. It is due to an inherited defect of iron transport across the intestinal cells such that excessive iron is absorbed from a normal diet. Pathologically excessive iron is deposited in many tissues especially the myocardium, the liver, the adrenal glands, and the pancreas. The effects of excess iron are usually only manifest after many years, commonly in the fourth decade. Myocardial involvement gives rise to congestive cardiac failure, pancreatic involvement causes diabetes mellitus, and hepatic involvement causes cirrhosis, as illustrated here. Excessive iron, stored as haemosiderin, causes liver cell death.

In this micrograph, liver cells contain enormous amounts of iron which is stained blue by Perls stain. The iron pigment is present in hepatocytes, Kuppfer cells lining the sinusoids and in macrophages in the portal areas.

Excessive iron may also be stored in the liver due to dietary excess or frequent blood transfusion. In these instances there is marked storage in Kuppfer cells before hepatocytes become involved. This is termed *secondary haemosiderosis*.

## Fig. 13.8 Cirrhosis *(illustrations opposite)*
**(a) alcoholic cirrhosis** (MP)
**(b) cryptogenic cirrhosis** (MP)
**(c) cryptogenic cirrhosis** (van Gieson stain; MP)
**(d) cirrhosis due to chronic active hepatitis** (MP)

*Cirrhosis* is the end result of continued damage to liver cells from a great many causes. It is characterized by fibrous septa which cut across the liver lobules and the formation of nodules of regenerating liver cells. Portal tracts are interconnected by broad bands of fibrous tissue.

The effects of this altered liver architecture and cellular damage are twofold. First there may be reduced liver cell function with consequences listed in Fig. 13.1 and second, there is disturbance of blood flow through the liver from portal vein to hepatic vein. The effect of this vascular obstruction is an increase in portal venous pressure. Anastamoses open up between the portal circulation and the systemic venous system resulting in large dilated veins called *varices*. The most important site of varices is in the lower oesophagus but they can occur elsewhere. These dilated thin-walled varices are liable to rupture and this is a common fatal event in patients with cirrhosis.

The classification of cirrhosis is based on the disease which caused the underlying liver damage. The most important causes are chronic alcohol abuse, chronic aggressive hepatitis, biliary cirrhosis (primary and secondary to obstruction), and a large percentage where no underlying disease can be found, known as *cryptogenic cirrhosis*.

The diagnosis of cirrhosis is confirmed by liver biopsy, usually using a needle, and histological examination is directed towards identifying the nature of any underlying disease process as well as establishing evidence of cirrhosis.

In micrograph (a) there is evidence of cirrhosis with broad fibrous bands **F** connecting portal areas **P**; the intervening nodules of liver cells **L** show marked fatty change; this is an example of alcoholic cirrhosis.

Micrograph (b) shows a typical cirrhotic pattern with bands of fibrous tissue **F** disrupting the lobular architecture; there is no inflammation, fatty change or specific features. If there are also no clinical pointers to the aetiology, this is classified as cryptogenic cirrhosis. Micrograph (c) is from the same case, this time stained by a method which emphasises the fibrosis (stained red).

Cirrhosis following chronic aggressive hepatitis is illustrated in micrograph (d). The portal tracts **P** contain large numbers of chronic inflammatory cells and in some areas these inflammatory cells spill over the limiting plate into nodules of hepatocytes. There are also focal areas of inflammation **I** in the liver parenchyma. The portal tracts show evidence of fibrosis and fibrous bands **F** containing chronic inflammatory cells have formed bridges between adjacent portal areas. These features are all characteristically seen in chronic aggressive hepatitis (see Fig. 13.5).

In the treatment of cirrhosis the physician attempts to control the underlying liver disease which is the cause of the progressive fibrosis. Repeated liver biopsy is used to monitor the progress of the disease.

Older classificastions of cirrhosis grouped the diseases according to the size of the regeneration nodules seen at postmortem or laparotomy. In *macronodular cirrhosis* large nodules up to several centimetres in diameter are present. *Micronodular cirrhosis* is characterized by uniform small nodules of regeneration up to one centimetre in diameter. While useful to describe macroscopic features, this classification does not help in assessing disease type or progress.

In active cirrhosis there is evidence of continuing damage to liver cells whereas in inactive cirrhosis there is no evidence of continuing liver damage.

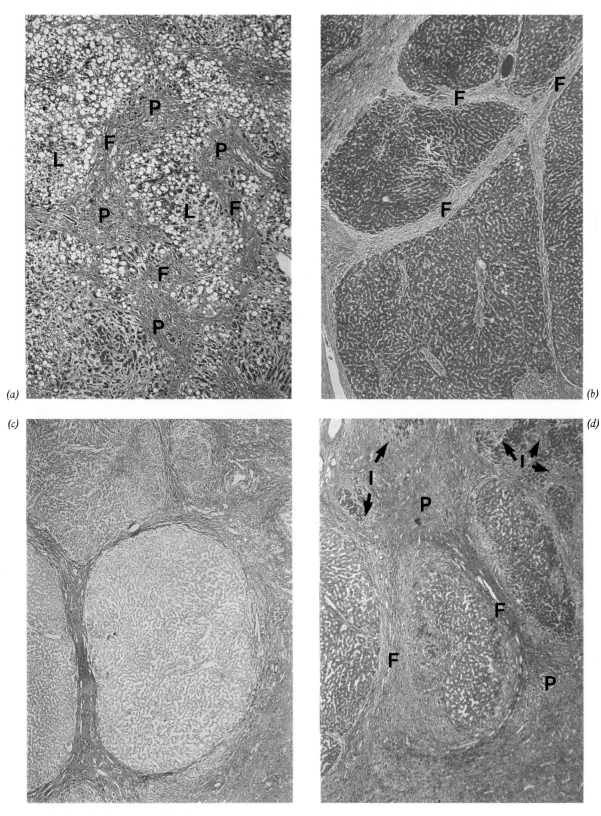

*(a)*

*(b)*

*(c)*

*(d)*

**Fig. 13.8   Cirrhosis**

### Fig. 13.9    Hepatocellular carcinoma (HP)

Primary carcinoma of the liver is a relatively uncommon
condition compared to secondary malignant deposits; pre-
existing cirrhosis, hepatitis B infection and certain carcinogens
in food appear to be important predisposing factors. In Britain,
most hepatocellular carcinomas arises in cirrhotic livers,
however, the condition is much more common in certain
African and Asian countries due to other causes.

The tumour may form a single massive nodule, multiple
small nodules or exhibit a diffuse infiltrating pattern. In this
example, the tumour cells resemble normal hepatocytes; in
some places they are arranged in cords **C**, in others in a duct-
like pattern **D**. In well differentiated tumours, bile may be
present in the tumour cells.

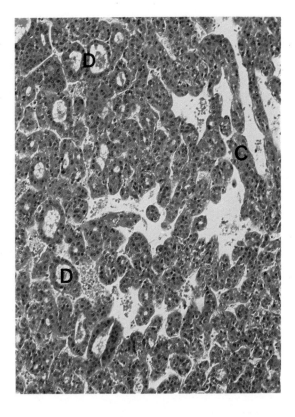

### Fig. 13.10    Cholangiocarcinoma (HP)

Cholangiocarcinoma arises from bile duct epithelium and may
be extrahepatic (in the extrahepatic bile ducts) or intrahepatic
in location. Histologically, a dense fibrous stroma is a
conspicuous feature. The malignant epithelium forms small
gland-like structures and the cells are often very pleomorphic.

These tumours may spread along intrahepatic portal tracts or
may form large nodular growths in the liver.

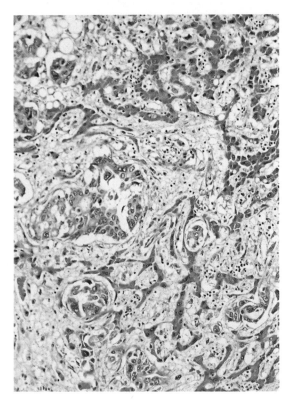

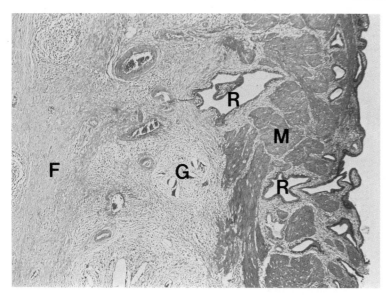

## Fig. 13.11 Chronic cholecystitis (LP)

Many gall bladders containing stones are removed surgically because of abdominal pain. On histological examination, there is evidence of low grade chronic inflammation with marked muscle hypertrophy **M** and an infiltrate of lymphocytes and plasma cells in the submucosal layer. Irregular gland-like mucosal pockets extend deep into the thickened muscle layer and are known as *Rokitansky-Aschoff sinuses* **R**.

Outside the muscle layer, aggregates of histiocytes form around inspissated bile forming *bile granulomata* **G**. There is fibrosis **F** and mild chronic inflammation beneath the serosa.

If bile becomes inspissated and concentrated within the gall bladder, it may cause an acute chemical cholecystitis with a more neutrophilic inflammatory component.

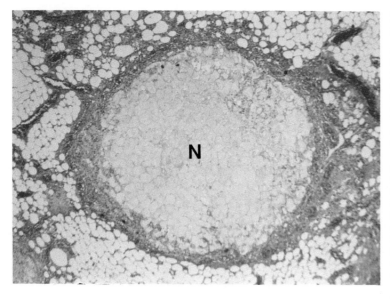

## Fig. 13.12 Fat necrosis in acute pancreatitis (MP)

*Acute pancreatitis* is a condition in which there is sudden destruction of the pancreatic gland due to liberation of the digestive pancreatic enzymes. This results in a massive chemical peritonitis causing severe abdominal pain and shock. The two important predisposing conditions are alcoholism and biliary tract disease (usually stones).

Histologically, there is extensive haemorrhagic necrosis of pancreas and surrounding tissues. Release of pancreatic enzymes gives rise to a characteristic feature termed *fat necrosis*. With the naked eye, numerous chalky-white spots are seen in peripancreatic and omental fat. Histologically, they represent foci of necrotic adipose tissue **N**, surrounded by a darker staining rim of inflammatory cells.

Acute pancreatitis has a poor prognosis, particularly in the elderly. Serum amylase levels are markedly raised due to release from the damaged pancreatic gland and have a useful diagnostic value.

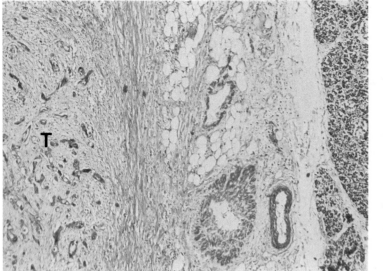
(a)

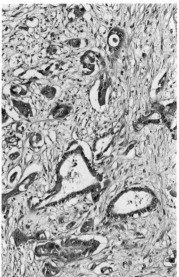
(b)

## Fig. 13.13 Adenocarcinoma of the pancreas
**(a)** LP
**(b)** HP

These tumours virtually all arise from the pancreatic ductal epithelium and are of great importance because of their insidious manner of growth, often remaining undetected until a very advanced stage. The majority of tumours arise in the head of the gland where they tend to obstruct the bile duct thus presenting early with painless jaundice. Macroscopically, the tumours are hard and white.

Micrograph (a) shows tumour **T** with normal pancreas on the right. Note the characteristic tortuous, irregular glands in a dense fibrous stroma. At higher magnification in micrograph (b) the tumour is seen to have a ductular arrangement, the cells having pleomorphic nuclei with a high nucleus to cytoplasmic ratio.

# 14. Urinary system

## Introduction

The main functions of the kidneys are the excretion of nitrogenous by-products of body metabolism, and the maintenance of water and electrolyte homeostasis. The structural unit responsible for these functions, the nephron, has two components, the glomerulus and the renal tubule. The glomerulus consists of a highly specialized capillary network from which water, electrolyte ions and nitrogenous waste products are filtered into the lumen of the renal tubule. The ultrafiltrate then passes along the tubular system where selective reabsorption of water and electrolytes occurs leaving unwanted water and electrolytes, together with nitrogenous waste materials such as urea, creatinine etc. to pass out of the kidneys as urine.

From a functional and pathophysiological viewpoint, the glomerulus is a relatively passive structure whereas the renal tubule is made up of highly metabolically active cells. Thus glomerular function tends to be disrupted by pathological phenomena which alter (often in a subtle way) glomerular structure, whereas disorder of renal tubular function is more often brought about by some metabolic insult to the tubular cells such as hypoxia, exposure to circulating toxins etc. Nevertheless, both nephron components are utterly dependent for their normal function on adequate perfusion of the kidney by circulating blood and if this is disrupted there are serious consequences to both nephron components. In addition, the components of the nephron are so intimately related both structurally and functionally, that any pathological lesion affecting one component will usually have an impact on the other; for example, primary glomerular lesions lead to secondary tubular change and conversely primary tubular failure eventually disrupts glomerular function. The kidneys have a considerable degree of functional reserve but when disease processes damage sufficient numbers of nephrons to outstrip the homeostatic ability of the remaining nephrons, renal failure ensues.

## Renal impairment syndromes

For simplicity, renal disorders can be divided into two main types: *total* in which all functions of the nephron are impaired, or *partial* (selective) in which only certain functions are disturbed. The syndromes of total renal impairment are known clinically as *chronic* and *acute renal failure*. Partial renal dysfunction is the hallmark of the clinical conditions known as the *nephritic syndrome*, the *nephrotic syndrome*, the *mixed nephritic-nephrotic syndrome* and their minor or precursor stages namely *renal haematuria* (i.e. haematuria arising from the kidney parenchyma as opposed to the collecting system) and *persistent proteinuria*.

In **chronic renal failure**, there is progressive retention of nitrogenous metabolites (uraemia) due to insufficient glomerular filtration. Concomitant failure of tubular function produces widespread abnormalities in biochemical homeostasis including salt and water retention, metabolic acidosis, and other electrolyte imbalances including hyperkalaemia. Many renal lesions can produce the chronic renal failure syndrome but all have as their common basis the *slowly progressive, irreversible destruction of almost all nephron units*, both glomerular and tubular components. The primary lesion may be disease of the vessels (e.g. hypertension or vasculitis), glomerular (e.g. glomerulonephritis), or tubular, or there may be destruction of the whole nephron secondary to diseases such as pyelonephritis, urinary outflow obstruction etc. A kidney in which all nephrons have been irreversibly damaged is small and shrivelled and is known as an *end-stage kidney* (see Fig. 14.11).

In **acute renal failure,** there is abrupt cessation of activity of the nephrons, usually manifest initially as a marked fall in urine production (*oliguria*) which may even be total (*anuria*). Disturbances of fluid and electrolyte balance soon follow, particularly a rise in the serum potassium level and metabolic acidosis; if nephron failure persists, features of nitrogen retention develop. Again, many different types of lesion can produce acute renal failure, but all have as their common basis the *acute, sometimes reversible, cessation of nephron activity*. The initiating lesion may be primarily vascular as in hypovolaemic shock where there is hypoxic injury or necrosis of tubular epithelial cells (see Fig. 1.2), glomerular, as in some forms of glomerulonephritis, or tubular as in papillary necrosis (see Fig. 14.10). The important difference from chronic renal failure is that the acute syndrome is sometimes reversible and normal nephron function may be restored if the pathological stimulus is removed either spontaneously or as a result of treatment.

The **acute nephritic syndrome** (formerly inaccurately called acute glomerulonephritis) is characterized by haematuria and oliguria, oedema (often periorbital) and a rise in blood pressure and blood urea concentration, usually transient. It generally results from such primary glomerular lesions as have the effect of obstructing the glomerular capillary lumina. When glomerular blood flow is reduced, glomerular filtration also falls causing the oliguria, rise in blood pressure and retention of nitrogenous metabolites. Swollen and damaged glomerular capillary endothelial cells are usually responsible for the obstruction of the glomerular capillary lumina and this, with the concomitant glomerular basement membrane damage, permits leakage of red blood cells and some protein into the urine. *Acute glomerulonephritis* is the general term applied to glomerular lesions of this type and an example is illustrated in Fig. 14.3.

The **nephrotic syndrome,** in contrast, is characterized by severe proteinuria which leads to a fall in serum protein concentration (hypoalbuminaemia) and consequent marked osmotic oedema of peripheral tissues. Many types of renal lesion can produce heavy proteinuria and the nephrotic syndrome, but most have as their basis a disturbance of glomerular capillary basement membrane function permitting the leakage of plasma proteins across the filtration barrier and into the urine. In most cases of nephrotic syndrome, there is some detectable structural abnormality of the glomerular basement membrane, either alone, or as part of a disease process affecting other glomerular components such as the mesangium or endothelial cells. Such structural abnormalities commonly arise from deposition of immune complexes as in *membranous nephropathy* (see Fig. 14.2) and lupus nephritis, infiltration by amyloid (see Fig. 14.2), and nonspecific thickening as in diabetes mellitus (see Fig. 4.7). In some cases of the nephrotic syndrome, particularly in children, there is no structural abnormality detectable in the basement membrane, at least by any techniques currently available, and the term *minimal change nephropathy* has been therefore applied.

In the **mixed nephritic-nephrotic syndrome** the patient exhibits some of the features of both syndromes. It is mainly seen in association with glomerular lesions with both a proliferative (capillary lumen-obstructing) and membranous (protein-leaking) component. The most common lesion of this type is the *mesangiocapillary glomerulonephritis* also known as *membranoproliferative glomerulonephritis* (see Fig. 14.6).

The glomerular lesions described above may subside spontaneously or with treatment. However if they progress, glomerular blood flow is obstructed, glomerular filtration ceases and the tubules associated with affected glomeruli undergo atrophy; thus entire nephrons may become permanently and irreversibly damaged. When sufficient nephrons have been destroyed, the clinical features of the disease will evolve from the nephritic or nephrotic syndrome into the syndrome of chronic renal failure. By way of illustration, a patient with the nephrotic syndrome due to diabetic glomerular disease may slowly develop the features of chronic renal failure as individual nephrons are progressively converted into functionless units by glomerular hyalinization and tubular atrophy. In a similar manner, a patient who initially presents with the acute nephritic syndrome due to a rapidly progressive crescentic glomerulonephritis (see Fig. 4.4) may quickly progress to the syndrome of acute renal failure as the glomeruli are rapidly destroyed by the disease process. Some of the more important clinical and pathological features of the various patterns of renal impairment are summarized in Fig. 14.1.

The above discussion about glomerular disorders was intended to demonstrate the association between structural derangement of the glomerulus and the functional consequences and their clinical manifestations. In practice the situation is less simple since, despite intense clinical and pathological study using electron microscopy, immunofluorescence and other techniques, understanding is far from complete. It is now believed that many of these primary glomerular disorders have an immunological basis since immunoglobulins and immune complexes can be demonstrated in the glomerular basement membranes and mesangium in many of these renal lesions (see Fig. 14.2b). In response to damaging stimuli, the glomerulus appears to react in one or more of the following ways:

(a)  swelling or proliferation of the normally flat endothelial cells lining the glomerular capillary lumina;
(b)  proliferation of the epithelial cells investing the outer surface of the glomerular capillary tuft (the podocytes) and the cells lining the inner surface of Bowman's capsule;
(c)  thickening of the glomerular basement membranes or
(d)  proliferation of the cells of the mesangium and excessive production of acellular mesangial material.

Irreversible glomerular damage whatever the cause is usually followed by progressive replacement of the vascular glomerular tuft by mesangial material leading to the condition of *glomerular hyalinization* also illustrated in Fig. 14.7 and 14.8. Many of the subtleties of these glomerular disorders are difficult to visualize in standard H & E stained paraffin sections and require specially prepared thin sections stained by special techniques.

Primary lesions of the glomerulus are often referred to by the loose term 'glomerulonephritis', a word incapable of accurate definition. Its use persists in the classification and nomenclature of primary active proliferative and destructive lesions of the glomerulus (see Figs. 14.3 to 14.6); the term 'chronic glomerulonephritis', formerly used in an imprecise way to describe what is now called end-stage kidney, has fortunately been largely discontinued.

## Systemic causes of renal disease

Many systemic diseases may lead to the destruction of sufficient numbers of nephrons to cause impairment of renal function, particularly diseases producing structural abnormalities in small blood vessels. The kidney is especially vulnerable to the effects of arterial hypertension as seen in Figs 10.1 and 10.2, and irreversible damage to nephrons may result either acutely as in accelerated hypertension or progressively over a period of years in essential benign hypertension; both these forms of *hypertensive nephrosclerosis* are illustrated in Fig. 14.8. Renal disease is also an important complication of diabetes mellitus which particularly affects small renal arterioles and glomerular capillaries; the important features of *diabetic nephropathy* are shown in Fig. 14.7.

The tubular components of the nephron may be primarily damaged as a result of hypovolaemic shock, by inorganic and organic toxins, or as the result of infection. In hypokalaemic states and intoxication, tubular epithelial cells may exhibit marked cytoplasmic degenerative changes or frank necrosis leading to the pathological term *acute tubular necrosis* and producing the clinical syndrome of acute renal failure. Tubular epithelial cells have considerable powers of recovery and regeneration, and acute renal failure may be reversible under such circumstances if the patient can be sustained in the interim by dialysis and other supporting measures.

Pyogenic infections of the pelvicalyceal system (*pyelitis*) and renal parenchyma (*pyelonephritis*) are usually caused by Gram-negative bacilli which are normally commensals in the lower intestinal tract; they gain access to the kidney either by ascending infection from the lower urinary tract or by blood stream spread. Acute pyogenic pyelonephritis is illustrated in Fig. 14.9. Tuberculous pyelonephritis may also arise by similar routes of spread and is shown in Fig. 3.12. Acute pyelonephritis, diabetes and analgesic abuse predispose to another form of necrosis affecting the tubular component of the nephron, this time confined to the collecting tubules and ducts of the renal papilla; this condition is known as *papillary necrosis* and is illustrated in Fig. 14.10.

## Tumours of the urinary system

The most common tumour of the kidney in adults is the *renal adenocarcinoma* derived from the tubular epithelial cells; it is illustrated in Fig. 14.12 and one of its important methods of spread is shown in Fig. 6.6. The kidney is the site of an important malignant tumour of children, the *nephroblastoma*, also known as *Wilms' tumour* (see Fig. 14.13), an example of an embryonal tumour. The pelvicalyceal system is lined by transitional epithelium (urothelium) which is continuous with that of the ureter and bladder. Tumours of the urothelium (*transitional cell carcinoma*) are common and of particular interest because of the possible role of chemical carcinogens such as aniline dyes in their pathogenesis (see Figs 6.12 and 14.14).

**Fig 14.1  Renal impairment syndromes: summary of general principles**

| Syndrome | Main clinical and biochemical features | Basic pathophysiology | Common causes |
|---|---|---|---|
| Acute renal failure | Oliguria (anuria)<br>Hyperkalaemia<br>Acidosis<br>Uraemia (rapid rise) | Abrupt, often reversible, cessation of all nephron activity | Acute damage to *all* tubules e.g. acute tubular necrosis of anoxic or toxic cause (Fig. 1.2)<br><br>Acute damage to *all* glomeruli e.g. rapidly progressive crescentic glomerulonephritis (Fig. 14.4) |
| Chronic renal failure | Uraemia (slow inexorable rise)<br>Chronic electrolyte disturbances (acidosis, hyperkalaemia) | Slowly progressive cessation of nephron activity following irreversible destruction | End stage kidney (Fig. 14.11) due to many causes including primary glomerular diseases, hypertension (Fig. 14.8), diabetes (Fig. 14.7) and congenital disorders e.g. polycystic kidney. |
| Nephritic syndrome | Haematuria<br>Oedema<br>Transient uraemia and hypertension | Obstruction to blood flow through glomerular capillary lumina, usually due to blockage by proliferating capillary endothelial cells, leading to decreased glomerular filtration rate and increased blood pressure and blood urea | Acute glomerulonephritis (Fig. 14.3) |
| Nephrotic syndrome | Proteinuria<br>Hypoalbuminaemia<br>Oedema | Structural abnormality of glomerular capillary basement membrane leading to leakage of protein into urine | Immune complex deposition in basement membrane e.g. membranous nephropathy (Fig. 14.2)<br><br>Diabetic thickening of basement membrane (Fig. 14.7)<br><br>Amyloid deposition in basement membrane (Fig. 4.2) |
| Mixed nephritic-nephrotic syndrome | Nephrotic syndrome with some nephritic features usually haematuria | Combined abnormality of glomerular basement membranes and capillary lumina | Mesangiocapillary glomerulonephritis (Fig. 14.6) |

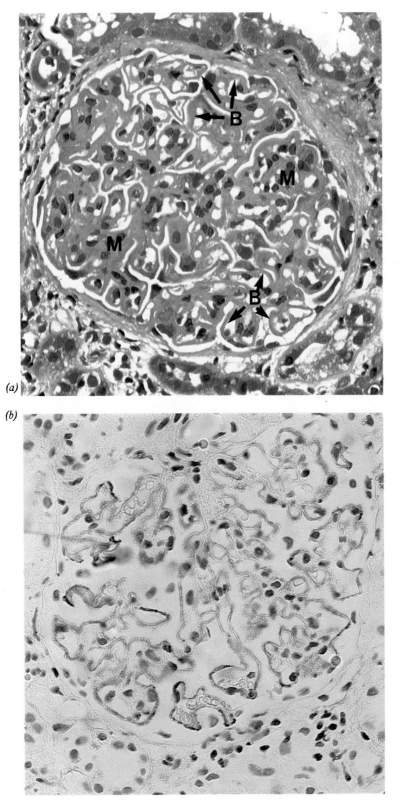

*(a)*

*(b)*

### Fig. 14.2   **Membranous nephropathy**

(a) H & E (HP)
(b) Immunoperoxidase method (HP)

In this condition the glomerular basement membranes are diffusely and fairly uniformly thickened, often reaching 5 or 6 times normal thickness. With the H & E stain, the basement membranes **B** appear thick, eosinophilic and sometimes slightly refractile. There is no associated endothelial or epithelial (podocyte) proliferation although there may be a slight increase in mesangial material **M** in severe and long standing cases. Much of the basement membrane thickening appears to be due to the presence of immune complexes which can be demonstrated by electron microscopy or, as in micrograph (b), by immunohistochemical methods; in micrograph (b) the brown stain represents immunoglobulin (in this case IgG) incorporated in the glomerular basement membranes.

In *membranous nephropathy*, the filtration properties of the glomerular basement membrane are somehow disrupted, allowing leakage of plasma proteins, especially albumin, into the urine; the condition usually presents clinically as severe proteinuria, often with the nephrotic syndrome.

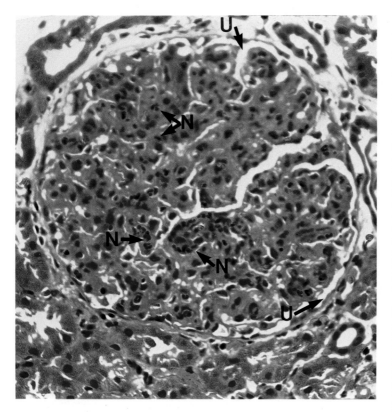

### Fig. 14.3   Acute proliferative ('endocapillary') glomerulonephritis (HP)

This form of glomerulonephritis most commonly occurs in children and often follows a streptococcal infection, usually of the throat. The typical histological features are a marked proliferation of the endothelial cells lining the glomerular capillaries, and infiltration of the glomerular tuft by neutrophils; this latter feature explains one of the synonyms for this condition, *acute exudative glomerulonephritis*. In this high power micrograph, note the increased cellularity of the tuft due to proliferation of endothelial cells (and probably also, some mesangial cells) which have virtually obliterated the capillary lumina; the urinary space **U** remains clear since there has been no proliferation of podocytes. Note also the increased numbers of neutrophils **N** in the glomerular tuft.

An important feature of this condition is the involvement of all segments of the glomerulus which distinguishes this disease from focal glomerulonephritis shown in Fig. 14.5. The obstruction of glomerular capillary lumina diminishes glomerular filtration and causes leakage of erythrocytes and this condition usually presents with haematuria, transient hypertension and oedema in the acute nephritic syndrome.

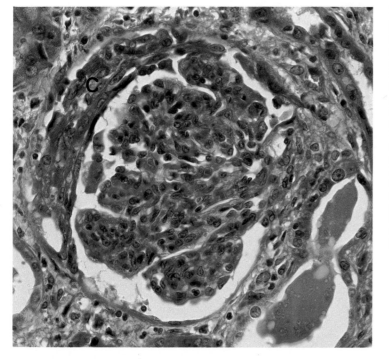

### Fig. 14.4   Acute crescentic glomerulonephritis (HP)

Sometimes the changes illustrated and described in Fig. 14.3 are accompanied by proliferation of podocytes and the epithelial cells lining Bowman's capsule. Uneven proliferation of Bowman's capsule epithelial cells around only part of the circumference of Bowman's capsule produces a so-called *crescent* **C**. The significance of this change is that continued proliferation of the crescent may obliterate the glomerular tuft, leading to irreversible glomerular destruction and subsequent nephron atrophy. If a large proportion of glomeruli show crescent formation there is rapidly progressive renal impairment and total renal failure ensues in a short time.

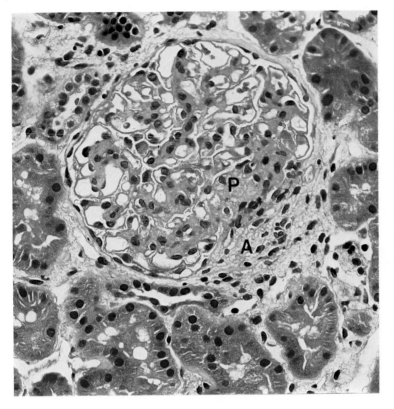

**Fig. 14.5   Focal segmental glomerulonephritis** (HP)

In the types of glomerulonephritis discussed in Fig. 14.3 and 14.4 the pathological changes affect all segments (*global*) of all glomeruli (*diffuse*). In contrast, there are a number of glomerular disorders such as *Henoch-Schönlein purpura, IgA mesangial disease* and many others in which endothelial and epithelial proliferation only involves some segments (*segmental*) of some glomeruli (*focal*).

This micrograph of old Henoch-Schonlein disease provides such an example. Note the segmental area of proliferation **P** in the glomerular tuft, largely the result of increase in size and number of mesangial cells and (at the later stage shown here) increase in acellular mesangial material; there is also proliferation and swelling of endothelial cells and irregular basement membrane thickening. Note the normality of the remaining segments of the glomerular tuft. Sometimes the abnormal segment of the tuft becomes adherent to Bowman's capsule to form a *tuft adhesion* **A** as in this example.

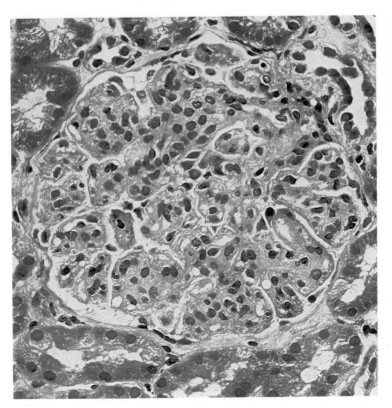

**Fig. 14.6   Mesangiocapillary (membranoproliferative) glomerulonephritis**

In this condition, all segments of all glomeruli undergo both mesangial and endothelial cell proliferation and marked widespread basement membrane thickening. The latter is due to a combination of extensive immune complex deposition and interpositioning of mesangial material between basement membrane laminae. Unfortunately neither of these basement membrane features are discernible in H & E stained paraffin sections, and special stains or electron microscopy are necessary to demonstrate them adequately. More easily seen, as in this micrograph, is the expansion of each segment of the tuft producing an exaggerated lobular appearance of the glomerulus and accounting for the now outdated term of *lobular glomerulonephritis* by which this condition was formerly known. The combination of basement membrane abnormality and cellular proliferation usually results in the nephrotic syndrome, often with some superadded features of the nephritic syndrome (e.g. haematuria).

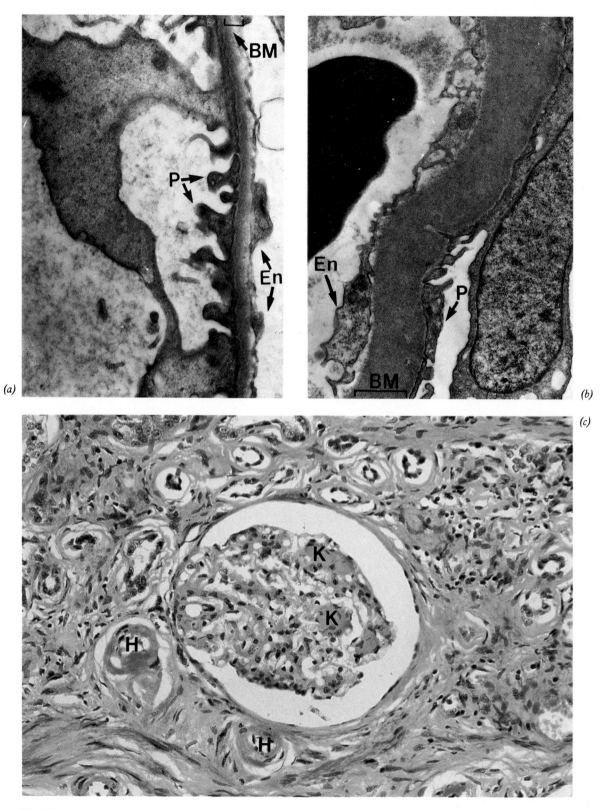

Fig. 14.7 Diabetic nephropathy

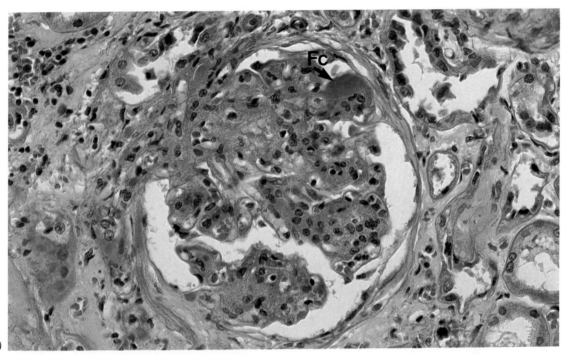

*(d)*

## Fig. 14.7   Diabetic nephropathy *(illustrations (a), (b) and (c) opposite)*
**(a) normal glomerular basement membrane** (EM)   **(b) diabetic basement membrane** (EM)
**(c) nodular diabetic glomerulosclerosis** (HP)   **(d) diffuse diabetic glomerulosclerosis** (HP)

Diabetes mellitus may affect the kidney in a variety of different ways both specific and nonspecific.

Since the kidneys are highly vascular organs they are subject to the same exaggerated atherosclerotic changes found elsewhere in the body in larger arterial vessels. One result of this is to predispose the kidney to chronic ischaemic changes. Diabetes is also associated with increased incidence and severity of bacterial infections, which, in the urinary system, means a greatly increased incidence of pyelonephritis and infections of the lower tract. Acute papillary necrosis (Fig. 14.10) is a severe renal complication of diabetes, particularly in the presence of associated pyelonephritis.

More specifically, characteristic changes occur in the glomeruli (*diabetic glomerulosclerosis*), and in the walls of afferent and efferent arterioles. Among the early glomerular changes is a uniform and homogeneous thickening of the glomerular capillary basement membrane, best seen by electron microscopy; this feature is illustrated in micrograph (b), with the normal shown for comparison in micrograph (a). In both electron micrographs, note the glomerular capillary basement membrane **BM** invested by thin endothelial cell cytoplasm **En** on the inner aspect, and by epithelial cell (podocyte) foot processes **P** externally. In diabetes, the basement membrane may be up to 4 or 5 times normal thickness.

In more advanced glomerular involvement, the basement membrane thickening is associated with an increase in mesangial cells and matrix. The mesangial matrix increase is often segmental and localized to produce characteristic acellular nodules, often with compressed mesangial cell nuclei pushed to their periphery; these nodules are called *Kimmelstiel-Wilson nodules*. This pattern of diabetic glomerular involvement is shown in micrograph (c), and is called *nodular diabetic glomerulosclerosis;* note the Kimmelstiel-Wilson nodules **K**. In another pattern the mesangial cell and material increase

is diffuse and global, not segmental and nodular, producing the change called *diffuse diabetic glomerulosclerosis,* illustrated in micrograph (d). Both patterns may occur in the same kidney, and nodule formation may be superimposed upon the diffuse change within the same glomerulus. In both patterns, there is escape of plasma protein across the thickened but leaky glomerular capillary wall into the urinary space; occasionally inspissated protein may be deposited on the outer surface of the glomerular tuft (*fibrin caps*) or on the inner surface of Bowman's capsule (*capsular drops*). A fibrin cap **Fc** is demonstrated in micrograph (d), associated with diffuse diabetic glomerulosclerosis. These features are also seen in chronically ischaemic glomeruli and are not specific to diabetic glomerular disease.

A frequent feature of diabetic renal disease is hyalinization of afferent and efferent arteriole walls, a further manifestation of the predisposition of the diabetic kidney to vascular disease ranging from large renal artery atherosclerosis to capillary wall basement membrane thickening. This arteriolar hyalinization **H**, well shown in association with nodular diabetic glomerulosclerosis in micrograph (c), may also extend into the vascular hilum of the glomerulus. The combination of arterial atherosclerosis and arteriolar hyalinization progressively reduces the blood flow to the glomeruli thus chronic ischaemic changes, such as hyalinization of glomeruli and periglomerular fibrosis, are common associated findings in diabetic renal disease.

The initial glomerular basement membrane changes result in proteinuria and even the nephrotic syndrome, but with progressive diabetic glomerulosclerosis and chronic ischaemic nephron atrophy, the features of chronic renal failure may supervene. Acute pyelonephritis or renal papillary necrosis (see Figs 14.9 and 14.10) may precipitate acute renal failure.

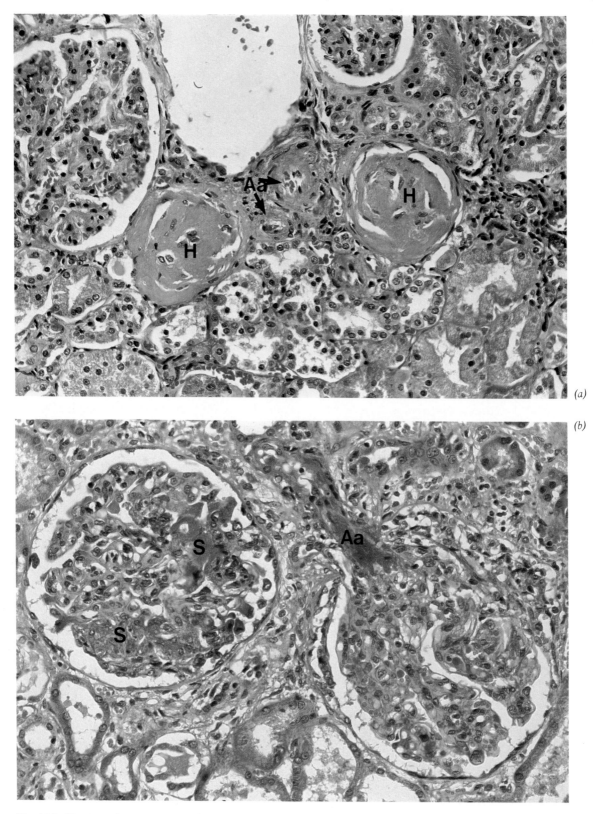

**Fig. 14.8  Hypertensive nephrosclerosis**

## Fig. 14.8    Hypertensive nephrosclerosis *(illustrations opposite)*
## (a) benign hypertensive nephrosclerosis (HP)
## (b) malignant hypertensive nephrosclerosis (HP)

The vessel changes in systemic hypertension have been discussed and illustrated in some detail in Figs 10.1 and 10.2. The kidney is particularly vulnerable to the damaging effects of these vessel changes and renal failure is an important complication of untreated hypertension.

The pathological changes in the kidney depend on the severity and rate of progress of the hypertension. In *benign (essential) hypertension,* where the hypertension is of gradual onset and progression and reaching only moderately elevated diastolic pressures, the large and medium sized renal arteries show marked thickening of their walls by a combination of medial hypertrophy, elastic lamina reduplication, and fibrous intimal thickening (see Fig. 10.1a); arterioles show hyaline thickening of their walls (see Fig. 10.1b). These changes reduce the calibre of all renal afferent vessels and the resulting chronic ischaemia leads to progressive *sclerosis* (hyalinization) of the glomerulus and subsequent disuse atrophy of the tubular component of the nephron. Micrograph (a) shows a clump of glomeruli, two of which have become converted into hyaline amorphous pink staining masses **H** as a result of chronic ischaemia following hyalinization of the walls of their afferent arterioles **Aa;** the other glomeruli are as yet unaffected. Slowly progressive loss of functioning nephrons may eventually lead to chronic renal failure and the morphological state known as end-stage kidney (see Fig. 14.11).

In contrast, in *malignant (accelerated) hypertension,* where the rise in blood pressure is rapid and severe, the arterial and arteriolar changes are different. Large and medium sized arteries may show only concentric thickening of the intima by loose, rather myxomatous, fibroblastic tissue (see Fig. 10.2a), and there is no elastic lamina reduplication or significant medial hypertrophy. Small arteries may show marked concentric fibroblastic intimal thickening so that the lumen is often virtually obliterated. Arterioles frequently show patchy acute necrosis of their walls with the accumulation of amorphous, brightly eosinophilic proteinaceous material *(fibrinoid)* in the damaged walls (see Fig. 10.2b). This change is known as *fibrinoid necrosis* and as seen in the micrograph (b) often affects the afferent arterioles **Aa** at the glomerular hila and may extend into the glomerular tuft to affect some segments **S** of the glomerular capillary network. These small vessel changes are acute in onset and may produce an abrupt reduction in blood supply to the nephrons, often producing glomerular micro-infarction and tubular epithelial necrosis. The effect is to produce a catastrophic reduction in glomerula filtration, and the patient may develop acute oliguric or anuric renal failure. Not infrequently, the patient with long standing benign hypertension may suddenly develop an accelerated phase, and the histological changes in the kidney may be those of mixed benign and malignant nephrosclerosis.

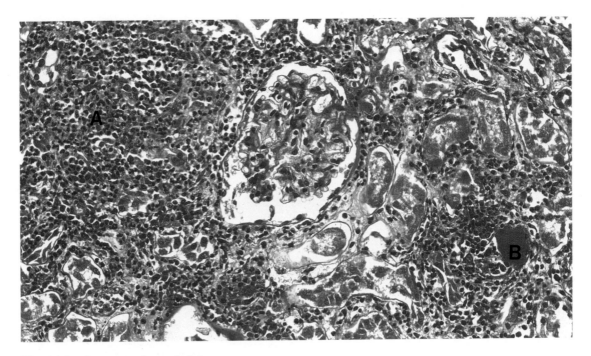

## Fig. 14.9    Acute pyelonephritis (HP)

Acute suppurative bacterial infections of the kidney usually follow ascending infection from the lower urinary tract, particularly when there is obstruction to urinary outflow such as in benign prostatic hyperplasia or pressure from the fetus in pregnancy; in such cases, coliform organisms are the most frequent infecting agent. Infection may arise in the kidney by the haematogenous route during episodes of bacteraemia.

In established *acute pyelonephritis* there may be extensive infiltration of the kidney by neutrophil polymorphs, often with abscess formation. In the micrograph, note the extensive infiltration of the kidney by small dark staining neutrophils, early abscess formation **A,** and a clump of purple staining bacteria **B.**

## Fig. 14.10    Renal papillary necrosis (LP)

This low power photomicrograph shows the condition known as *papillary necrosis* or *necrotizing papillitis*. The tip of the papilla **P** undergoes necrosis of a coagulative type, with preservation of ghost-like outlines of the papillary tubules and collecting ducts. In the early stages there is a neutrophil inflammatory response at the junction **J** between normal and necrotic papilla but this largely disappears at a later stage when the necrotic papilla separates and is shed. This condition, which is probably ischaemic in nature, often occurs in association with acute pyelonephritis particularly when accompanied by an obstructive lesion in the lower urinary tract. It may also be seen with or without overt infection in *diabetic nephropathy* and in *analgesic nephropathy*. If there is sudden loss of many papillae, the patient may develop acute renal failure.

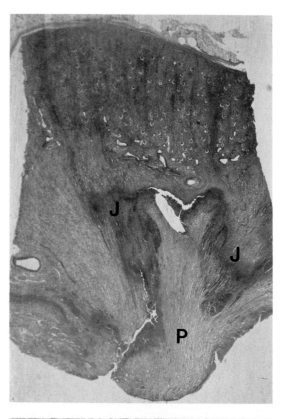

## Fig. 14.11    End-stage kidney (MP)

Many progressive renal diseases of greatly differing pathogenesis are followed by progressive nephron destruction paralleled clinically by insidious deterioration of renal function culminating in death due to chronic renal failure. At necropsy, the kidneys are usually found to be small and hard with symmetrical atrophic thinning of the cortex and poor demarcation of cortex from medulla. This condition is known as *end-stage kidney* and both in gross and histological appearance there is often little clue to the original renal pathology. In the cortex, there is widespread replacement of glomerular tufts by avascular, acellular hyaline material **H** (*hyalinization*). The cortical tubules **T** also become shrunken and atrophic and the relatively expanded interstitial spaces **I** undergo fibrosis; some atrophic tubules may become cystically dilated with *casts* of inspissated proteinacious material **P** which is highly eosinophilic. The shrunken cortex is sometimes marked by scars, formerly attributed to chronic pyelonephritis; infection is now believed to contribute to only a small proportion of cases and most of the scars are probably ischaemic in origin. The term chronic pyelonephritis should be confined to cases where renal scarring is associated with evidence of active or recurrent infection.

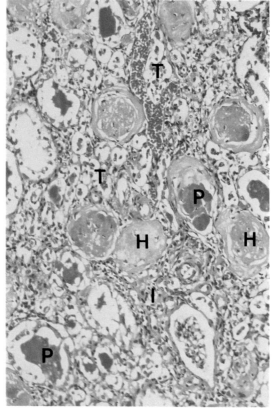

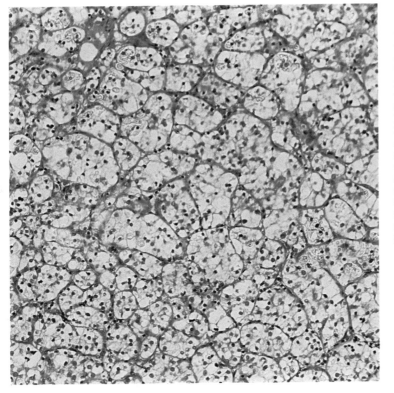

## Fig. 14.12   Renal tubular carcinoma (HP)

The most common malignant tumour of the kidney is the *renal adenocarcinoma* derived from renal tubular epithelium. The tumour cells are large and polygonal in shape and, as in this example, often with characteristically clear cytoplasm, the result of cytoplasmic glycogen and lipid accummulation. In other histological variants, the tumour cell cytoplasm is granular and pink staining, more closely resembling the tubular epithelium from which these tumours are derived. Renal tubular carcinoma tends to breach the walls of intrarenal venous tributaries and to grow as solid cords along the lumen of the renal vein towards and into the inferior vena cava (see Fig. 6.6).

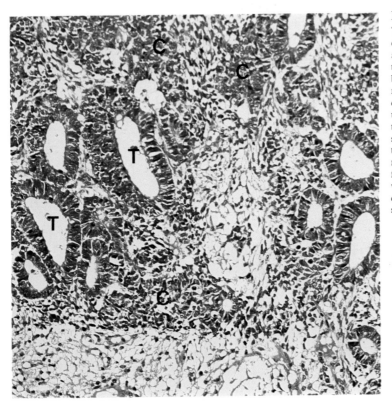

## Fig. 14.13   Nephroblastoma (HP)

The kidney is the site of one of the most common of the embryonal tumours, the *nephroblastoma* or *Wilms' tumour*. This tumour of infants and children is believed to originate from embryonic renal blastema, and, although largely composed of primitive and undifferentiated cells **C,** usually shows a tendency in some areas to form tubular structures **T** resembling primitive renal tubules; occasionally, structures resembling immature glomeruli are found. There are many histological variants of this tumour, some of which contain primitive tissue cells such as skeletal muscle cells (rhabdomyoblasts).

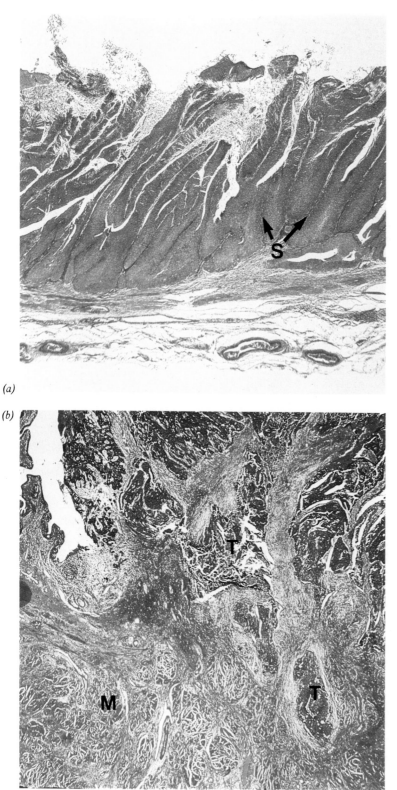

*(a)*

*(b)*

## Fig. 14.14  Transitional cell carcinoma
**(a) well differentiated** (LP)
**(b) poorly differentiated** (LP)

The urinary collecting system, including the pelvicalyceal system, the ureters, bladder and much of the urethra, is lined by a specialized type of epithelium known as transitional epithelium or urothelium. Tumours of the urothelium are common and all are regarded as malignant despite the fact that many are well differentiated histologically and show no evidence of invasion when first detected.

As in the pelvicalyceal tumour shown in microgrph (a), well differentiated tumours commonly arise as frond-like papillary outgrowths from the urothelial surface and have a slender connective tissue stroma **S** supporting the layers of neoplastic cells.

In less well differentiated tumours, some semblance of this papillary pattern is retained but it is lost in the most poorly differentiated tumours, usually in the bladder. The less well differentiated tumours often appear as sessile ulcerated plaques and, as shown in micrograph (b), the tumour **T** extends deeply through the bladder submucosa and muscular wall **M.**

Urothelial tumours are frequently multifocal in origin, and there is a strong link between their development and exposure to certain industrial chemicals such as aniline dyes.

The prognosis of urothelial tumours depends on their location, the histological pattern, the degree of cytological differentiation, and the extent of local invasion when the tumour is first detected. The cytology of transitional cell tumours is shown in more detail in Fig. 6.12.

# 15. Lymphoreticular system

## Introduction

The lymphoreticular system encompasses that diffuse mass of tissue in the body responsible for nonspecific cellular defence mechanisms and the immune system. The nonspecific defence functions are mainly performed by phagocytic cells of the *macrophage-monocyte system* which act as scavengers for extraneous particles including bacteria and viruses which breach the body's surface protective mechanisms, as well as mopping up any debris from normal cellular and tissue turnover, and wear and tear. The monocyte component comprises the monocytes of circulating blood which are also known to spend some, if not most, of their existence sequestered as macrophages (histiocytes) in connective tissues throughout the body. Other macrophages are thought to be relatively fixed within the tissues and some of these are located on the 'reticular' supporting structure in certain organs such as lymph nodes. The endothelial cells lining the whole vascular system appear to have a limited phagocytic ability which in some organs such as the liver and spleen is so enhanced as to make clear distinction between endothelium and macrophage-monocyte system difficult; the Kuppfer cells lining the liver sinusoids are a classical example. This explains the old term *reticulo-endothelial system* applied to the macrophage-monocyte system.

Many extrinsic particles, particularly viruses and bacteria, are recognized as foreign, i.e. antigenic, and excite an immune response which is highly specific for one or more of the biochemical constituents of the foreign material i.e. the antigens. The cells responsible for the immune mechanism are the lymphocytes which mediate their activity in one of two main ways:
(i) the *cell mediated response,* involving the activity of T lymphocytes which are either directly or indirectly cytotoxic.
(ii) the *humoral response* which involves the activation of B lymphocytes which transform into antibody-secreting plasma cells; interaction of antibody with antigen leads to destruction of the antigen.

Although the immunological response is primarily performed by lymphocytes, other cells of the system may be involved in processing antigen prior to activation of the specific immune mechanisms; cells of the reticulo-endothelial system also often execute final antigen destruction in a more specific manner, either by phagocytosis of the products of T lymphocyte activity or by engulfing antigen-antibody complexes.

The macrophage-monocyte (reticulo-endothelial) system is thus inextricably linked with lymphocytes making up the immune system, to give a functional entity often described as the *lymphoreticular system.*

Although some of the lymphoreticular system exists in the form of distinct organs such as the spleen, thymus and lymph nodes, much of the cellular constituents are scattered diffusely throughout the body in the connective tissues especially that underlying the epithelium of the gastro-intestinal and respiratory tracts.

The haemopoietic system, mainly located in bone marrow, also contains a large element of the lymphoreticular system since it is responsible for the production of monocytes and some lymphocytes.

## Reactive disorders of lymph nodes

The lymphoreticular system is remarkably labile and quickly responds to the presence of foreign material; lymph nodes draining the affected area are commonly the first element to be involved. The lymph node response is known as *reactive hyperplasia* and may involve one or more of the principal cellular contituents of the node, depending on the nature of the foreign material encountered:

(a) in a predominantly cell-mediated response, there is hyperplasia of the paracortical (parafollicular) region of the node, mainly occupied by T lymphocytes (*parafollicular* or *paracortical hyperplasia*);
(b) in a predominantly humoral response, there is hyperplasia of the cortical follicles mainly composed of B lymphocytes, and germinal centres containing proliferating B lymphocytes often develop (*follicular hyperplasia*);
(c) other foreign materials evoke intense phagocytic activity leading to dilatation of subcapsular and medullary sinuses with increased numbers and activity of the phagocytic sinus-lining cells; this is known as *sinus hyperplasia* or *sinus catarrh.*

Examples are shown in Fig. 15.1. Certain foreign agents stimulate specific and typical reactive patterns in lymph nodes, for example toxoplasmosis, drugs etc. These specific patterns of reactivity allow a diagnosis of disease to be made on lymph node biopsy. In addition, lymph nodes are classically involved by the so called specific chronic granulomatous inflammations such as tuberculosis, sarcoidosis and syphilis which are described in Chapter 3.

## Malignant disorders of the lymphoreticular system

Apart from reactive changes in which the lymphoreticular system is mounting an immune response to some foreign agent, the most common disorder encountered in the lymphoreticular system is the development of neoplastic proliferation of the various cell lines. Such conditions are collectively known as *lymphomas* and despite the suffix -oma, all are malignant in that they may become widely disseminated.

*Hodgkin's disease* is one of the most important and common of these diseases although the exact cell of origin is uncertain. Hodgkin's disease exists in a number of different forms each with a different clinical course and prognosis; these are illustrated in Fig. 15.2.

The nomenclature of the other lymphomas has developed over many years and there is a variety of different classifications and terminological systems used in different centres and countries. As a result, the same pathological entity may rejoice in several different names, and international authorities cannot yet agree on a consistent form of classification and terminology. Several general principles can be extracted from the various classifications which are useful in predicting the likely prognosis of the lymphoma.

(i) Lymphomas may be classified according to pattern of growth as being either *follicular* or *diffuse*. In the follicular pattern the cells form aggregates which resemble lymphoid follicles but without germinal centres, whereas, in the diffuse pattern, there is diffuse distribution of cells with no evidence of follicular aggregation. The pattern of growth appears to correspond to the degree of differentiation of the neoplastic cells; follicular lymphomas are generally more highly differentiated and have a better prognosis than the diffuse pattern lymphomas.

(ii) Lymphoma cells may be classified according to size into *small cells* and *large cells*. Some systems extend the classification of cells further by use of enzyme markers, electron microscopy and immunohistochemical study to include likely cell type (B, T or histiocyte) and functional state (immunoblast, plasma cell-like etc). In general, classification based purely on size allows a useful prediction of behaviour to be made, large-celled lymphomas behaving in a more malignant fashion than small-celled lymphomas. The interpretation of lymphoma histology in lymph nodes is sometimes rendered difficult because the neoplastic cells are usually intimately mixed with benign reactive lymphoid cells which can look very similar in appearance. Fig. 15.3 sets out some of the more commonly used systems of nomenclature and attempts to show how each tumour entity derives its various synonyms.

The most common form of lymphoma is that which is derived from lymphocytes, the *lymphocytic lymphoma*; these occur in a spectrum of malignancy which, as described above, is subdivided according to pattern of growth and cell type, either large or small. Examples are illustrated in Fig. 15.4.

The *leukaemias* are malignant neoplasms of the various white cell types in circulating blood and their precursors in the bone marrow, and as such are considered to be part of the spectrum of neoplasms of the lymphoreticular system. *Chronic lymphocytic leukaemia* is a disease of middle aged and elderly adults in which the bone marrow and circulating blood are flooded by neoplastic proliferation of small lymphocytes similar to those seen in small cell lymphocytic lymphoma. *Acute lymphoblastic leukaemia* is a disease of children in which the marrow becomes overwhelmed by the rapid neoplastic proliferation of immature cells of the lymphoid series which spill over into the circulating blood; the main clinical effects of this disease result from the destruction of normal haemopoietic tissue causing severe anaemia and deficiency of neutrophils and platelets thus predisposing to overwhelming infection and severe coagulation disorders.

*Chronic myelocytic leukaemia* and *acute myeloblastic leukaemia*, both usually diseases of adults, are neoplasms of the granulopoietic series; fairly mature neutrophils, metamyelocytes and myelocytes predominate in the chronic form, whilst primitive myeloblasts predominate in the more rapidly fatal acute form.

Chronic myeloid leukaemia appears to be part of the spectrum of diseases known as *myeloproliferative disorders*. Also included in this group are *polycythaemia rubra vera* and *myelofibrosis*. The former is a neoplastic proliferation of erythrocyte precursors resulting in production of vast excesses of erythrocytes whereas in the latter the blood-forming areas of bone marrow are replaced by fibrous tissue, leading to defective and inadequate blood formation and compensatory development of haemopoietic tissue in extramedullary sites such as spleen and liver (see Fig. 15.6). The interesting feature of these conditions is that they may transform into chronic myeloid leukaemia which may then undergo *blast transformation* into acute myeloblastic leukaemia. Other forms of leukaemia (including monocytic leukaemia) are relatively rare. The leukaemias are generally considered as haematological disorders rather than the province of histopathologists, chronic lymphocytic leukaemia in bone marrow is shown in Fig. 15.5 to emphasize the pathological relationship to the lymphomas.

An important lymphoreticular tumour is *myeloma*, a neoplasm of antibody-producing plasma cells. This may occur as a solitary osteolytic plasma cell tumour in the bone, as multiple osteolytic tumours scattered throughout the skeleton, or as a diffuse infiltration of the bone marrow by plasma cells (see Fig. 15.7).

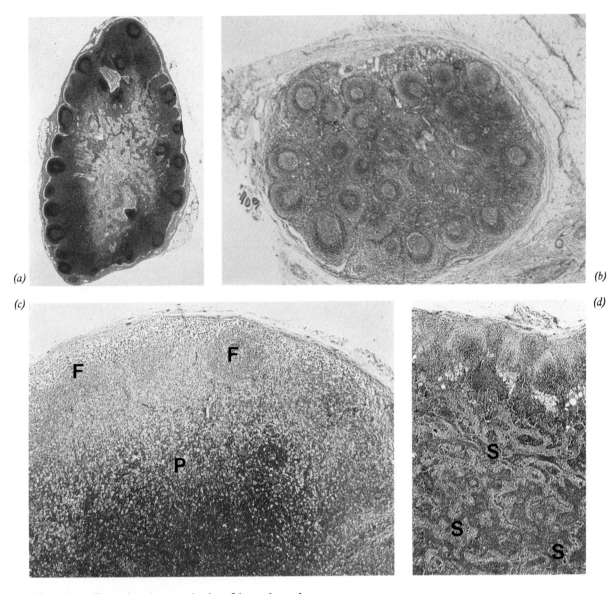

## Fig. 15.1   Reactive hyperplasia of lymph nodes
**(a) normal lymph node** (LP)
**(b) follicular hyperplasia** (LP)
**(c) paracortical hyperplasia** (MP)
**(d) sinus hyperplasia** (MP)

Damage or inflammation in any tissue may excite a reactive response in the lymphoreticular cells of lymph nodes draining the affected area. There are three basic patterns of response, namely *follicular hyperplasia, paracortical hyperplasia* and *sinus hyperplasia*, which may be seen separately or in combination according to the nature of the stimulus.

In follicular hyperplasia, illustrated in micrograph (b), there is an increase in number and size of cortical lymphoid follicles, each developing a predominantly humoral immune response since the cortical follicles are known to be sites of B lymphocyte proliferation. Compare this with a normal lymph node shown in micrograph (a).

In paracortical (parafollicular) hyperplasia as seen in micrograph (c), the lymphoid follicles **F** are small and insignificant, often pushed to the periphery of the node beneath the capsule by the mass of proliferating lymphocytes in the paracortical zone **P**, the domain of T lymphocytes. This pattern of hyperplasia is often seen in viral infections.

In sinus hyperplasia, shown in micrograph (d), there is no great increase in the lymphoid component of the node, but the medullary sinuses **S**, are extremely prominent by virtue of dilatation and hyperplasia of the sinus-lining cells. This pattern is usually seen in nodes draining an area of tissue damage in which endogenous particulate matter, lipid and fluid are released; examples include nodes draining an area of chronically inflamed skin or a degenerating tumour.

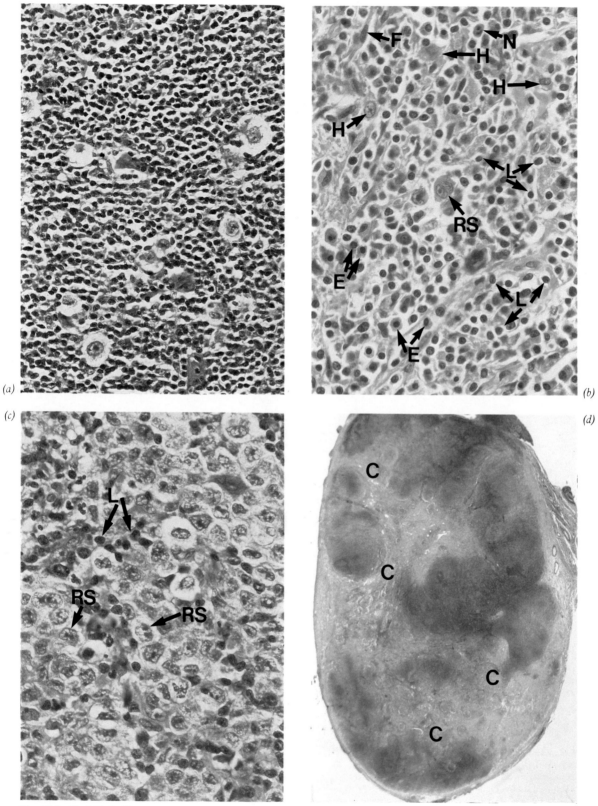

(a)

(b)

(c)

(d)

Fig. 15.2  Hodgkin's disease

## Fig. 15.2  Hodgkin's disease *(illustrations opposite)*
### (a) lymphocyte predominant pattern (HP)   (b) mixed cellularity pattern (HP)
### (c) lymphocyte depleted pattern (HP)   (d) nodular sclerosing pattern (LP)

*Hodgkin's disease* is a malignant neoplasm of the lymphoreticular system which usually becomes manifest initially by lymph node enlargement but later by splenomegaly, hepatomegaly and bone marrow involvement. The nature of the tumour cell line is not known but the cell population is usually mixed, with neoplastic cells being surrounded by benign reactive cells. Present in the tumour are lymphocytes, large pale staining histiocyte-like cells, eosinophils and some fibroblasts. Some of the large pale staining cells are pleomorphic and may assume multinucleate giant cell forms. Characteristic of Hodgkin's disease is the *Reed-Sternberg cell,* a binucleate form in which the two nuclei are often mirror images of each other in shape. Various histological subtypes of Hodgkin's disease occur, each with a slightly different pattern of behaviour and prognosis.

The group with the best prognosis is the *lymphocyte predominant pattern* seen in micrograph (a). In this type, the lymphocytes (which are structurally normal) form extensive sheets within which are scattered large pale staining cells including occasional Reed-Sternberg cells.

The next most favourable prognosis applies to the most common form, *mixed cellularity Hodgkin's disease* shown in micrograph (b), in which there is a numerically even distribution of lymphocytes **L** and histiocyte-like cells **H**; occasional eosinophils **E**, neutrophils **N** and fibroblasts **F** are scattered about. Classical Reed-Sternberg cells **RS** are also present.

The type with the worst prognosis is *lymphocyte-depleted Hodgkin's disease* illustrated in micrograph (c) in which the dominant cell type is the pale staining histiocyte-like cell often showing numerous pleomorphic multinucleate forms including Reed-Sternberg cells **RS**; lymphocytes **L** and other reactive cells are scanty.

Most commonly, Hodgkin's disease destroys the normal architecture of the lymph node completely producing a homogeneous appearance in which no trace of the original corticomedullary demarcation and follicular pattern remains. However, one form of Hodgkins disease, the *nodular sclerosing pattern* seen in micrograph (d), results in the deposition of broad irregular bands of collagenous fibrous tissue **C** which separates the cellular Hodgkin's tumour mass into islands imparting a nodular appearance to the cut surface of the node. The cellular pattern in the nodules is usually of a mixed cellularity type but lymphocyte-depleted and lymphocyte-predominant types may also occur in this pattern. The nodular sclerosing pattern usually indicates a comparatively good prognosis. There is some dispute as to whether the nodular sclerosing variant of Hodgkin's disease should be regarded as a distinct entity or merely as a variation of the more normal diffuse pattern.

The prognosis of Hodgkin's disease is related to the histological type and also to the extent of involvement of the lymphoreticular system as a whole. Treatment regimes differ according to histological type and stage (extent of involvement). Investigation usually involves biopsy examination of lymph nodes, bone marrow, spleen and liver, access to the latter often necessitating a so called 'staging' laparotomy.

## Fig. 15.3  Classification of lymphomas

| British system (National lymphoma investigation) | Rappaport system | Traditional system |
|---|---|---|
| *Follicular pattern* | *Nodular pattern* | |
| Follicle centre cells small | Lymphocytic, poorly differentiated | |
| Follicle centre cells mixed | Mixed | Follicular lymphoma |
| Follicle centre cells large | Histiocytic | |
| *Diffuse pattern* | *Diffuse pattern* | |
| Lymphocytic, well differentiated | Lymphocytic, well differentiated | |
| Lymphocytic, intermediate differentiation | Lymphocytic, poorly differentiated | Lymphosarcoma |
| Lymphocytic, poorly differentiated | | |
| Lymphocytic, mixed | Mixed | |
| Undifferentiated large cells | Undifferentiated | Reticulum cell sarcoma |
| Histiocytic | Histiocytic | |
| Plasma cell | — | |
| Unclassified | — | |

*Note:* these classifications are abridged for simplicity. While there are broad similarities between the linked names, there are both areas of overlap and exclusion in certain terms.

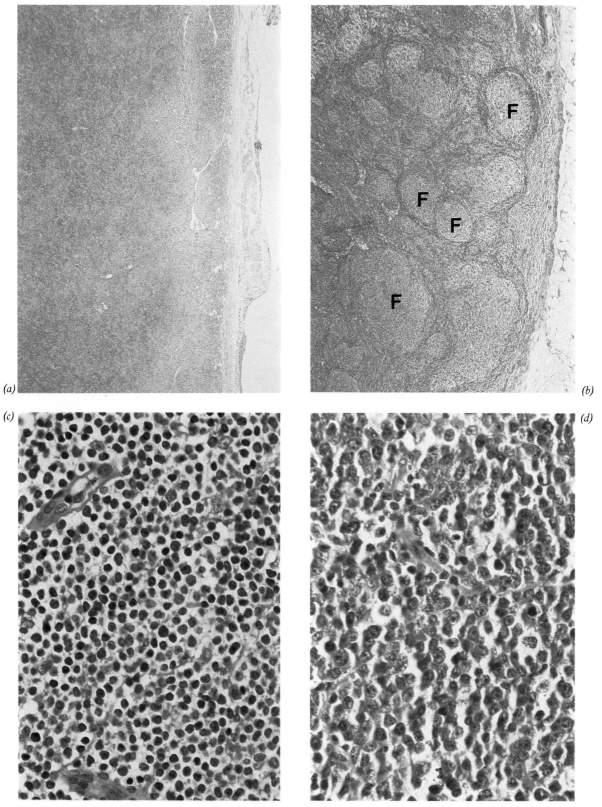

Fig. 15.4   Lymphocytic lymphoma

## Fig. 15.4   Lymphocytic lymphoma *(illustrations opposite)*
**(a) diffuse pattern** (LP)   **(b) small cell lymphoma** (HP)
**(c) small cell lymphoma** (HP)   **(d) large cell lymphoma** (HP)

As described in the chapter introduction, lymphocytic lymphomas may be subdivided by pattern of growth into follicular and diffuse types, and also by size of cell into small and large cell variants. These micrographs show four variants of lymphocytic lymphoma based upon these criteria.

Note in the *diffuse pattern* shown in micrograph (a) how the normal architecture of the node has been completely effaced and replaced by uniform sheets of neoplastic lymphocytes; in contrast, in the *follicular pattern* illustrated in micrograph (b) the neoplastic cells are aggregated into irregular follicles **F**, larger and more irregular than normal follicles and devoid of germinal centres.

Within both the follicular and diffuse patterns, there is further subdivision into small and large cell variants which are illustrated at higher magnification in micrographs (c) and (d) respectively. In the *small cell variant,* the tumour cells are like small lymphocytes with round darkly staining nuclei and only an insignificant rim of surrounding cytoplasm. The *large cell variant* exhibits less uniformity of nuclear shape, size and staining intensity, most nuclei being large and with an open chromatin pattern.

Consistent with the general principles outlined earlier, follicular pattern lymphocytic lymphomas have a better prognosis than the diffuse pattern variants and the small cell types have a better prognosis than the large cell types.

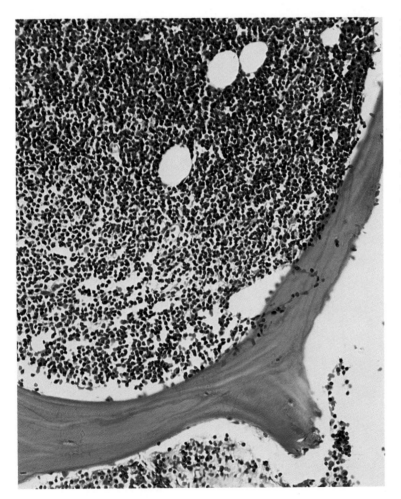

## Fig. 15.5   Bone marrow in chronic lymphocytic leukaemia (HP)

In *chronic lymphocytic leukaemia,* the bone marrow becomes infiltrated by small lymphocytes similar to those seen in small cell lymphocytic lymphoma (see Fig. 15.4c) and very large numbers of similar cells appear in the peripheral circulation. Although the occupation of the marrow is extensive, destruction of the normal haemopoietic marrow elements is not as rapid or severe as in acute lymphoblastic leukaemia and the condition runs a less fulminating course.

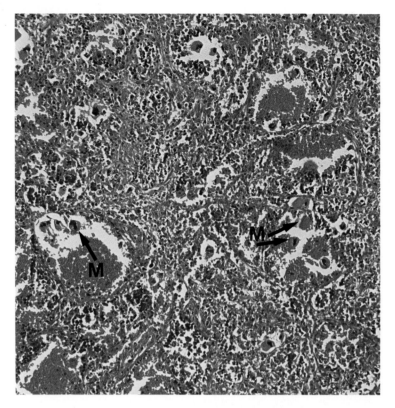

### Fig. 15.6   Spleen in myelofibrosis (MP)

The replacement of haemopoietic bone marrow by progressive fibrosis in *myelofibrosis* leads to loss of capacity to produce erythrocytes, leucocytes and platelets. This is partly compensated for by extramedullary haemopoiesis, when other organs of the lymphoreticular system acquire again their fetal potential for haemopoiesis.

The spleen is the principal organ involved in this compensatory process and becomes greatly enlarged. Histologically the red pulp of the spleen is markedly expanded by the presence of immature erythropoietic and granulopoietic tissue, with many megakaryocytes **M.**

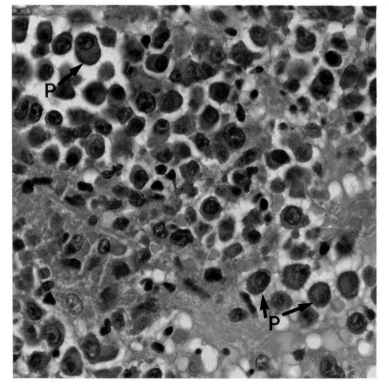

### Fig. 15.7   Myeloma (HP)

*Myeloma* is a tumour of plasma cells which may present with solitary, multifocal or diffuse bone marrow involvement. In this example from a patient with diffuse marrow involvement, note the presence of increased numbers of plasma cells **P** which, in normal marrow, are only a very minor constituent.

Significant destruction of normal blood-forming marrow usually only occurs at a late stage in the natural history of the disease when bone marrow replacement by neoplastic plasma cells can become very extensive.

Almost all myelomas are derived from a single clone and therefore the tumours produce a vast excess of a single monoclonal antibody which can be easily detected in circulating blood; light chains of the monoclonal antibody may appear in the urine (Bence-Jones protein).

# 16. Female reproductive system

## Disorders of the lower genital tract

The vulva is subject to many of the conditions affecting skin elsewhere in the body, including various inflammatory conditions such as dermatitis (see Figs 20.5 and 20.6), but is also an important site for specific infective lesions which are transmitted sexually, including the chancre of primary syphilis. Many vulval inflammatory lesions lead to intense itching, so the histological features of these conditions are complicated by the effects of trauma from scratching. In elderly post-menopausal women, the vulval mucosa tends to become thickened and white as a result of epithelial atrophy and subepithelial fibrosis, a condition known pathologically as *lichen sclerosus et atrophicus* (see Fig. 16.1). Many pathological lesions may produce the clinical appearance of *leukoplakia*, including chronic inflammatory disease e.g. neurodermatitis, the early stages of lichen sclerosus, and some forms of vulval *carcinoma in situ*; in the last condition, marked epithelial dysplasia is the classic histological feature (see Fig. 5.6). The most important malignant tumour of the vulva is *squamous carcinoma* (Fig. 16.2).

The *vagina* is rarely the site of important primary lesions of histopathological interest, although it may more often be secondarily involved in endometriosis (see Fig. 16.13) and malignant tumours of the cervix or endometrium.

The *cervix* frequently shows chronic inflammatory changes, *chronic cervicitis* (Fig. 16.3), which may also be associated with polypoid hyperplasia of the endocervical mucosa sometimes with the formation of a large pedunculated polyp containing distended endocervical glands and stroma (see Fig. 16.4). Clinically, the most important lesions of the cervix are epithelial dysplasia, carcinoma in situ, and squamous carcinoma all of which originate at the cervical squamocolumnar junction; these related conditions and their pathogenesis are considered in detail in Fig. 16.5.

## Disorders of the uterus and Fallopian tubes

The uterine endometrium undergoes monthly cyclical changes under the influence of hormonal stimuli during the period between menarche and menopause, normally only being suspended in pregnancy. Before menarche the endometrial glands and stroma are compact and inactive, a state they return to after the menopause. At menarche, around the menopause, and for the first few cycles after a pregnancy, the endometrium shows a mixture of inactive and normal functional patterns. Under the influence of oral contraceptive drugs and intrauterine contraceptive devices, the endometrium assumes various other histological patterns.

Excessive or uncoordinated hormonal stimulation of the endometrium may produce diffuse endometrial hyperplasia. Two patterns are recognized, *simple (cystic) hyperplasia* and *adenomatous (atypical) hyperplasia*; these are illustrated in Fig. 16.7. Localized areas of polypoid hyperplasia forming *endometrial polyps* are common and often contain cystically dilated endometrial glands (see Fig. 16.6). The most common malignant tumour of the endometrium is *endometrial carcinoma*, an adenocarcinoma derived from endometrial glands (see Fig. 16.8).

Endometrial infection is uncommon, but may follow genital tuberculosis or mechanical obstruction to the endocervical canal e.g. by tumour, often leading to a distension of the endometrial cavity by pus (*pyometria*).

The myometrium is the site of one of the most common benign connective tissue tumours, the *leiomyoma* (see Fig. 16.9 and also Fig. 6.4a and b); in the myometrium these smooth muscle tumours become progressively more collagenous as they enlarge, giving rise to the colloquial term *fibroid*.

The myometrium may also contain islands of ectopic endometrium which may be subject to the usual cycle of proliferative and secretory changes under the influence of ovarian hormones; such changes may give rise to pain and other menstrual disturbances. When involving the uterine muscle, this ectopic endometrium is known as *adenomyosis* (Fig. 16.10); such ectopic endometrial tissue may also be found in various other sites throughout the genital tract and abdomen when it is described by the more general term *endometriosis* (Fig. 16.13).

The Fallopian tubes may become infected by any of the pyogenic bacteria, including gonococcus, and the acute inflammation may be complicated by obstruction of the tubal lumen, leading to the chronic suppurative inflammation and abscess formation. These conditions, known as *acute salpingitis*, *chronic salpingitis* and *tubo-ovarian abscess* respectively, are discussed with Figure 16.11. Along with tuberculous infection of the Fallopian tube (see Fig. 3.14) they constitute an important cause of female infertility due to tubal lumen obliteration. Scarring of the tube and other disorders may prevent the free passage of a fertilized ovum into the endometrial cavity and implantation may occur in the oviduct leading to *tubal ectopic pregnancy* (Fig. 16.12); this usually culminates in massive haemorrhage caused by the placenta eroding through the tubal wall.

## Disorders of the ovary

Under the influence of pituitary gonadotrophins, the ovary undergoes cyclical changes providing for the development and release of a mature ovum at the mid point of each monthly menstrual cycle, and for the production of the ovarian hormones which control the menstrual cycle. During the proliferative phase of the menstrual cycle, certain ovarian follicles enlarge culminating in maturation of one follicle which discharges its single ovum into the Fallopian tube (ovulation); the follicle, until this time also responsible for production of oestrogens, now develops into the corpus luteum responsible for producing progesterone until the beginning of the next menstrual cycle when the follicle atrophies to form the redundant collagenous corpus albicans. This regular sequence of changes is normally only interrupted by the advent of pregnancy, during the first trimester of which the corpus luteum persists. On occasions however, the sequence is aborted at some stage and small *follicular* or *luteal cysts* may form. Some small cysts may also form by inclusion of islands of surface 'germinal' epithelium of the ovary; these are known as *germinal inclusion cysts*. These three types of cysts are shown in Fig. 16.14.

A wide range of tumours may arise in the ovary, both cystic and solid. Neoplastic cysts are common, and include *serous* and *mucinous cystadenomas*, and their malignant equivalents, *serous* and *mucinous cystadenocarcinomas*. These lesions are illustrated in Figures 16.15 and 16.16. A bizarre type of ovarian cyst is the *dermoid cyst*, an example of a benign teratoma, characterized by a large cystic component containing a wide variety of tissues (see Fig. 16.17).

Endometriosis may also affect the ovary (see Fig. 16.13), and one form of malignant tumour of the ovary is the so called endometrioid carcinoma, histologically resembling the adenocarcinoma of the endometrium (see Fig. 16.8). Many other primary tumours may arise in the ovary, derived from germ cells e.g. *dysgerminoma*, the ovarian equivalent of the testicular seminoma (see Fig. 18.2), follicular cells (e.g. *granulosa cell* and *theca cell tumours* (Fig. 16.18) and from stromal connective tissue e.g. fibroma. Some primary ovarian tumours secrete excess quantities of hormone independent of pituitary control; as an example, theca cell tumours may secrete excess oestrogens and induce diffuse endometrial hyperplasia or even endometrial carcinoma. The ovary may occasionally be the site of metastatic carcinoma spread from other primary sites; a well known example is the so called *Krukenberg tumour* in which there is infiltration of the ovary by mucin-secreting adenocarcinoma of signet ring pattern (see Figs 6.13 and 12.8) usually derived from stomach or colon, and possibly reaching the ovary by transcoelomic spread.

Details of the various structural and functional abnormalities of the placenta, decidua, membranes and umbilical cord are generally outside the scope of this book, however, hydatidiform mole (Fig. 16.19) and choriocarcinoma (Fig. 16.20) are included as examples of disorders of placental growth.

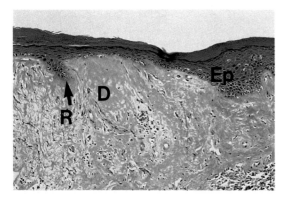

### Fig. 16.1  Lichen sclerosus et atrophicus (HP)

This condition of unknown aetiology presents clinically as thin, smooth, whitish plaques around the vulva often with narrowing of the introitus. Histologically there is marked thinning and atrophy of the epidermis **Ep** with virtual disappearance of rete pegs **R** and skin appendages. The epidermal atrophy is associated with hyalinization of the underlying dermis **D**, seen as homogenous pink staining. Dermal vessels may show perivascular accumulation of lymphocytes and some plasma cells.

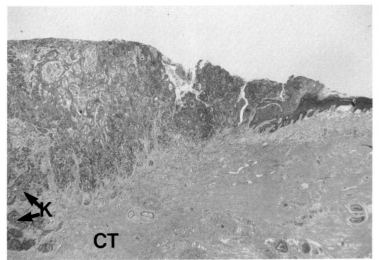

### Fig. 16.2 Squamous carcinoma of vulva (MP)

*Vulval carcinoma*, which most commonly occurs in the very elderly, presents as raised indurated areas which eventually undergo central ulceration. These tumours are almost always slow growing, highly differentiated squamous carcinomas and exhibit abundant keratin pearl formation **K** (see also Fig. 6.11). The tumour may originate in labia majora, labia minora or clitoris, and may spread deeply into underlying connective tissue **CT** and thence via lymphatics to superficial inguinal lymph nodes.

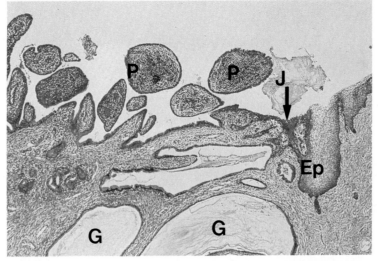

### Fig. 16.3 Chronic cervicitis (MP)

This micrograph shows some of the features of long standing chronic inflammation of the cervix, *chronic cervicitis*. The ectocervical squamous epithelium **Ep** is normal except for slight thickening. The major changes are seen in the endocervix immediately above the squamocolumnar junction **J**; here there is micropolyposis, the core of each tiny polyp **P** showing a heavy chronic inflammatory cell infiltrate, mainly lymphocytic. Deeper endocervical glands **G** show cystic dilatation. Long standing inflammation may lead to squamous metaplasia of the surface endocervical epithelium.

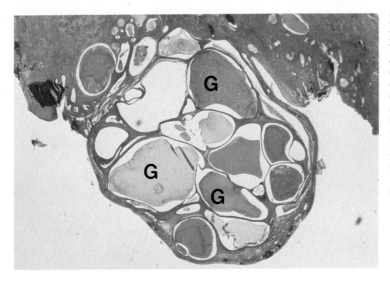

### Fig. 16.4 Endocervical polyp (LP)

This micrograph shows an early benign *endocervical polyp* arising from the endocervical canal. The polyp is composed of cystically dilated glands **G** of varying sizes, each distended by mucin and lined by columnar endocervical mucin-secreting epithelium. As the polyp enlarges it may develop a fibrous stroma between the cystic glands, and surface ulceration may follow extrusion through the external os.

Cervical polyps are an important cause of abnormal vaginal bleeding.

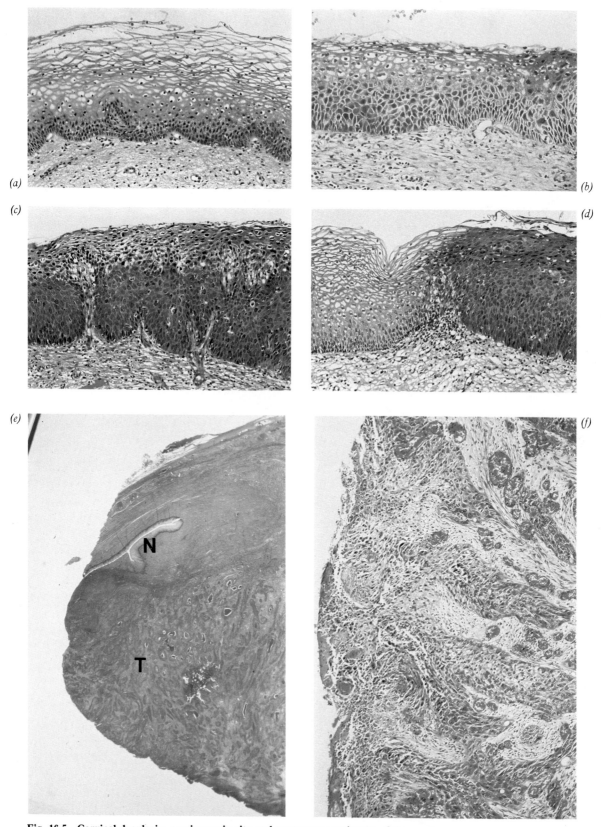

**Fig. 16.5  Cervical dysplasia, carcinoma in situ and squamous carcinoma of the cervix**

# Fig. 16.5 Cervical dysplasia, carcinoma in situ and squamous carcinoma of the cervix

*(illustrations opposite)*

**(a) normal ectocervix** (HP)  **(b) mild-moderate dysplasia** (HP)
**(c) moderate-severe dysplasia** (HP)  **(d) carcinoma in situ** (HP)
**(e) invasive carcinoma** (LP)  **(f) poorly differentiated carcinoma** (HP)

The vagina and vaginal aspect of the cervix are covered by stratified squamous epithelium which is well adapted to withstand the normal vaginal environment. The endocervical canal on the other hand is lined by a simple columnar mucin-secreting epithelium; at a microscopic level this is deeply folded so as to form gland-like invaginations into the cervical stroma which are responsible for the elaboration of normal cervical mucus.

The junction between stratified squamous and columnar epithelium normally lies at the external os. The volume of the cervical stroma expands under the influence of hormones during each menstrual cycle, at menarche and during pregnancy, and this causes eversion of the vaginal end of the endocervical canal thus exposing some of the simple columnar epithelium to the vaginal environment. This exposed epithelium appears red in relation to the surrounding stratified squamous epithelium and hence became inaccurately known as a *cervical erosion*; more appropriate is the term *cervical ectropion*. Under the influence of the vaginal environment the ectropic columnar epithelium may undergo squamous metaplasia (see Fig. 5.5) to form stratified squamous epithelium indistinguishable from the lining epithelium native to the vagina. This metaplastic area, described as the *transformation zone*, appears to be unstable and susceptible to dysplastic changes possibly induced by external factors; it is speculated that herpes virus type II and spermatozoa could be involved.

The dysplastic changes may well regress if these uncertain predisposing factors are eliminated. However, it is believed that some undergo irreversible neoplastic change with the development of *carcinoma in situ*. Furthermore, a proportion of untreated cases of carcinoma in situ are thought to transform into frank *invasive squamous carcinoma*.

The development of invasive squamous carcinoma may thus be prevented by intercepting the dysplastic process at some earlier stage and cervical cytology has been developed as a method of screening and monitoring this process in the population of women at risk. Once significant dysplastic changes have been demonstrated cytologically, histological examination of biopsy specimens is used to define accurately the degree of dysplasia and to plan appropriate treatment.

Recently the CIN (cervical intraepithelial neoplasia) classification has been developed for this purpose. CIN grade I corresponds to mild dysplasia, CIN grade II to moderate dysplasia, and CIN grade III includes severe dysplasia and carcinoma in situ. Grade I and grade II lesions are usually managed conservatively, but grade III lesions must be eliminated by such methods as local surgery and laser cautery. Invasive carcinoma demands radical excision.

Micrographs (a) to (d) illustrate the spectrum of cervical epithelial appearances from normal stratified squamous epithelium through to carcinoma in situ. Micrograph (e) shows an example of invasive cervical carcinoma and its cytological features are shown in micrograph (f).

As seen in micrograph (a), normal ectocervical epithelium has a typical stratified squamous form with all cell division

being confined to a single basal layer of small darkly staining cuboidal cells. As the cells undergo maturation, their eosinophilic cytoplasm expands greatly and the cells are pushed upwards into a stratum equivalent to the prickle cell layer of the skin. Beyond this, the cells undergo progressive degenerative changes, their nuclei becoming first pyknotic then undergoing karyorrhexis and karyolysis (see Fig. 1.4); the cytoplasm becomes progressively flattened until the cells are finally shed from the surface.

In mild dysplasia as shown in micrograph (b), the basal and prickle cell layers are thickened and exhibit an increased degree of cellular pleomorphism with the nuclei being abnormally large and prominent in the prickle cell layer and mitoses being evident beyond the basal layer; the surface layer is thinned but the surface cells are relatively normal. At the right of the micrograph, the dysplastic changes are more marked and extend almost to the surface; there, the mild dysplasia (CIN grade I) has given way to moderate dysplasia (CIN grade II).

Micrograph (c) shows a moderate degree of dysplasia at the left of the field, the hyperchromatic dysplastic cells extending more than half way towards the surface and mitotic figures being evident far beyond the basal layer. At the right of the field, the changes are more severe with dysplastic cells extending almost to the surface and leaving little semblance of stratification; this would be classified as CIN grade III.

Micrograph (d) illustrates an abrupt transition from normal stratified squamous epithelium on the left to highly dysplastic epithelium on the right. The pleomorphic dysplastic cells, including mitotic forms, extend right to the surface and there is almost complete loss of stratification. These features meet all the criteria for malignant change; the basement membrane however remains intact and there is no evidence of invasion of the underlying stroma so this lesion is classified as carcinoma in situ (CIN grade III). The abnormal nucleated surface cells in this lesion were detected in a cervical smear; alerted to the presence of dysplasia, the clinician then obtained this biopsy to establish the exact diagnosis.

A critical feature of the dysplastic examples just discussed is that the basement membrane remains sharply defined and intact. With any evidence of microinvasion or more extensive spread into underlying tissues, the lesion is defined as *invasive carcinoma*.

Invasive carcinoma is illustrated in micrograph (e). Note that purple staining tumour **T** has replaced most of the cervical stroma and muscle although a portion of normal vaginal epithelium **N** remains at the tumour margin. The surface of the tumour is ulcerated and this accounts for the frequent presenting feature of post-coital bleeding.

The surface of this tumour is shown at high magnification in micrograph (f). The lesion consists of islands of darkly staining pleomorphic cells invading the loose cervical stroma; the tumour is poorly differentiated since there is no evidence of pink staining keratin formation, characteristic of well differentiated squamous carcinoma (see Fig. 6.11).

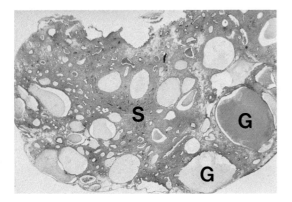

### Fig. 16.6   Endometrial polyp (LP)

*Endometrial polyps* are an important but innocuous cause of abnormal uterine bleeding at or near the menopause; they are pedunculated and often multiple. Most are composed of cystically dilated glands **G** in a typical loose endometrial stroma **S** and covered by a layer of flattened endometrial surface cells. The glands and stroma in some polyps are responsive to ovarian hormones, and thus show evidence of proliferative, secretory or hyperplastic activity accordingly.

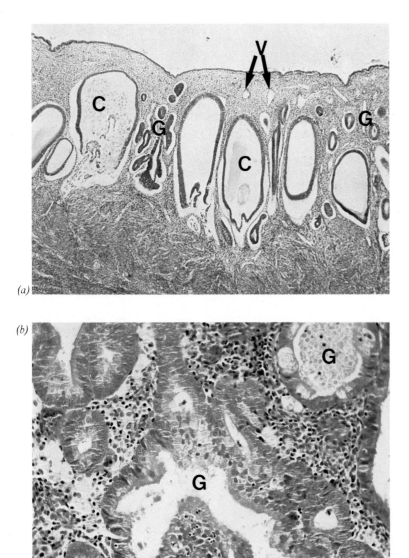

*(a)*

*(b)*

### Fig. 16.7   Endometrial hyperplasia
### (a) simple (cystic) hyperplasia (MP)
### (b) adenomatous (atypical) hyperplasia (HP)

*Endometrial hyperplasia* appears to be a response to excessive or uncoordinated ovarian hormone production and may be either cystic or adenomatous in form. In *simple (cystic) hyperplasia* as shown in micrograph (a), the endometrial lining becomes thickened with the formation of numerous tiny cysts **C** scattered among normal looking endometrial glands **G** which may themselves be increased in number; the cysts result from dilatation of endometrial glands. The intervening stroma frequently contains prominent thin walled blood vessels **V**; heavy uterine bleeding is the most common presenting symptom.

In *adenomatous hyperplasia*, shown in micrograph (b) at higher magnification, the glands **G** are very numerous and often tightly packed; few show cystic dilatation but many are irregular in shape and size, often with papillary infoldings. Adjacent glands are often so closely packed that there appears to be no intervening stroma (architectural atypia). An important histological feature in this type is that many of the glandular cells show marked cytological atypicality with nuclear and cytoplasmic pleomorphism and increased mitotic activity. Some foci are histologically indistinguishable from well differentiated endometrial adenocarcinoma (see Fig. 16.8). Both types of hyperplasia may also follow excess oestrogen secretion and the specimen shown in micrograph (b) was associated with the theca cell tumour shown in Fig. 16.18.

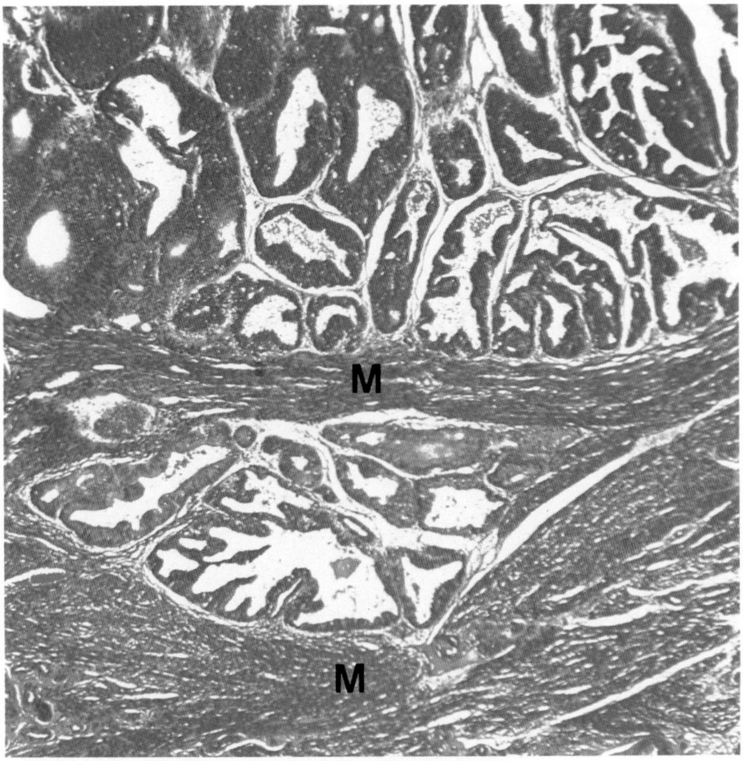

### Fig. 16.8    Endometrial adenocarcinoma (MP)

The most common malignancy of the body of the uterus is this malignant tumour of the endometrial glands; it usually occurs in post-menopausal women. Well differentiated forms bear many histological similarities to the atypical adenomatous hyperplasia shown in Fig. 16.7 (b) but malignancy can be recognized by the invasion of the underlying myometrium **M**, as in this micrograph. The luminal surface also extends out irregularly to distend the uterine cavity. Distorted, irregular, glandular patterns are frequent, and focal squamous metaplasia is seen in some forms. The tumour spreads by local invasion through the myometrium and via lymphatics to iliac and para-aortic lymph nodes.

### Fig. 16.9    Leiomyoma (fibroid) of myometrium (LP)

This benign tumour of myometrial smooth muscle is a very common cause of abnormal or excessive uterine bleeding and pelvic discomfort. It provides a good illustration of the growth pattern of benign tumours within solid organs and is also illustrated in Fig. 6.4. The tumour is composed of fascicles of smooth muscle cells but larger tumours also show foci of fibroblastic collagen formation **C**, particularly towards the centre of the tumour. Gradual expansion of the tumour compresses the surrounding myometrium **M**, leading to atrophy of normal myometrial smooth muscle cells and leaving only the scanty collagenous stroma which becomes compacted to form a distinct pseudocapsule **P**. Some tumours arise near the endometrial cavity and may protrude into the cavity to produce a polypoid submucous fibroid. Secondary changes may also occur, including extensive collagenization and calcification (especially with increasing age), liquefactive necrosis to form fluid-filled areas of cystic degeneration, and, very rarely, sarcomatous change. To an extent, the growth of these tumours is hormone-dependent, since they almost always shrink and partially regress after the menopause.

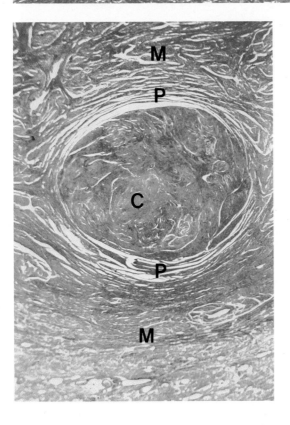

### Fig. 16.10   Adenomyosis of the uterus (MP)

*Adenomyosis* is the term applied to a condition in which islands
of ectopic endometrial glands **G** and stroma **S** are found
embedded deep within the myometrium **M**, often at a
considerable distance from the normal endometrium. Their
presence is often associated with symmetrical increase in
myometrial bulk thus enlarging the uterus; occasionally they
stimulate a more localized increase in smooth muscle to
produce a leiomyoma-like mass containing endometrial islands,
a lesion called an *adenomyoma*.

This ectopic endometrium is responsive in the normal
manner to ovarian hormones but being abnormally confined by
surrounding tissues may give rise to pain. Ectopic
endometrium may occur anywhere in the pelvic region when it
is known by the term *endometriosis* (see Fig. 16.13).

### Fig. 16.11   Acute salpingitis (MP)

In *acute salpingitis* the tubal mucosa **M** becomes hyperaemic,
oedematous, and infiltrated with neutrophil polymorphs
and the lumen becomes filled with purulent exudate **P**
containing abundant neutrophils. Blockage of the tubal lumen
often follows, preventing drainage and leading to distension of
the tube by pus (*pyosalpinx*). Sometimes the inflammation
produces adhesions between tube, fimbriae and ovary, and
extension of suppuration to these areas may produce multiple
locules of pus, the *tubo-ovarian abscess*. Without the
intervention of antibiotics, the combination of adhesions and
suppuration rarely permits total resolution of the acute
inflammation and a state of chronic inflammation generally
ensues. This state, known as *chronic salpingitis*, may persist for
many years resulting in fibrosis and tubal obstruction and is an
important cause of female infertility.

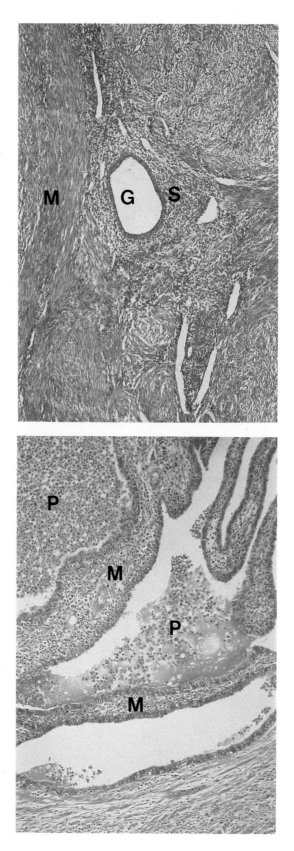

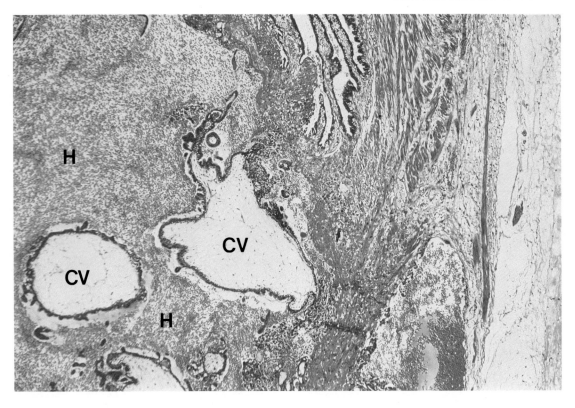

## Fig. 16.12   Tubal ectopic pregnancy (MP)

The Fallopian tube is the most frequent location for inappropriate implantation of the fertilized ovum, *ectopic pregnancy*. The tubular lumen becomes filled with developing embryo, placenta and associated membranes including chorionic villi **CV** and decidual tissue. The tubal wall is often deeply congested and thinned, and stromal cells in the mucosa near the implantation site may show decidual change.

Ectopic pregnancies usually become dramatically apparent by severe haemorrhage **H** into the lumen (*haematosalpinx*), often followed by tracking of blood into the peritoneal cavity; tubal ectopics therefore most often present as acute abdominal emergencies; only very rarely does the pregnancy continue to near normal term.

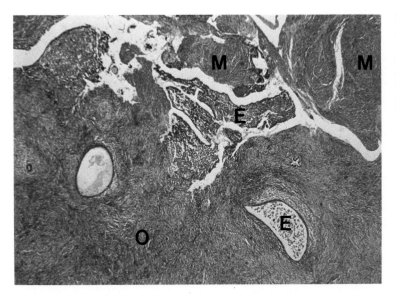

## Fig. 16.13   Pelvic endometriosis (MP)

The Fallopian tube, paratubular connective tissues and ovaries are a frequent site for the condition known as *endometriosis*, in which islands of ectopic endometrial glands and stroma are found outside the uterine body.

This micrograph shows islands of endometriosis **E** in both ovarian stroma **O**, and pink staining smooth muscle **M** of Fallopian tube wall. Fibrosis secondary to the endometriosis has led to adhesion of the ovary to the tube, forming an ill defined tubovarian mass. Endometriosis affecting the serosal surfaces may also lead to adhesion between tube, ovary, uterus and loops of bowel. Isolated endometriosis may also occur within the myometrium when it is known as adenomyosis (see Fig. 16.10).

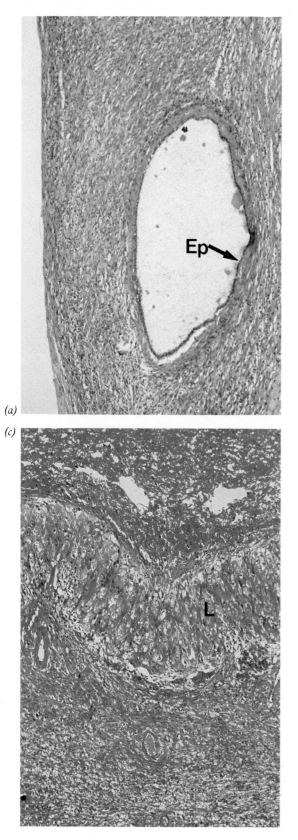

*(a)*

*(c)*

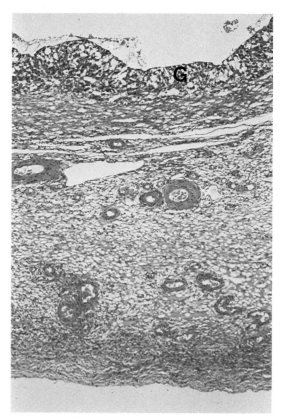

*(b)*

### Fig. 16.14  Physiological and developmental cysts of ovary
**(a) germinal inclusion cyst** (MP)
**(b) follicular cyst** (MP)
**(c) luteal cyst** (MP)

The most common type of ovarian cyst is the so-called *germinal inclusion cyst* illustrated in micrograph (a); these cysts are commonly multiple, small and mainly located near the ovarian surface. Although formerly considered to be follicular cysts (i.e. derived from effete Graafian follicles), they are lined by the same flattened 'germinal' epithelium **Ep** as the ovary surface, and are thus now considered to be 'germinal' inclusion cysts.

True *follicular cysts*, as illustrated in micrograph (b), are less common than was formerly believed. They are derived either from incompletely formed Graafian follicles or from follicles which have ruptured but not undergone transition to corpora lutea. Follicular cysts are lined internally by granulosa cells **G** which usually form a thicker layer than do the flattened cells lining the germinal inclusion cyst; continuing enlargement of the follicular cyst however leads to atrophy of the lining cells so that distinction between a large follicular cyst and a germinal inclusion cyst may be difficult.

The *luteal cyst* is probably derived from a corpus luteum which has not undergone atrophy to a corpus albicans. The cyst is usually ovoid with a slightly irregular outline; microscopically it contains clear or brownish fluid and is lined by a yellow coloured layer of variable thickness. Histologically, as shown in micrograph (c), the yellow layer is composed of plump luteal cells **L** with lipid-rich cytoplasm.

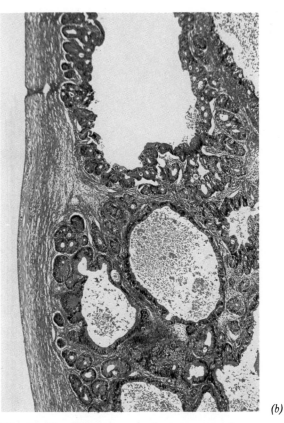

(a)

(b)

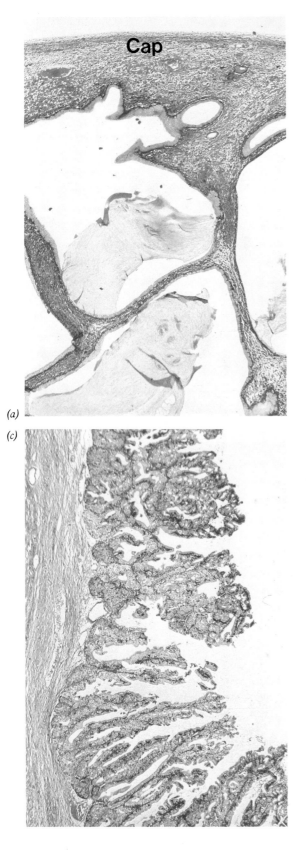

(c)

### Fig. 16.15   Mucinous cystic tumours of ovary
**(a) benign mucinous cystadenoma** (MP)
**(b) mucinous cystadenocarcinoma** (MP)
**(c) mucinous tumour of borderline malignancy** (MP)

Both benign and malignant forms of this tumour develop as large masses virtually replacing the ovary, and taking the form of multiloculated cysts, the cystic spaces containing thick mucoid material. The *benign cystadenoma*, as shown in micrograph (a), has a smooth outer surface since the tumour exhibits no tendency to invade through the capsule **Cap**. The cystic locules are lined by tall columnar epithelium with uniform basal nuclei and copious mucin-containing cytoplasm at the luminal aspect.

The malignant variant, *mucinous cystadenocarcinoma* illustrated in micrograph (b) is much less common. The tumour is more solid, with smaller cystic spaces. The cells are usually recognizably columnar, but the nucleus occupies much more of the cell, and the remaining cytoplasm usually contains much less mucin than its benign counterpart. The cytoplasm is therefore less pale staining and may even be quite eosinophilic, as in this example. Cytological criteria apart, evidence of malignancy in these tumours is usually demonstrated by invasion of tumour cells through the capsule (not shown in this micrograph) at some point on the circumference of the tumour. Some mucinous tumours, apparently benign to the naked eye, show some evidence of cytological atypia and may encroach on the capsule without penetrating it; they are regarded as showing *borderline malignancy* and their prognosis is better than the overtly malignant tumours; an example is shown in micrograph (c).

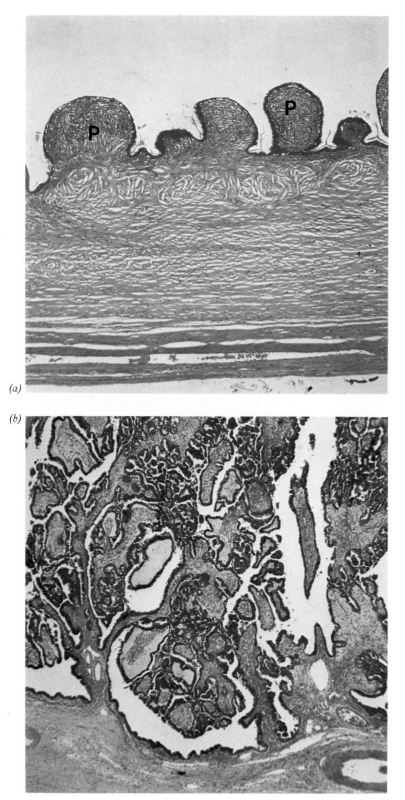

*(a)*

*(b)*

### Fig. 16.16   Serous ovarian cystic tumours
### (a) serous cystadenoma (MP)
### (b) serous papillary cystadenocarcinoma (MP)

Like the mucinous cystic tumours, the serous tumours may also develop into very large cystic masses replacing the ovary. In the *benign serous cystadenoma* the cysts are multilocular, though usually less so than the mucinous tumours, and are filled with a clear watery (serous) fluid. The benign cysts are lined by columnar epithelium, often ciliated in places, but the epithelium may be partly flattened in the larger, tense cysts. A characteristic feature of benign serous cystadenomas as seen in micrograph (a) is the presence of variable numbers of small rounded or papilliferous ingrowths **P** composed of a variably dense stroma covered by tall columnar epithelium.

In the malignant variant as shown in micrograph (b), the papillary ingrowths are more numerous and papilliferous and tend to fill the cystic cavity. The benign tumours have a smooth serosal surface, since the epithelial components show no tendency to invade and breach the capsule, whereas the malignant variant eventually invades through the capsule, often producing warty outgrowths on the serosal surface. The overtly malignant variety also shows marked cellular atypia and the cells become heaped up into irregular masses. Some of the papillary growths contain spherical, concentrically laminated calcified bodies in their stroma; these *psammoma bodies* are typical of papillary tumours of the ovary, although they are also seen in papillary tumours of the thyroid and in meningiomas (see Fig. 22.9). As with the mucinous equivalent, tumours of borderline malignancy occur.

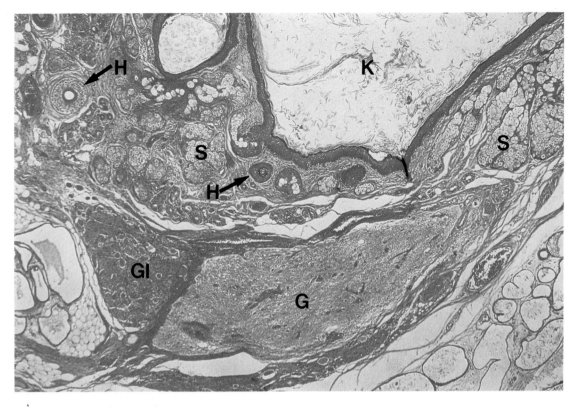

### Fig. 16.17   Benign cystic teratoma (MP)

This tumour, formerly known as *dermoid cyst of the ovary,* is an example of a benign, well differentiated teratoma in which ectodermal elements usually predominate. The lesion takes the form of a unilocular, thin walled cyst filled with a thick, yellowish, pasty material composed of masses of degenerating keratin **K**, often containing hair. This is produced by the lining epithelium of the cyst which is keratinizing stratified squamous epithelium resembling skin. At one end of the cyst can usually be found a raised area within which are other teratomatous components including hair follicles **H**, sebaceous glands **S** and occasionally teeth. Although ectodermal derivatives particularly skin and skin appendage components predominate, mesodermal (e.g. cartilage and smooth muscle)

and endodermal (e.g. respiratory and gut epithelium) elements are a minor component in some tumours. Neuroectodermal tissues may also be found and in the example illustrated, note the area of glial tissue **G** and a ganglion **Gl** alongside.

Cystic teratomas are most common in young women, and in that group are almost always benign; malignant change can occur in some previously benign teratomata, particularly in long standing tumours in elderly women. The component which most commonly shows malignant change is squamous epithelium. Benign cystic teratomas are a different entity from the solid malignant ovarian teratomas of children and pubertal girls which behave in a malignant manner from the outset.

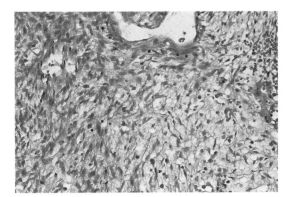

### Fig. 16.18   Theca cell tumour (thecoma) (MP)

This is but one example of a number of ovarian tumours which may secrete hormones. Theca cell tumours are spherical solid tumours with a yellowish cut surface appearance. The tumour is composed of plump spindle cells resembling those of a cellular fibroma, but differing in that the cell cytoplasm contains fine lipid droplets (responsible for the yellow colour of the tumour); the cells are loosely packed in some areas and tightly in others. The lipid droplets do not stain with the H&E method as here but can be demonstrated by applying a lipid stain (e.g. oil red O) to a frozen section of the tumour. This tumour secretes excessive amounts of oestrogens and may be associated with endometrial hyperplasia (see Fig. 16.7) or even endometrial carcinoma.

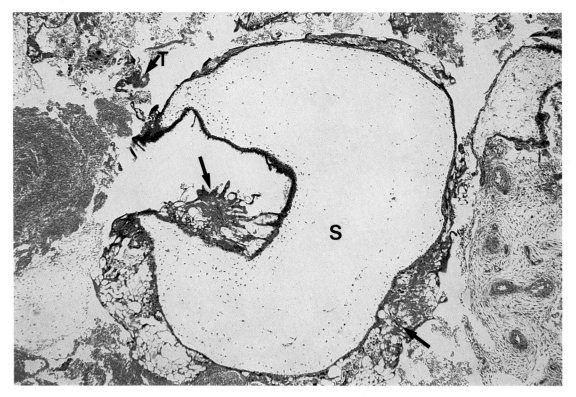

## Fig. 16.19   Hydatidiform mole (MP)

The condition known as *hydatidiform mole* arises in a small proportion of nonproductive pregnancies. The fetus fails to develop but the membranes remain viable; the chorionic villi become markedly swollen and expanded as a result of hydropic swelling of the villous stromal core **S** which contains none of the vessels usually present in functional villi. These cyst-like translucent swellings are invested by a layer of cytotrophoblast and syncytiotrophoblast, which in normal chorionic villi are a single layer thick. In hydatidiform mole, the layers of the trophoblast become thickened (arrowed) and there may be disconnected masses of trophoblast cells **T** lying apparently free of the main tumour mass and showing features of cellular pleomorphism. Hydatidiform moles exhibit a wide spectrum of behaviour; some are eradicated by simple curettage, others persist despite repeated curettage, and a small number develop into undoubtedly malignant choriocarcinoma (see Fig. 16.20).

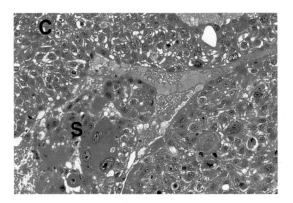

## Fig. 16.20   Choriocarcinoma (HP)

*Choriocarcinoma* is a malignant tumour derived from trophoblast cells of a normal or abnormal pregnancy, most frequently the latter; a few may develop from a hydatidiform mole. They are composed of highly dysplastic masses of cytotrophoblast cells **C** and syncytiotrophoblast cells **S**, showing no evidence of chorionic villus formation. This tumour is remarkably invasive, readily breaching the myometrium and metastasizing widely via lymphatics and the blood stream; the lungs are a common site of metastasis. Haemorrhage and necrosis in the tumour are common.

Choriocarcinoma may also develop as a component of a teratomatous tumour; the most commonly seen example of this is in malignant teratoma of the testis (see Fig. 18.3) where the presence of a choriocarcinomatous component puts the tumour into the poor prognostic category (MTT — malignant teratoma trophoblastic).

# 17. Breast

## Introduction

The female breast, being dependent on a variety of hormones for its normal activity, exhibits considerable structural and functional variation through life. Apart from the overt changes occurring at puberty, pregnancy, lactation and menopause, more subtle changes also occur within the normal menstrual cycle; as a corollary, hormonal disturbances probably underlie various disorders of the breast, notably *fibroadenosis*, but probably also play some part in the pathogenesis of more serious conditions such as breast tumours. Likewise, the male breast normally remains rudimentary unless breast enlargement, *gynaecomastia* (see Fig. 17.7), is induced by exogenous or endogenous hormone imbalance; the latter may result from the use of certain drugs e.g. spironolactone.

Clinically, the importance of many breast disorders lies in the need to distinguish them with certainty from malignant tumours so that the patient may be reassured or appropriate surgical treatment instituted promptly.

Infections of the breast are uncommon and mainly occur during lactation, the organisms (usually *Staphylococcus aureus*) gaining access through cracks and fissures in the nipple and areola; the resulting *bacterial mastitis* is often followed by the development of a *breast abscess* which may become chronic and require surgical drainage. More commonly, inflammation of the breast follows trauma which may be of sufficient severity to produce a condition known as *fat necrosis* (see Fig. 17.1).

The most frequent disorder of the female breast is *fibroadenosis* (see Fig. 17.2), also known by a variety of other terms including *cystic mammary dysplasia* and *fibrocystic disease*; the condition is characterized by a variety of proliferative and other changes affecting all components of the mammary unit (lobule, ducts and supporting stroma) probably in response to subtle disturbances of hormone levels, particularly oestrogen.

The most common benign tumour of the breast is the *fibroadenoma* (Fig. 17.3), a localized proliferation of breast ducts and stroma. Such lesions occur most frequently in isolated form in young women ('breast mice'), but nodules of histologically identical tissue may also be a component of fibroadenosis; fibroadenoma may therefore be a form of hormone-dependent nodular hyperplasia rather than a true benign tumour. The only other benign tumour of much clinical significance is the benign *intraduct papilloma* (Fig. 17.4), usually occurring as a solitary lesion in one of the larger mammary ducts. Histologically similar papillary lesions may also be multifocal, occupying some of the ectatic (dilated) ducts as a component of some patterns of fibroadenosis (see Fig. 17.3); here the lesion is known as *florid duct papillomatosis* and may represent hormone-induced hyperplasia rather than a true neoplasm.

Malignant tumours of the female breast are common, with a peak incidence in the decade before the menopause. Most are adenocarcinomas arising from the epithelium of either the mammary lobules (*lobular carcinoma*) or the mammary ducts (*ductal carcinoma*); the range of histological appearances is illustrated in Fig. 17.5 and Figs 6.4 (c) and (d). In some cases the development of invasive breast cancer may be preceded by carcinoma in situ in which the malignant cells proliferate within the mammary ducts or lobules but do not breach the basement membrane (*intraduct or intralobular carcinoma*). Carcinoma of the breast does occur in males but is extremely uncommon.

In some cases of breast carcinoma, both in situ and invasive, malignant cells may spread within mammary and lactiferous ducts onto the surface of the nipple resulting in *Paget's disease of the nipple* (see Fig. 17.6).

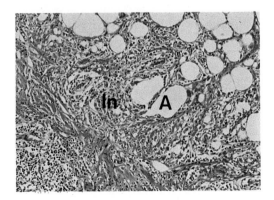

### Fig. 17.1 Fat necrosis (MP)

Trauma to the breast, sometimes apparently quite trivial, may result in necrosis of mammary adipose tissue. Following a typical initial acute inflammatory response, the continuing presence of necrotic adipose tissue **A** excites a chronic inflammatory cell infiltrate **In**, in which lipophages (macrophages containing lipid) and plasma cells may be present in large numbers. Fibrous proliferation at the margins of the damaged area produces a hard, often irregular, breast lump which may resemble a breast carcinoma on palpation.

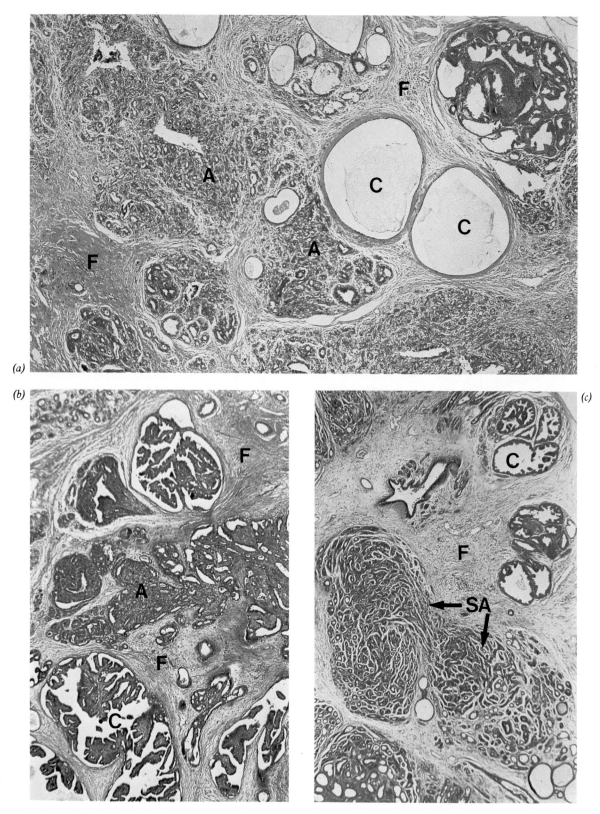

*(a)*

*(b)*

*(c)*

**Fig. 17.2    Fibroadenosis of breast**

**Fig. 17.2   Fibroadenosis** *(illustrations opposite)*
**(a) typical lesion** (MP)
**(b) adenosis and florid duct papillomatosis** (MP)

This condition is common in the breasts of mature women, increasing in frequency and severity towards the menopause, and is probably effected by hormone imbalance. Although here referred to as *fibroadenosis*, it has attracted many descriptive synonyms including *fibrocystic disease, benign cystic hyperplasia, benign cystic mastopathy* and *cystic mammary dysplasia*. In essence, the changes are the result of various different patterns of distortion and overgrowth of the functional breast unit, including ducts, lobules and supporting fibrous stroma. The epithelial components show hyperplastic overgrowth (*adenosis*) and the fibrous tissue increases (*fibrosis*).

This sequence of micrographs shows the wide range of changes which may be present. A frequent feature is marked dilatation of the ducts, to produce cystic lesions of various sizes, often large; such cysts **C** can be seen in each of these micrographs. Although the cysts are usually simple and lined by flattened ductular epithelium as in micrograph (a), they may be lined by large cells with strongly eosinophilic cytoplasm as in micrograph (c), a feature known as *apocrine metaplasia* because of the resemblance to apocrine sweat glands. Sometimes the cystically dilated ducts are filled by papillary ingrowths from the wall as in micrograph (b), a condition known as *florid duct papillomatosis* and similar in

**(c) apocrine metaplasia and sclerosing adenosis** (MP)

appearance to the usually solitary duct papillomas which may occlude the larger mammary and nipple ducts (see Fig. 17.4).

The changes which may occur in the mammary lobules are essentially those of hyperplastic proliferation of lobular acini (*adenosis*) and of the terminal part of the mammary duct within the lobule (*terminal duct hyperplasia*). Examples of lobular acinar adenosis **A** are shown in each of these micrographs. In all cases, the proliferating epithelial tissue is surrounded by fibrous tissue **F** of variable density. In addition, there may be proliferation of fibrous tissue within the lobules of proliferating acini, splitting the acini apart and compressing them into elongated strips. This change, known as *sclerosing adenosis* **SA** is seen in micrograph (c); histologically it may be difficult to distinguish from some invasive patterns of carcinoma. Some areas of fibroadenosis occasionally contain ill-defined nodules which are histologically identical to benign fibroadenoma (see Fig. 19.3).

At its simplest, fibroadenosis may show only replacement of mammary adipose tissue by dense fibrous tissue with the only epithelial component being ectatic mammary ducts; this is particularly seen in women after the menopause, and is sometimes merely described as *mammary fibrosis*.

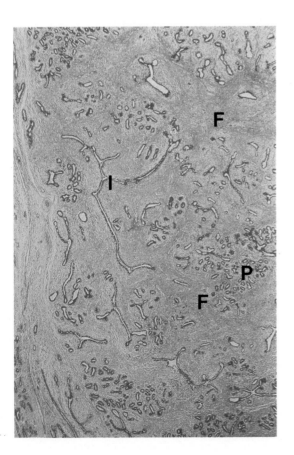

**Fig. 17.3   Fibroadenoma** (MP)

This condition commonly arises in the breasts of young women (under 30) as a solitary lesion but may occur as a component of fibroadenosis (see Fig. 17.2) particularly in older women approaching the menopause. It is usually considered to be a benign tumour but may well represent a nodular form of benign mammary hyperplasia (fibroadenosis). The mass is well circumscribed by a condensation of connective tissue and is composed of both epithelial and fibrous stromal components. The epithelial components form glandular structures lined by mammary duct-type epithelium, whilst the stromal component is a loose, cellular form of fibrous tissue **F**. In very large masses, the stroma may be myxomatous.

Two patterns of growth are seen, often in the same lesion. In the *pericanalicular pattern* **P**, the epithelial component takes the form of rounded ducts which remain small and undistorted with the stroma arranged round them in a roughly symmetrical and regular manner. By contrast, in the *intracanalicular pattern* **I**, the ducts appear elongated but actually represent sections cut through flattened spaces compressed by the stromal component which appears to proliferate in an irregular nodular manner; in general, this latter pattern is more prominent in the larger fibroadanomata. In both patterns of fibroadenoma, hormonal changes such as occur in pregnancy and lactation, may induce marked proliferation of the epithelial component.

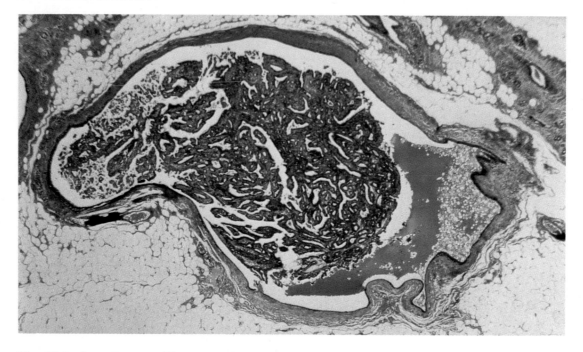

**Fig. 17.4   Intraduct papilloma** (LP)

Papillomas of mammary duct epithelium may arise as solitary or multiple lesions; solitary lesions as shown here are usually located in the larger lactiferous ducts near the nipple and present with blood-stained discharge from the nipple. The lesions are usually small, consisting of a delicate pink staining supporting stroma covered by a single or double layer of cuboidal or low columnar epithelial cells resembling those lining the mammary duct from which the papilloma has arisen; with larger lesions, the duct is often dilated. Multiple duct papillomata (florid duct papillomatosis) occur as a component of fibroadenosis (see Fig. 17.2). Malignant change is rare.

**Fig. 17.5   Carcinoma of the breast** (*illustrations opposite*)
**(a) intraduct** (HP)                       **(b) intralobular** (HP)
**(c) infiltrating ductular** (HP)      **(d) infiltrating lobular** (HP)

Carcinoma of the breast may originate in the epithelium of the mammary ducts or the breast lobular glands (*ductular* and *lobular carcinoma* respectively) although the vast majority (perhaps 80%) are probably of ductal origin. Most tumours of either type show evidence of invasive behaviour when first diagnosed but both ductular and lobular carcinomas may have an in situ stage exhibiting the cytological characteristics of malignancy yet showing no evidence of invasive behaviour, being still confined by the epithelial basement membrane of the duct or lobule.

In noninfiltrating *intraduct carcinoma*, proliferating ductal epithelium fills and distends the ducts. In micrograph (a), note a small lobular duct filled with tumour **T** and surrounded by normal acini **A**. The tumour cells are large and pale staining with large nuclei and prominent nucleoli; there may be evidence of increased mitotic activity and some abnormal mitotic figures. Sometimes duct distension is marked and the tumour cells at the centre undergo necrosis (*comedo pattern*). Note that there is no infiltration of malignant cells into surrounding stroma **S** and that the epithelial basement membrane is unbroached. Infiltration eventually supervenes, however, the tumour becoming an *infiltrating ductular carcinoma* and as shown in micrograph (c), cords of tumour cells **T** then spread out from their ductal origin into the surrounding fibrous stroma **S**.

In noninfiltrating *intralobular carcinoma* as shown in micrograph (b), the normal lobular mammary architecture is maintained but the mammary lobules are increased in size as a result of proliferation of lobular epithelial cells with the cytological characteristics of malignancy. The cells fill and expand the acini of the mammary lobule, but the basement membrane remains intact and the general architecture of the lobule thus remains undisturbed. In *infiltrating lobular carcinoma* as shown in micrograph (d), the tumour cells **T** broach the basement membranes of the acini and spill out into the surrounding stroma **S**, whence they infiltrate into the fibroadipose breast tissue, often in narrow columns.

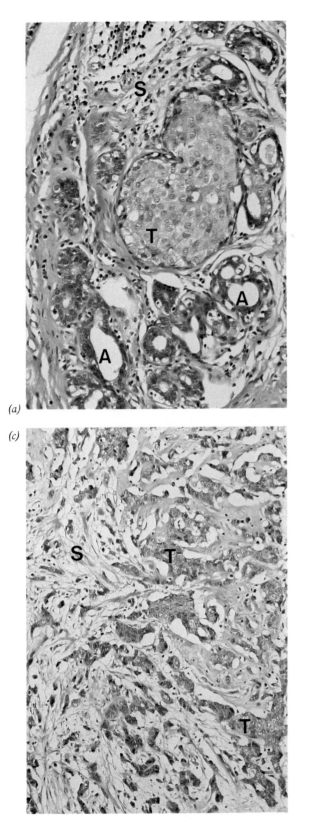

Fig. 17.5 Carcinoma of the breast

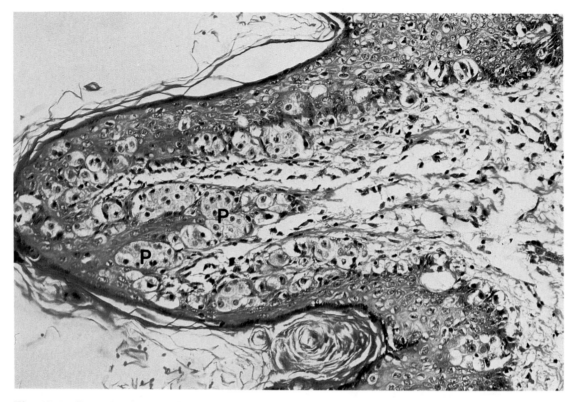

## Fig. 17.6    Paget's disease of the nipple (HP)

Some patients with carcinoma of the breast (usually of ductal origin) develop reddening and thickening of the skin of the nipple and areola, often followed by fissuring and ulceration. In this condition, known as *Paget's disease of the nipple*, the epidermis of the nipple and areola becomes infiltrated by large pleomorphic epithelial cells with hyperchromatic nuclei and pale cytoplasm. These cells, known as *Paget cells* **P**, are breast carcinoma cells which are presumed to have spread along the epithelium of the mammary and nipple ducts to the surface from an intraduct or infiltrating ductular carcinoma which is invariably present in the underlying breast tissue. This is not a primary change of the epidermal cells of the nipple skin but represents *intraepithelial spread* of malignant cells.

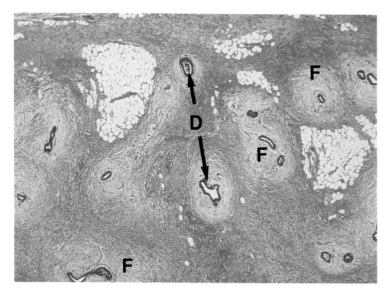

## Fig. 17.7    Gynaecomastia of male breast (MP)

The male breast is normally rudimentary and inactive, consisting merely of scanty fibroadipose tissue containing occasional atrophic mammary ducts lined by a single layer of flat cuboidal epithelium. Occasionally, under conditions of relative oestrogen excess, either endogenous (e.g. puberty, old age) or exogenous (e.g. stilboestrol therapy for carcinoma of prostate), male breast tissue undergoes hyperplasia resulting in *gynaecomastia*. The simple mammary ducts **D** become enlarged, often with thickening of the epithelial layer and a concomitant increase in periductal fibrous tissue **F** which may be markedly collagenous. Gynaecomastia may also be induced by certain drugs (e.g. spironolactone, cimetidine).

# 18. Male reproductive system

## Introduction

Inflammation of the testis (*orchitis*) may result from virus infections, as in mumps, and the testis may also be the site of a gumma in the tertiary stage of syphilis (see Fig. 3.19). Bacterial infections are usually complications of infections of the lower urinary tract or following surgical instrumentation. A particular form of orchitis is *granulomatous orchitis* (see Fig. 18.1) which may follow an episode of trauma to the testis, or sperm retention as, for example, after vasectomy. The most important pathological lesions of the testis are the tumours *seminoma* and *teratoma* illustrated in Figs 18.2 and 18.3 respectively; both are highly malignant tumours. Venous infarction of the testis due to *torsion* is an important cause of testicular pain in childhood and young adulthood and is illustrated in Fig. 18.4.

Like the testis, the epididymis may become infected by pyogenic bacteria in association with lower urinary tract infection and surgical instrumentation; when infection occurs, both the testis and epididymis are commonly involved together, a condition known as *acute epididymo-orchitis*. The epididymis is occasionally the site of metastatic tuberculous infection, *tuberculous epididymitis*, (see Fig. 3.15), usually secondary to active pulmonary or renal tuberculosis; the testis is rarely involved.

The prostate gland frequently undergoes *benign nodular hyperplasia* in elderly men, probably due to an alteration in hormone balance. This important lesion, shown in Fig. 18.5, produces obstruction to bladder outflow as a result of pressure on the prostatic urethra; in turn, the obstruction may produce pressure effects on the proximal conducting system of the urinary tract, leading to *hydroureter* and *hydronephrosis* with pressure atrophy of the renal parenchyma. As with other abnormalities of the tract, prostatic hyperplasia also predisposes to infection and stone formation. Invasive *carcinoma of the prostate* is a common and important malignant tumour in men; it is dealt with in Fig. 18.6. Small foci of tumour with the histological characteristics of prostatic adenocarcinoma but exhibiting little tendency to enlarge, invade or spread, are commonly seen as an incidental finding at autopsy or in prostates removed for benign hyperplasia in the very elderly; such lesions are called *latent carcinomas*.

The most important pathological lesion of the penis is *squamous carcinoma* (see Fig. 18.7) which is usually located on the glans or prepuce; the glans penis is also the site of a form of noninvasive carcinoma in situ known as *erythroplasia of Queyrat* illustrated in Fig. 18.8. It probably represents a form of dysplasia falling just short of frank carcinoma, a concept dealt with in Chapter 6.

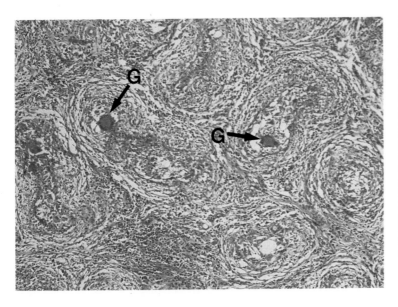

### Fig. 18.1 Granulomatous orchitis (MP)

This form of inflammatory disease of the testis most commonly follows trauma to the testis or surgery to the spermatic cord. The testis becomes uniformly firm and enlarged and has a homogenous pallid cut surface appearance. Histologically, there is diffuse chronic inflammatory cell infiltration, mainly lymphocytes and plasma cells, with numerous granulomata containing giant cells **G**. These inflammatory changes are associated with destruction and atrophy of seminiferous tubules which in this micrograph have been almost entirely destroyed. The cause of this inflammation is not known but it may represent a type of abnormal response to extruded spermatozoa.

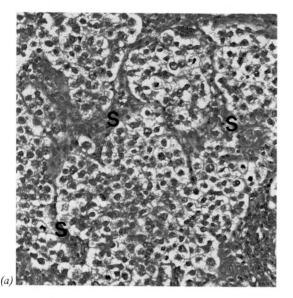

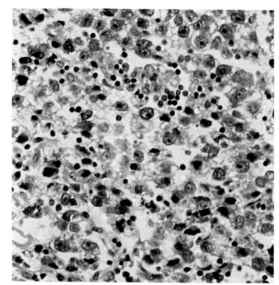

*(a)*

*(b)*

## Fig. 18.2   Seminoma
### (a) well differentiated (HP)
### (b) poorly differentiated (HP)

*Seminoma* is the most common tumour of the testis, with a peak incidence from 30 to 45 years. On cut surface, the tumour is pale, creamy-white and homogenous with a faint lobular pattern; necrosis and haemorrhage are rare unless the tumour is very large. Histologically, most seminomas show the classical appearance illustrated in micrograph (a). The tumour consists of sheets of uniform, tightly packed, polygonal cells with clear cytoplasm and a round central nucleus; the cells are divided into clumps by fine fibrous septa **S** in which there is a variable accumulation of small lymphocytes. Less differentiated histological variants occur, as shown in micrograph (b); the tumour cells are more variable in size and shape with pleomorphic nuclei and showing greater mitotic activity. Seminoma is a malignant tumour and tends to spread via lymphatics, initially to iliac and para-aortic lymph nodes.

## Fig. 18.3   Teratoma of testis *(illustrations opposite)*
### (a) differentiated teratoma (MP)
### (c) malignant teratoma intermediate (MP)
### (b) malignant teratoma undifferentiated (HP)
### (d) malignant teratoma undifferentiated with seminoma (HP)

*Testicular teratomas* are slightly less common than seminomas with a younger peak incidence at between 20 and 35 years. Teratomas are thought to be derived from multipotent cells capable of differentiating into derivatives of all three germ layers, mesoderm, ectoderm and endoderm; this feature is best seen in well differentiated teratomas as illustrated in micrograph (a). In general, teratomas have a partly cystic cut surface appearance, and necrosis and haemorrhage are extensive, even in quite small tumours; this offers a most useful means of distinguishing it from the homogeneous seminoma. Teratomas of the testis are malignant and spread early via the blood stream, often to the lung. Among the teratomas however there is a wide range of malignant behaviour, the aggressiveness of the tumour, tendency to metastasize and prognosis varying according to the histological form of the tumour. A number of histological classifications exist, the nomenclature used here being that of the Testicular Tumour Panel and Registry of the Pathological Society of Great Britain and Ireland.

   (a) *Differentiated teratoma (TD).* This type shows the least aggressive behaviour and has the best prognosis. It contains any of a wide variety of differentiated tissues closely resembling those of the mature adult body; derivatives of mesoderm (e.g. cartilage **C**, smooth muscle **M**), ectoderm (e.g. squamous epithelium) and endoderm (e.g. respiratory epithelium **R**) may all be present. This form closely resembles the benign cystic teratoma of the ovary (see Fig. 16.17) and is most common in children.

   (b) *Malignant teratoma undifferentiated (MTU).* In this histological variant, no differentiated elements are seen and the poorly differentiated tumour cells are arranged in carcinoma-like patterns, often part glandular or tubular, and sometimes in solid patternless masses. No differentiated organoid elements such as cartilage are present. This type is also known as *embryonal carcinoma* (particularly in the USA) and has a bad prognosis. A sub-variant of undifferentiated teratoma contains areas with the histological and biochemical features of malignant syncytio- and cytotrophoblast; this type is called *malignant teratoma trophoblastic (MTT)* or *choriocarcinoma.*

   (c) *Malignant teratoma intermediate (MTI).* As its name implies, this form is histologically intermediate between the differentiated and undifferentiated types. Part of the tumour **U** is of the undifferentiated (embryonal carcinoma) type, whilst other areas show some tendency to differentiation into organoid structures, though rarely as well differentiated as in a differentiated teratoma; in this example there is some immature cartilage **C** and formed epithelium **E**.

   (d) *Teratoma with seminoma (MTU+S).* Sometimes seminomatous areas coexist with teratomatous areas in one tumour, one or other type predominating, In this micrograph, note the pale staining cells of the seminoma component **Sem** contrasting with the darker staining cells of undifferentiated teratoma **T**.

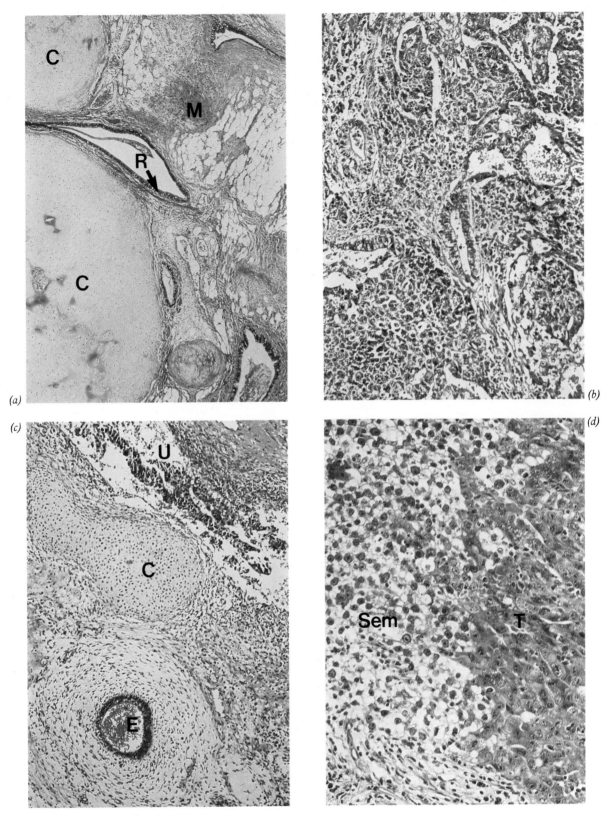

*(a)*

*(b)*

*(c)*

*(d)*

Fig. 18.3    Teratoma of testis

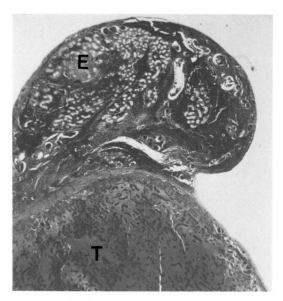

### Fig. 18.4   Torsion of the testis (LP)

The arterial supply and venous drainage of the testis pass in the long course of the spermatic cord to and from the major vessels in the abdomen and pelvis. The spermatic cord is liable to twist, leading to compression of the thin walled veins and obstruction of venous drainage from the testis. If this state persists for several hours or more without correction, the testis **T** and epididymis **E** may become deeply congested and subsequently undergo *venous infarction*, in which necrosis is associated with severe congestion and extravasation of blood. The histological changes are similar to those seen in venous infarction of the bowel following volvulus or strangulation, and described in Fig. 9.6.

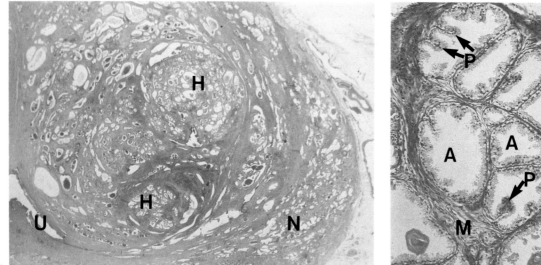

*(a)*                                                                                                   *(b)*

### Fig. 18.5   Benign prostatic hyperplasia
### (a) (LP)    (b) (HP)

*Benign prostatic hypertrophy* is a common condition affecting elderly men in which the inner paraurethral components of the prostate gland undergo nodular glandular hyperplasia accompanied by hyperplasia of the intervening fibromuscular stroma of the gland. The peripheral glandular components of the prostate (making up the prostatic gland proper) are not involved in the hyperplastic process and become compressed and atrophic at the outer margin. At low magnification in micrograph (a), note the rounded nodules of hyperplastic prostatic tissue **H** in the inner (paraurethral) part of the gland, and the compressed nonhyperplastic zone **N** at the periphery. Since the paraurethral component of the prostate gland is involved, compression of the urethral lumen **U** is a frequent occurrence, being responsible for important clinical features of

this condition such as hesitancy, poor urinary stream and urinary retention. On cut surface, the typical hyperplastic prostate has a nodular microcystic appearance, the tiny cysts representing enormously dilated hyperplastic prostatic glandular acini.

At high magnification as in micrograph (b), the acini **A** are lined by tall prostatic epithelial cells with small basal nuclei; the cells have a regular arrangement but are sometimes thrown up into papillary folds **P**. Adjacent acini are separated by a variable amount of fibromuscular connective tissue **M** in which the muscular component may be hypertrophied; muscular hypertrophy is particularly prominent in the region of the bladder neck.

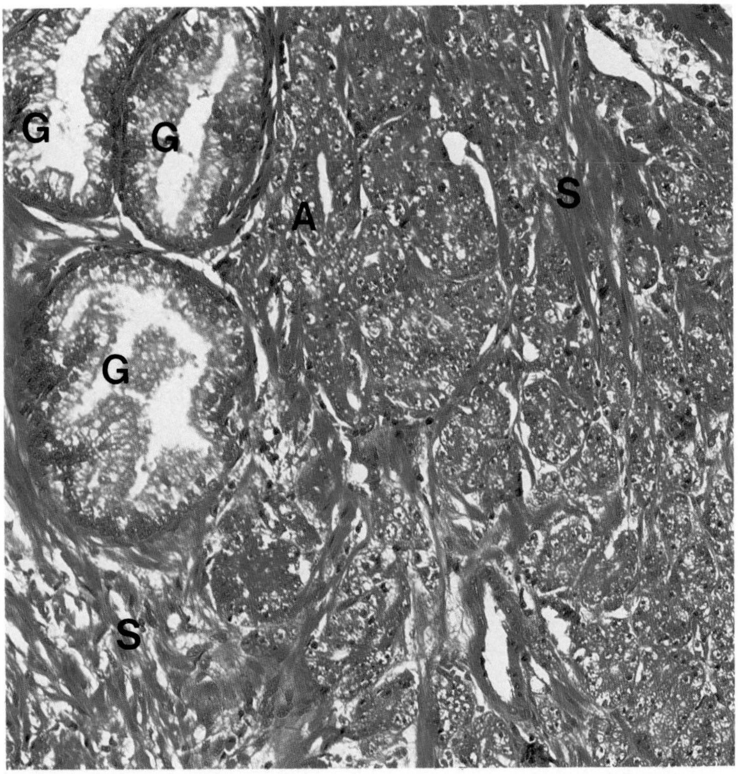

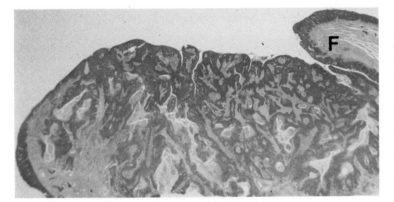

### Fig. 18.6  Carcinoma of the prostate (HP)

This common tumour usually arises in the peripheral component of the prostate gland, as opposed to benign prostatic hyperplasia, which characteristically develops in the paraurethral glandular component (see Fig. 18.5). This tumour, being derived from glandular cells of the prostatic acini, takes the form of an adenocarcinoma. In this moderately differentiated example, note that although much of the tumour is in the form of solid nests of cells, some acinar differentiation **A** remains. The tumour is seen adjacent to several normal benign glandular acini **G**, and is invading the pink staining fibromuscular stroma **S**. Arising, as it most frequently does, at the periphery of the gland, the tumour invades surrounding tissues at an early stage. Lymphatic spread to pelvic and para-aortic nodes, and haematogenous spread to bone particularly the lower vertebrae, are also significant modes of spread.

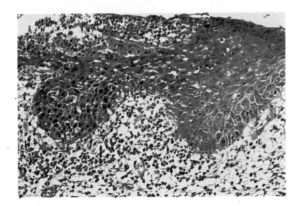

### Fig. 18.7  Squamous carcinoma of penis (LP)

This micrograph illustrates, at low magnification, a well differentiated keratinizing squamous carcinoma of the glans penis; part of the uninvolved foreskin **F** is included. In this example, islands of purple staining tumour extend deeply into the glans towards the urethra (not shown). Carcinoma of the penis is rare in circumcised men and chronic irritation and poor hygiene may be predisposing factors; metastatic spread is by lymphatics to superficial inguinal nodes.

### Fig. 18.8  Erythroplasia of Queyrat (HP)

This condition is a form of severe dysplasia or carcinoma in situ of the stratified squamous epithelium of the glans penis. In comparison with the more normal epithelium on the right, the abnormal cells are markedly dysplastic exhibiting a high nuclear-cytoplasmic ratio, pleomorphism, increased mitotic activity, and loss of stratification.

# 19. Endocrine system

## Pituitary gland

Structural defects of the pituitary gland are few, although functional abnormalities are potentially numerous, leading to under- or over- production of one or more of the many hormones produced by the pituitary and its target endocrine glands. Hypopituitarism may develop as a result of destruction of functioning pituitary cells by a large nonfunctioning *pituitary adenoma*. On the other hand, many pituitary adenomas are made up of functioning cells and may produce various hyperpituitarism syndromes such as acromegaly and Cushing's syndrome (see Fig. 19.1).

## Thyroid gland

The thyroid gland is the seat of many pathological processes which may lead to either diminished or excessive output of thyroxine. Hypothyroidism (myxoedema) may result from many causes some of which, for example *Hashimoto's disease* (see Fig. 19.2), have an autoimmune basis. By the time the thyroid is examined histologically in cases of long standing hypothyroidism, the thyroid often shows only shrinkage, fibrosis and destruction of most of the thyroid acini, with a sparse residual infiltrate of chronic inflammatory cells. This change, known as *primary atrophic thyroiditis* is analogous to the 'end-stage' of long standing kidney damage (see Fig. 14.11) and provides little evidence of the nature of the original thyroid abnormality.

Hyperthyroidism is usually the result of diffuse hyperplasia of the thyroid acinar cells most commonly in the condition known as Graves' disease (see Fig. 19.3); sometimes the hyperplasia is confined to a single *benign thyroid adenoma,* or to one or two nodules in an otherwise inactive *multinodular goitre* ('goitre' is the term now applied indiscriminately to almost any thyroid swelling). Nevertheless, the vast majority of thyroid adenomas and multinodular goitres are nonfunctional and do not lead to disturbances of thyroid hormone output. Examples are shown in Fig. 19.4. Three main forms of *thyroid carcinoma* occur; these are also nonfunctioning and are illustrated in Fig. 19.5. *Medullary carcinoma of the thyroid* is an uncommon malignant tumour of calcitonin-producing cells and is particularly notable for its production of amyloid (see Fig. 4.6).

## Parathyroid gland

The parathyroid glands show only two important pathological abnormalities, hyperplasia and benign adenoma (see Fig. 19.6); in both cases there are associated primary or secondary abnormalities of parathormone and calcium metabolism.

## Adrenal gland

The adrenal gland has two distinct morphological and functional components. The cortex secretes three groups of steroid hormones, namely glucocorticoids (e.g. cortisol), mineralocorticoids (e.g. aldosterone), and small quantities of sex hormones. The medulla (part of the APUD system) is responsible for the production of the catecholamines, adrenalin and noradrenaline. *Atrophy of the adrenal cortex* (see Fig. 19.7b) may result from primary autoimmune disease, but is now more commonly iatrogenic, the result of steroid therapy. Hyposecretion of adenocortical steroids, known clinically as *Addison's disease,* may also result from destruction of the gland by tuberculosis (see Fig. 3.13).

*Hyperplasia of the adrenal cortex* (see Fig. 19.7c and d), usually the result of prolonged stimulation of the adrenal cortex by pituitary ACTH or tumour-derived ACTH-like substance, may result in various hyperadrenalism syndromes such as *Cushing's syndrome* (excess cortisol production), *Conn's syndrome* (excess aldosterone production) or the *adrenogenital syndrome* (excess androgen production). These syndromes may also be caused by excess hormone production by a benign *adrenal cortical adenoma* (see Fig. 19.8) or its rare malignant counterpart, *adrenal cortical carcinoma*. Often, cortical hyperplasia is nodular rather than diffuse and it is impossible to distinguish between nodular cortical hyperplasia and multiple benign cortical adenomas.

The most important lesions of the adrenal medulla are tumours, the usually benign *phaeochromocytoma* (see Fig. 19.9) which produces excessive adrenalin and noradrenalin, and the malignant embryonal tumour of neuroblasts seen in childhood, the *neuroblastoma* (see Fig. 19.10). Both these tumours may also arise elsewhere in the abdomen in sites corresponding to embryological remnants of migrating adrenal medullary cell precursors.

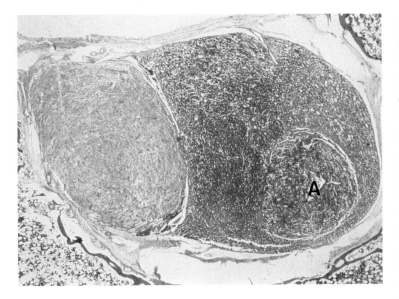

## Fig. 19.1 Pituitary adenoma (LP)

The micrograph shows a pituitary gland in situ in the pituitary fossa and cut in sagittal section. Within the substance of the anterior pituitary lies a small benign *pituitary adenoma* **A** composed of cells of a uniform type. The tumour is benign as evidenced by its well circumscribed, noninvasive, spherical appearance, and small enough to have caused no distortion of the pituitary outline or undue compression of adjacent normal pituitary cells. Such tumours are often nonfunctioning and would thus only become manifest either by impinging on vital local structures such as the optic chiasma causing visual disturbance, or by expanding to a size large enough to destroy the surrounding normal functioning tissue resulting in clinical hypopituitarism. In this particular case, the tumour cells secreted ACTH in gross excess and the patient died as a result of the metabolic and cardiac complications of *Cushing's disease*; in all his illness lasted no more than 7 or 8 weeks despite its 'benign' pathogenesis.

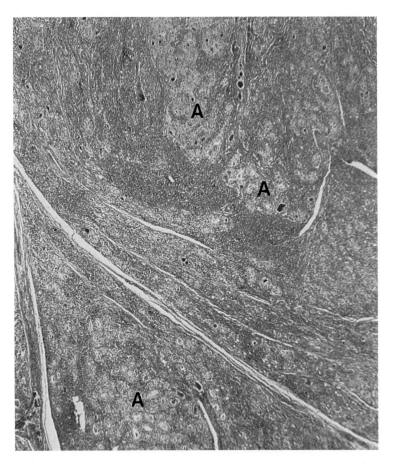

## Fig. 19.2 Hashimoto's thyroiditis (MP)

This disease is an autoimmune thyroiditis in which thyroid acini **A** are progressively destroyed by immunological processes and the gland becomes diffusely infiltrated by lymphocytes. In some areas, these small darkly staining cells tend to aggregate and often form typical lymphoid follicles with germinal centres. In the early stages of the disease, the extensive lymphoid infiltrate produces a diffusely enlarged firm thyroid gland with a pale cut surface appearance. As thyroid follicles are progressively destroyed over the years, the patient who at the outset is euthyroid or even slightly hyperthyroid, becomes increasingly hypothyroid (myxoed-ematous). When almost all thyroid acini are destroyed, the lymphoid infiltrate becomes less obvious and fibrosis supervenes, with progressive reduction in size of the gland.

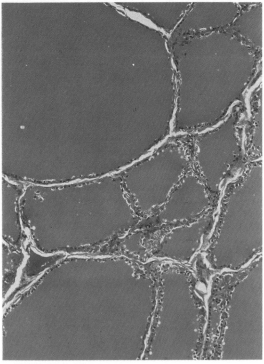

*(a)*

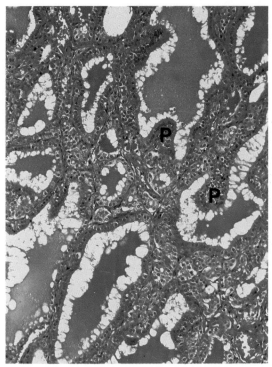

*(b)*

## Fig. 19.3 Thyrotoxic hyperplasia
### (a) normal thyroid (HP)
### (b) hyperplastic thyroid (HP)

Thyroid function is normally under the control of the hypothalamic-pituitary system via the release of TSH which stimulates thyroid acinar cells to liberate thyroxine. The resulting level of circulating thyroxine then regulates TSH production by a negative feedback mechanism.

Certain circumstances disrupt this balance resulting in prolonged excesss production of TSH or a functionally similar substance which then promotes hyperplasia and hypertrophy of thyroid acinar cells; this gives rise to the histological appearance known as *thyroid hyperplasia*. Depending on the underlying cause, the patient may be clinically euthyroid or thyrotoxic.

*Graves' disease* is by far the most common cause of pathological thyroid hyperplasia. In this autoimmune disease, a circulating immunoglobulin known as *long acting thyroid*

*stimulator (LATS)* is produced which binds to thyroid acinar cells mimicking the effects of TSH and resulting in excess secretion of thyroxine. The resulting glandular appearance is described as *thyrotoxic hyperplasia* and is illustrated in micrograph (b).

Compared to the normal thyroid shown in micrograph (a), the hyperplastic acinar cells are tall and have large nuclei reflecting a greater degree of metabolic activity. The acini themselves are smaller than normal because of the reduced amount of colloid resulting from increased thyroxine secretion. The hyperplastic acinar cells may crowd up on one side of the acini so as to project into the luman as papillary structures **P**. In Graves' disease, the thyroid may sometimes contain prominent lymphocytic aggregates (not shown in this specimen).

## Fig. 19.4 Thyroid adenoma and nodular goitre *(illustrations opposite)*
### (a) colloid adenoma (LP)
### (b) microfollicular adenoma (LP)
### (c) multinodular goitre (LP)

Thyroid adenomatous nodules are a common clinical finding and are often so numerous as to occupy the entire gland which may become considerably enlarged. Although described as 'adenomas' there is disagreement whether these should be regarded as true benign tumours, or as foci of hyperplasia, since identical lesions can arise in the thyroid as a result of dietary lack of iodine, congenital lack of enzymes or the activity of goitrogens. Whatever the pathogenesis, the nodules are usually spherical and of highly variable size; their internal structure may be of many different types, two of the more

common being illustrated here. Micrograph (a) shows the *colloid nodule* variety, in which the acini are markedly distended by normal looking colloid and the lining epithelium is much flattened; there is minimal interacinar stroma.

Micrograph (b) shows a *microfollicular adenoma*, composed of small tightly packed acini virtually devoid of luminal colloid giving the adenoma a more solid and compact appearance. Micrograph (c) shows a *multinodular goitre* which consists of numerous adenomatous nodules of varying size and histological type; the largest nodules **C** are usually of the colloid type.

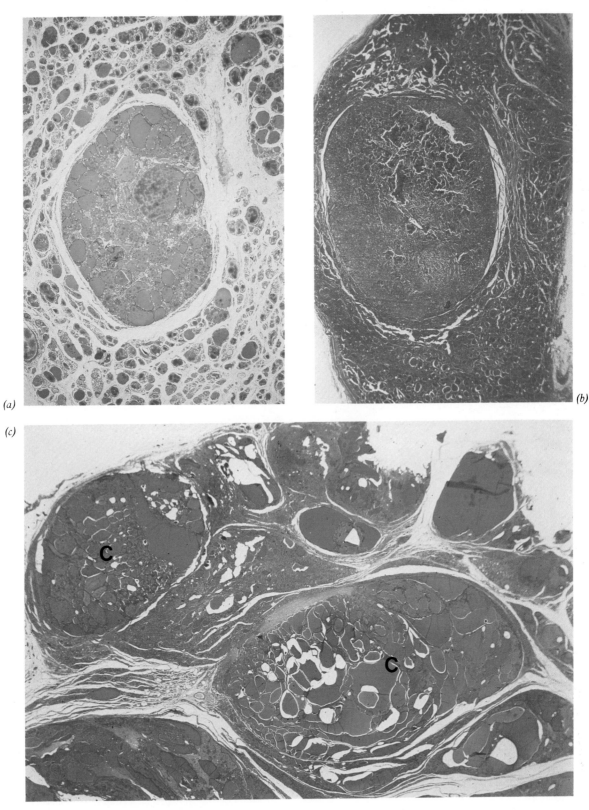

*(a)*

*(b)*

*(c)*

**Fig. 19.4    Thyroid adenoma and nodular goitre**

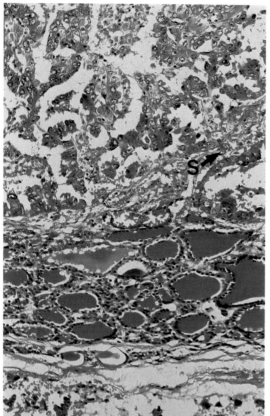

(a)

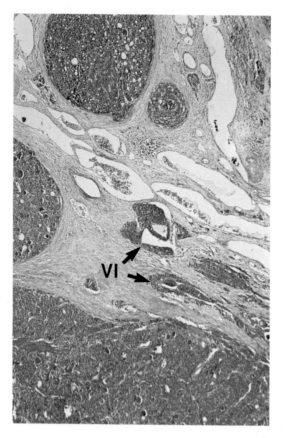

(b)

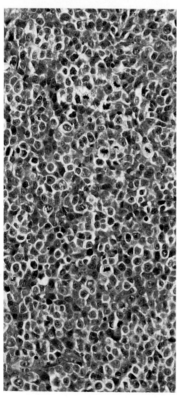

(c)

## Fig. 19.5 Carcinoma of thyroid
**(a) papillary** (HP)
**(b) follicular** (MP)
**(c) anaplastic** (HP)

Carcinoma of the thyroid takes three common histological forms, each with its own characteristic peak age incidence, mode of growth, pattern of spread, and prognosis. *Papillary adenocarcinoma* shown in micrograph (a) is the most common type, found particularly in young women under 40. The tumour is in the form of complex papillary structures each composed of a narrow stromal core **S** covered with a layer of glandular epithelium. The stromal cores sometimes contain small calcified laminated bodies known as *psammoma bodies* (not shown here). Note the normal thyroid tissue at the bottom of this field. The tumour tends to spread via lymphatics to regional nodes, and has the best prognosis of all thyroid cancers.

*Follicular carcinoma* illustrated in micrograph (b) has, as its name implies, a well structured follicular pattern and may be difficult to distinguish from a benign follicular adenoma (see Fig. 19.4) on cytological grounds alone; evidence of vessel invasion **VI** at the tumour edge provides clear evidence of malignancy. Bloodstream spread is the major method of metastasis, and lung and bone are common sites of secondary tumour deposits.

*Anaplastic carcinoma* as shown in micrograph (c) usually occurs in the very elderly and is composed of sheets of small, very poorly differentiated cells, largely occupied by a round, dark staining nucleus; such tumours may be histologically difficult to distinguish from large cell malignant lymphomas (see Fig. 15.4d). These tumours grow very rapidly and extensively invade local tissues, often presenting as a bulky mass in the neck associated with symptoms of tracheal compression.

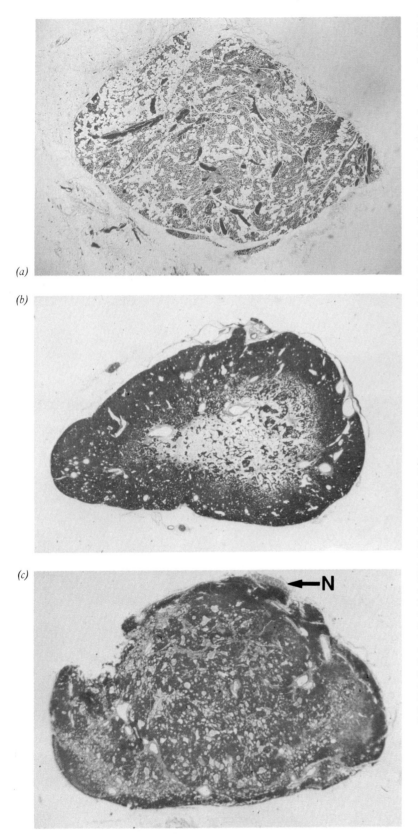

*(a)*

*(b)*

*(c)*

← **N**

### Fig. 19.6  Parathyroid hyperplasia and adenoma
### (a) normal parathyroid (LP)
### (b) hyperplastic parathyroid (LP)
### (c) parathyroid adenoma (LP)

The normal adult parathyroid gland contains small endocrine cells arranged in clumps or cords within highly vascular adipose tissue; with increasing age, more of the gland becomes replaced by adipose tissue. Should the need arise for a greater output of parathormone, for example in cases of excessive urinary calcium loss in chronic renal failure, the active hormone-secreting endocrine cells undergo hyperplasia replacing the parathyroid adipose tissue with endocrine cells; continued hyperplasia leads to symmetrical enlargement of the parathyroid gland as a whole. Compare the hyperplastic gland in micrograph (b) with the normal parathyroid in micrograph (a); the hyperplastic gland is only marginally larger than the normal gland, yet the hormonally-active endocrine component has increased two or threefold by replacing the adipose tissue component. If demand for excess parathormone persists, the gland may become markedly enlarged; these hyperplastic changes affect all four parathyroid glands uniformly.

In contrast, autonomous benign tumours of the parathryoid gland, *parathyroid adenomas*, usually only affect one of the four parathyroid glands, although occasionally they may be multiple. With only a single parathyroid gland to examine, it can be difficult to distinguish between parathyroid adenoma and *parathyroid hyperplasia*, however parathyroid adenoma occasionally has a small compressed fragment of normal parathyroid tissue stretched over part of its surface. In the small parathyroid adenoma shown in micrograph (c), a fragment of normal parathyroid tissue **N** can be seen at the periphery; the cellular arrangement in parathyroid adenoma is variable and the cells may be in the form of sheets or may be arranged in a microacinar pattern. With parathyroid adenoma, the noninvolved glands may show the *suppressed parathyroid pattern*, in which the endocrine component atrophies, to be replaced by adipose tissue; the gland may remain normal size.

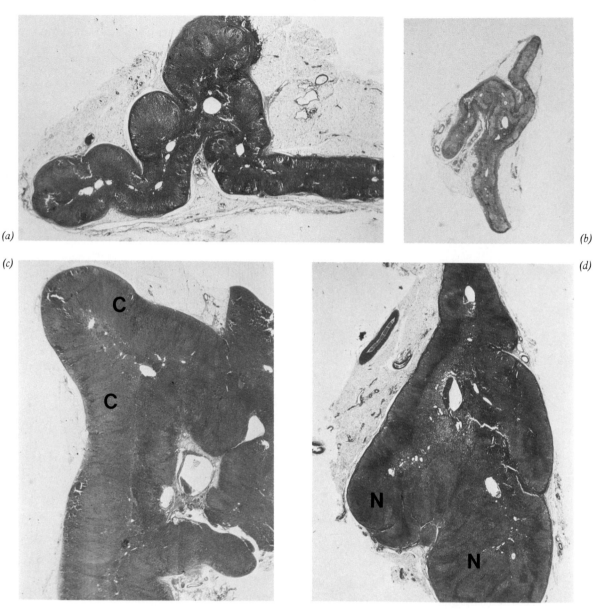

**Fig. 19.7   Adrenal cortical atrophy and hyperplasia**
**(a) normal** (LP)           **(b) atrophic** (LP)
**(c) diffuse hyperplasia** (LP)     **(d) nodular hyperplasia** (LP)

These micrographs, all taken at the same magnification, permit comparison of adrenal atrophy and hyperplasia with the normal. In *adrenal atrophy* as illustrated in micrograph (b), the marked reduction in size of the gland is due to reduction in the size of the cortex in which the characteristic subdivision into three zones becomes much less distinct. In this example, the atrophy was caused by the long term therapeutic administration of corticosteroids which suppress pituitary ACTH output.

Adrenal cortical hyperplasia occurs in either *diffuse* or *nodular forms* as illustrated in micrographs (c) and (d) respectively; the latter resembles multiple benign adenomata (see Fig. 19.8). In the diffuse form, the cortex **C** is uniformly and regularly thickened, often by cells of one type. In the much more common nodular form, the cortex contains adenoma-like nodules **N** of hyperplastic cortical cells, usually of zona fasciculata type. Adrenal cortical hyperplasia is usually caused by excess stimulation by ACTH from the pituitary e.g. from a pituitary adenoma (see Fig. 19.1) or by an ACTH-like substance e.g. from an oat cell carcinoma; rarely, it results from a congenital enzyme deficiency. The presence of cortical hyperplasia may be associated with various endocrine syndromes including *Cushing's syndrome* (hypersecretion of cortisol). Such syndromes may also occur with the solitary adrenal cortical adenoma (see Fig. 19.8) and with the rare adrenal cortical carcinoma.

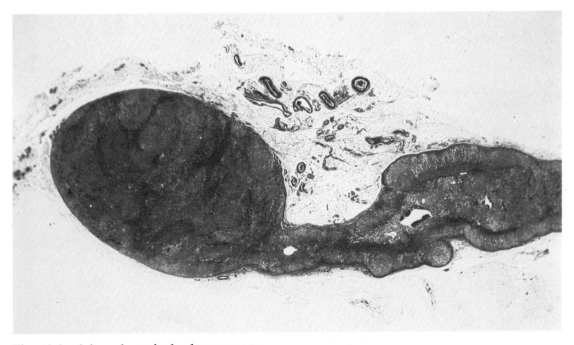

## Fig. 19.8   Adrenal cortical adenoma (LP)

Hyperadrenal syndromes may result from excessive secretion of hormones by a solitary benign *adrenal cortical adenoma*, the activity of which is independent of regulation by pituitary ACTH. These tumours form a circumscribed, spherical mass within the cortex and may be composed of a single cell type e.g. zona glomerulosa cells in Conn's syndrome, but more often contain a mixture of cortical cell types. Note how similar the adenoma is to the nodules in nodular cortical hyperplasia seen in Fig. 19.7 (d). Cortical adenomas are a fairly frequent incidental finding at necropsy, a fact which leads to the belief that most are nonfunctioning and asymptomatic. Almost all cortical adenomas have a yellow cut surface thereby distinguishing them from phaeochromocytomas which appear brown (see Fig. 19.9).

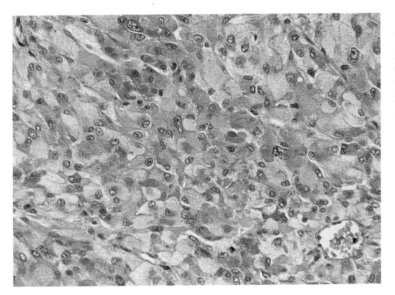

## Fig. 19.9   Phaeochromocytoma (HP)

Phaeochromocytoma is a benign tumour arising from cells of the adrenal medulla and capable of synthesizing and secreting adrenalin and noradrenalin. Most tumours are benign in terms of their growth characteristics but the excessive production of catecholamines often results in severe hypertension. Microscopically, the cut surface of the tumour is pale brown in colour, a useful distinguishing feature from the yellow coloured cortical adenoma (see Fig. 19.8). Histologically, the tumour is usually composed of nests of plump irregular cells, often with prominent granular cytoplasm. Nuclear and cytoplasmic pleomorphism is common but in these tumours is not necessarily an indication of malignancy; true malignant variants do occur, but diagnosis must be based on evidence of invasion and spread since purely cytological criteria are unreliable.

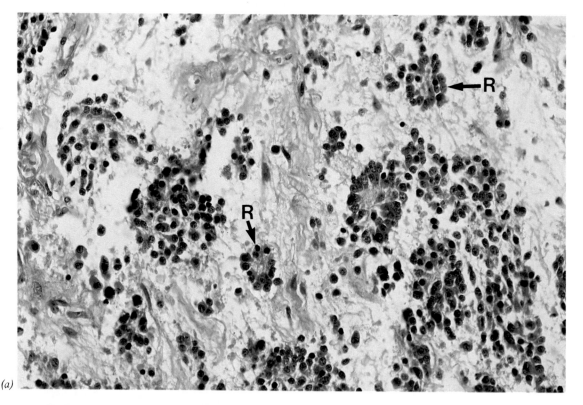

*(a)*

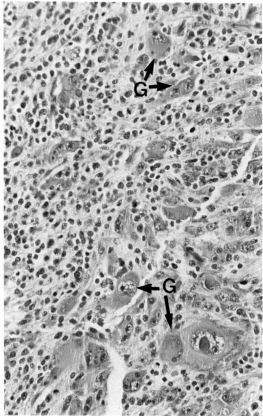

*(b)*

### Fig. 19.10 Adrenal embryonal tumours
**(a) neuroblastoma** (HP)
**(b) ganglioneuroblastoma** (HP)

*Neuroblastoma* is an example of an embryonal tumour (see Chapter 6) and is believed to be derived from primitive neuroblastic cells in the adrenal medulla. It occurs in children and is highly malignant, spreading mainly via the blood stream to internal organs especially the liver, and to the bones particularly those of the face and skull. The classical appearance of the neuroblastoma is shown in micrograph (a); there is usually extensive haemorrhage and necrosis, but the viable areas (as here) are composed of sheets of small undifferentiated tumour cells dominated by a densely stained nucleus surrounded by a very narrow irregular rim of cytoplasm. A characteristic feature is occasional clumps of cells arranged in the form of a rosette **R** surrounding a central zone of neurofibrils seen in transverse section; occasionally longitudinal bands of fibrils are present.

A somewhat less aggressive form of this tumour is known as the *ganglioneuroblastoma* and is illustrated in micrograph (b). These tumours exhibit some degree of differentiation, and ganglion cells **G** of varying degrees of maturity are found mixed with the small dark staining undifferentiated neuroblasts. Such tumours have a rather better prognosis than those composed entirely of the undifferentiated neuroblasts, although the outcome in such mixed tumours usually depends on the proportion and behaviour of the least differentiated, that is most malignant, component.

# 20. Skin

## Introduction

Many systemic diseases have manifestations, both clinical and pathological, in the skin. For example, skin rashes are a feature of many generalized viral infections such as measles, chicken pox and herpes. Systemic immunological diseases such as scleroderma, systemic lupus erythematosus and dermatomyositis, and some vasculitic disorders such as Henoch-Schönlein purpura, have major manifestations in the skin. In addition, the skin is the subject of many specific primary disorders, mainly inflammatory or neoplastic in nature.

While there are many different causes of tissue damage in the skin, it has only a limited repertoire of reactions to the damage; the most important of these patterns of reaction are illustrated in Figs. 20.1 to 20.4. Various skin disorders show these basic changes in different combinations and with varying degrees of severity. Few skin conditions have any absolutely pathognomonic histological features, and in most cases a precise diagnosis can only be made when the clinical history, macroscopic features, distribution and duration of the lesions are considered in conjunction with the histological appearances.

*Dermatitis* is a commonly used clinical term and is used to describe a wide variety of inflammatory skin conditions with many different causes. Histologically, nonspecific features of acute or chronic inflammation are seen (Figs 20.5 and 20.6) but in some cases there are other histological changes present which give a clue to the precise diagnosis or likeliest cause. Two specific and relatively common types of dermatitis, with characteristic histological features, are *lichen planus* (Fig. 20.7) and *psoriasis* (Fig. 20.8).

Viruses are responsible for many common skin lesions; some, like *viral warts* (Fig. 20.9), *keratoacanthoma* (Fig. 20.10) and *molluscum contagiosum* (Fig. 20.11) are probably primary skin lesions, whilst others, such as the vesicular lesions of herpes simplex, chicken pox and herpes zoster are merely the cutaneous manifestations of a more generalized viral illness, the last two being different manifestations of infection by the same virus. *Pyogenic granuloma* (Fig. 20.12) is a common, localized, nodular inflammatory lesion which frequently follows trauma.

Numerically, the commonest skin lesions of all are the ubiquitous pigmented lesions known colloquially as 'moles'. This nonspecific term encompasses a range of lesions called *naevi* characterized by the presence of aggregates of pigmented (melanin-producing) cells in various sites in the skin. Three important histological types, *junctional, intradermal* and *compound naevi*, are compared in Fig. 20.13. Clinically, the most important pigmented lesion is the *malignant melanoma* (Fig. 20.14), potentially a highly malignant tumour of epidermal melanocytes.

Epithelial tumours derived from the epidermis and its appendages are also common, the most frequent being the *basal cell carcinoma*, an invasive tumour of low grade malignancy derived from the basal cells. Basal cell carcinoma (Fig. 20.15) has characteristic histological features which enables it to be easily distinguished from *squamous cell carcinoma* (Fig. 20.16) a rather more aggressive malignant tumour derived from the prickle cell layer of the epidermis. The latter may be preceded by a type of carcinoma in situ in which the epidermal cells exhibit the cytological criteria of malignancy but show no evidence of invasive behaviour by broaching the epidermal basement membrane. Examples of this type of epidermal dysplasia include *solar ('senile') keratosis* and *Bowen's disease* (Fig. 20.17), analogous to the so-called erythroplasia of Queyrat of the penis (see Fig. 18.8) and carcinoma in situ of the cervix (see Fig. 16.5). Malignant lymphomas may involve the skin secondarily, however occasionally the skin is the site of the first manifestation of malignant lymphoma, a variant known as *mycosis fungoides* (Fig. 20.20).

Two common skin lesions which are difficult to classify are *epidermal cysts* (Fig. 20.18) and the so called *seborrhoeic keratosis* of the elderly (Fig. 20.19). The former, known to generations of clinicians by the inaccurate name *sebaceous cyst*, is probably an epidermal inclusion cyst, and the latter (also known as *seborrhoeic wart*) has formerly been widely regarded as a benign tumour of the basal cells of the epidermis, a belief perpetuated in the little used synonym, *basal cell papilloma*.

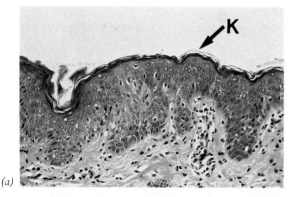

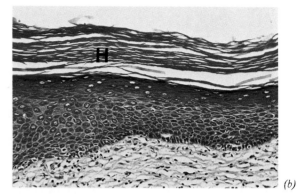

(a)

(b)

(c)

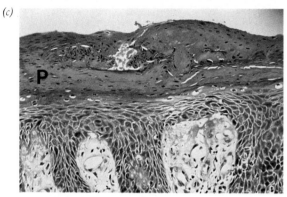

## Fig. 20.1 Abnormalities of surface keratin
**(a) normal keratin** (HP)
**(b) hyperkeratosis** (HP)
**(c) parakeratosis** (HP)

This series of micrographs compares the normal keratin **K** of thin skin seen in micrograph (a), with two common abnormalities of keratin, *hyperkeratosis* and *parakeratosis* shown in micrographs (b) and (c) respectively. In hyperkeratosis **H**, the keratin layer is thickened but otherwise normal (*orthokeratosis*). In parakeratosis **P** the keratin is also thickened, but shows the persistence of purple staining nuclear remnants; the granular layer is absent.

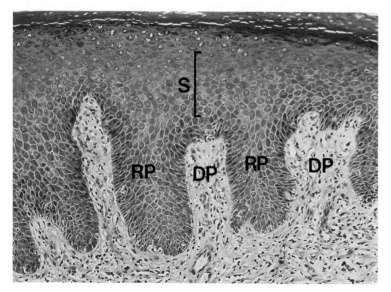

## Fig. 20.2 Abnormal epidermal thickening – acanthosis (HP)

*Acanthosis* is the term given to thickening of the epidermis usually due to an increase in the thickness of stratum spinosum **S** (prickle cell layer) and is a common feature of many skin conditions, particularly chronic inflammatory conditions (see Fig. 20.6). The thickening of the epidermal layer is particularly marked in the rete pegs **RP** which are expanded and elongated with prominent interdigitating dermal papillae **DP**.

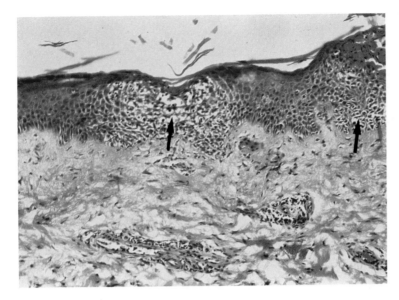

## Fig. 20.3 Intraepidermal oedema – spongiosis (HP)

Oedema of the epidermis causes separation of epithelial cells particularly in the prickle cell layer, a condition known as *spongiosis*. Accumulation of fluid between epidermal cells causes gaps to appear (arrow), which may coalesce with increased severity to form fluid-filled intraepidermal vesicles. Spongiosis with vesicle formation is a feature of acute dermatitis (see Fig. 20.5).

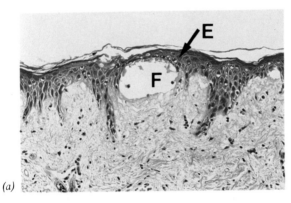

*(a)*

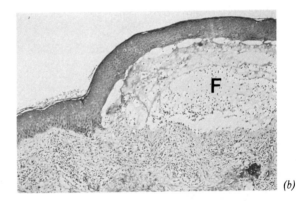

*(b)*

*(c)*

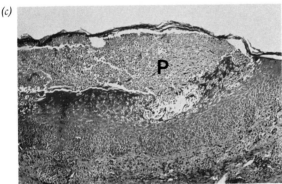

## Fig. 20.4 Other epidermal inflammatory reactions
**(a) vesicle** (HP)
**(b) bulla** (MP)
**(c) pustule** (HP)

Accumulations of fluid beneath or within the epidermis may cause small raised blebs on the skin; most are due to inflammation in the epidermis. When small, such lesions are termed *vesicles;* in micrograph (a), note the area of fluid accumulation **F** elevating and thinning the epidermis **E**. Larger collections of fluid are termed *bullae*. A bulla is shown in micrograph (b) at lower magnification than in (a); the collection of serous fluid **F** is much larger and may include small numbers of dark staining inflammatory cells. The term *pustule* is used to describe a collection consisting mostly of neutrophils with some serous fluid within or beneath the epidermis. Micrograph (c) shows a pustule **P** beneath the corneal layer of the epidermis.

Vesicles, bullae and pustules are further categorized as to location either *subepidermal, intra-epidermal* or *subcorneal*. Various disorders have characteristic sites of fluid accumulation in the skin.

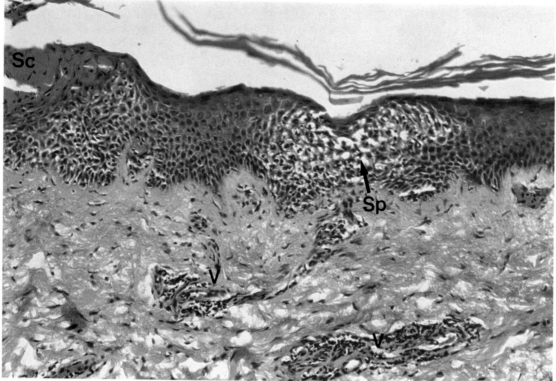

**Fig. 20.5   Acute dermatitis**

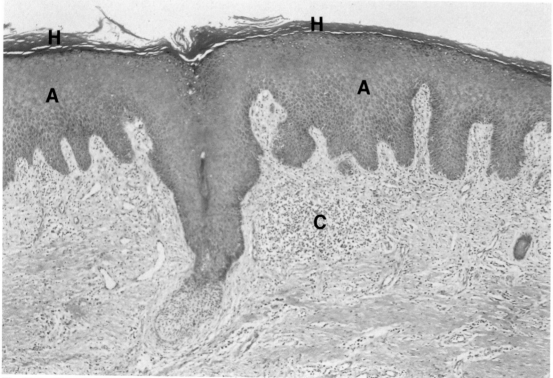

**Fig. 20.6   Chronic dermatitis**

SKIN 187

## Fig. 20.5 Acute dermatitis (HP; *illustration opposite above*)

In early *acute dermatitis* the major changes are epidermal, with fluid accumulating between the prickle cells (spongiosis). As the lesion progresses, the spongiotic areas may become converted into fluid-filled vesicles containing a few inflammatory cells, mainly lymphocytes and neutrophils, and there is variable diffuse infiltration of the epidermis by neutrophils. If the vesicles rupture onto the surface, crusts or scabs composed of fibrin and polymorph nuclei form. In the earlier stages, the upper dermis shows only oedema, but later there may be a mixed acute and chronic inflammatory cell infiltrate particularly around upper dermal blood vessels. In *subacute dermatitis,* the changes are identical but less severe,

with less obvious oedema and vesicle formation, and an inflammatory infiltrate which is proportionately more lymphocytic.

In this example of established acute dermatitis, note the central area of marked spongiosis **Sp** in the epidermis; there is considerable accumulation here of fluid containing polymorphs and this is the prelude to vesicle formation. The surrounding epidermis shows some early spongiotic change and a small diffuse infiltrate of inflammatory cells. At the extreme left, there is another area of spongiosis overlaid by scab **Sc**. In the dermis, the collagen is partly separated by oedema and a leucocytic infiltrate can be seen around the blood vessels **V**.

## Fig. 20.6 Chronic dermatitis (MP; *illustration opposite below*)

The histological features of a *chronic dermatitis* are seen in many skin rashes with varying causes. The characteristic feature is epidermal thickening due to acanthosis **A** and a variable degree of hyperkeratosis **H.** There is no infiltration of the epidermis by inflammatory cells, but the upper and mid dermis shows a moderate to heavy infiltrate of chronic

inflammatory cells **C**, mainly lymphocytes and plasma cells, particularly around blood vessels. The acanthosis and hyperkeratosis may produce the clinical appearance of *lichenification,* a feature recognized in the term *lichen simplex chronicus* applied to one of the variants of this chronic nonspecific dermatitic picture.

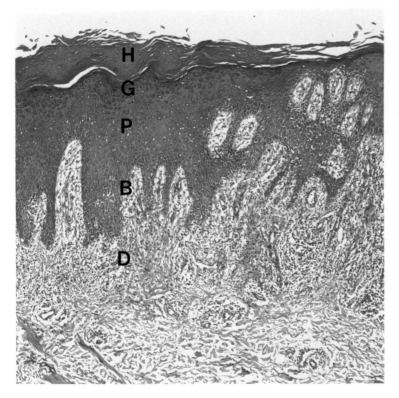

## Fig. 20.7 Lichen planus (MP)

*Lichen planus* is a clinically and histologically distinct type of dermatitis. In the epidermis there is hyperkeratosis **H,** and thickening of the granular layer **G,** whilst in the prickle cell layer **P,** acanthosis is seen. A characteristic feature is the disruption of the normally regular basal layer **B** by hydropic degeneration and destruction of basal cells leaving a ragged and irregular dermoepidermal junction. The dermis **D** shows a dense chronic inflammatory cell infiltrate mainly confined to the upper third. The combination of the heavy dermal infiltrate and the destruction of the basal layer may produce a jagged saw-tooth appearance of the rete pegs.

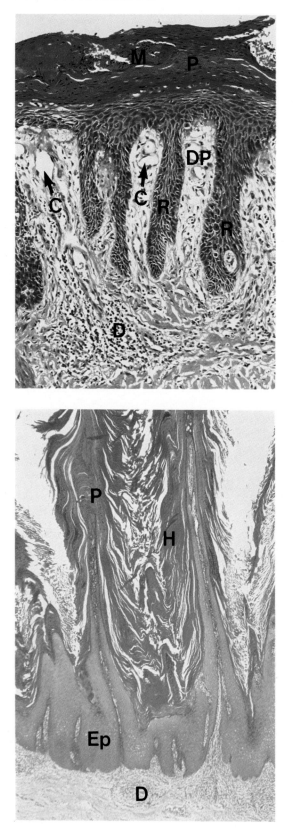

### Fig. 20.8 Psoriasis (HP)

*Psoriasis* is a chronic skin disease characterized by well demarcated, erythematous scaly lesions. Histologically, the major feature is acanthosis with greatly elongated narrow rete pegs **R.** Between the rete pegs, the epidermis is thinned over oedematous and prominent dermal papillae **DP** in which dilated capillaries **C** are prominent. The alternately thick and thin epidermis is covered by a parakeratotic layer **P** and may contain small aggregations of neutrophils forming microabscesses **M.**

There is a variable chronic inflammatory infiltrate in the upper dermis **D** and swollen dermal papillae.

### Fig. 20.9 Viral wart (verruca vulgaris) (MP)

The characteristic histological features of a viral wart on a nontraumatized area of skin is an exophytic papillary lesion in which an irregularly thickened epidermis **Ep** is covered by a thick layer of hyperkeratosis **H** in which there are parakeratotic spires **P** over the tips of the more prominent papillary epidermal outgrowths. The epidermal cells in an active viral wart usually show focal prominence of the granular layer, with some foci of large pale vacuolated cells in the upper stratum spinosum (not seen at this magnification). The dermis **D** shows a chronic inflammatory cell infiltrate. In skin areas prone to trauma, such lesions are less papillary, and may be dome-shaped (e.g. in juvenile warts of hands) or involuted (e.g. plantar warts of soles of the foot).

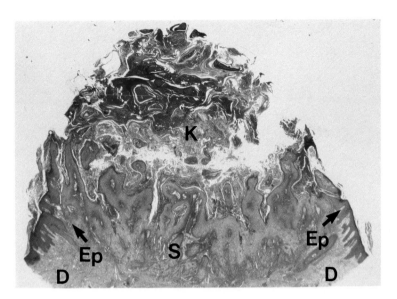

**Fig. 20.10    Kerato-acanthoma** (LP)

This lesion is of unknown aetiology but has many of the features of a viral condition. A localized proliferation of squamous cells **S** produces a nodule in the skin with a central crater containing large masses of keratin **K**.

At its periphery, the nodule has a collar of thin but normal epidermis **Ep** and the junction between normal and proliferating epidermis is abrupt. Cytologically, the proliferating squamous cells may exhibit marked atypia, with large swollen cells showing abnormal nuclei and increased mitotic activity, a feature which often leads to confusion with squamous carcinoma in biopsy specimens. The surrounding dermis **D** shows a heavy chronic inflammatory infiltrate with some inflammatory cells extending into the base of the lesion.

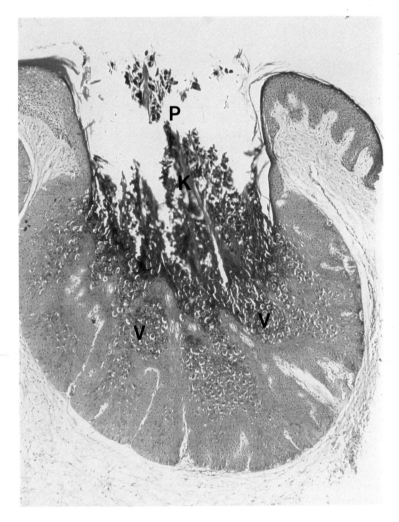

**Fig. 20.11    Molluscum contagiosum** (MP)

*Molluscum contagiosum*, like kerato-acanthoma, is a localized nodular thickening of epidermis; in this condition however, the viral aetiology is unquestioned since viral inclusion bodies **V** are easily visible, both in the proliferating epidermis, where they stain reddish, and in the overlying keratin plug **K**, where they stain blue-black. The keratinous plug extrudes through a central pit **P** at the apex of the dome-shaped nodule which is surrounded by normal epidermis.

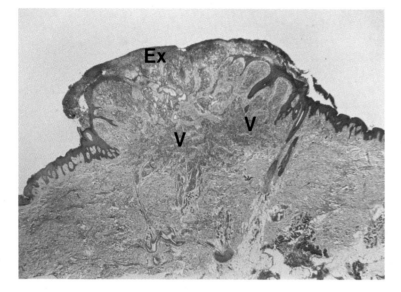

### Fig. 20.12   Pyogenic granuloma (LP)

The *pyogenic granuloma* is a common inflammatory lesion which may follow a minor penetrating injury e.g. rose thorn. It consists of a raised nodule of highly vascular tissue somewhat resembling a capillary angioma. This may represent an abnormal overgrowth of the vascular element of normal granulation tissue. At this magnification, the vascular tissue **V** appears as irregular blue stained areas. The surface of the lesion is frequently ulcerated as in this example in which the surface is covered by an inflammatory exudate **Ex.** A characteristic histological feature is a collar of proliferating epithelium at the margin of the lesion.

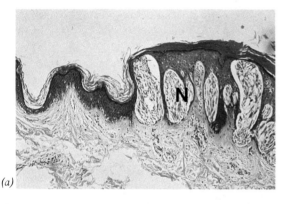

(a)

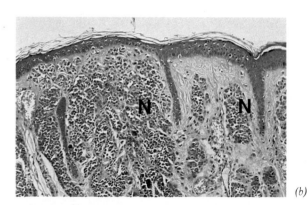

(b)

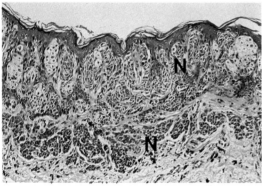

(c)

### Fig. 20.13   Benign naevi
### (a) junctional (HP)
### (b) intradermal (HP)
### (c) compound (HP)

The common *naevi*, moles, are benign accumulations of melanocytes; there are three distinct types. In the *junctional naevus* (micrograph a), large melanocytes aggregate in the basal layers of the epidermis (i.e. junction of dermis and epidermis) and may be so large that the overlying epidermis may be thinned; these *naevus cells* **N** have pale staining cytoplasm and may contain melanin. Junctional naevi occur most commonly before puberty.

In adults, *intradermal naevi* (micrograph b) are most common and in this type the naevus cells **N** form clumps in the upper dermis and are not present in the epidermis; these naevus cells are more compact and may also contain melanin pigment.

*Compound naevi* (micrograph c) are considered to represent a transition from junctional to intradermal forms and have naevus cells **N** both in the basal epidermis and in the upper dermis; with the passage of time the junctional component becomes less prominent and less active.

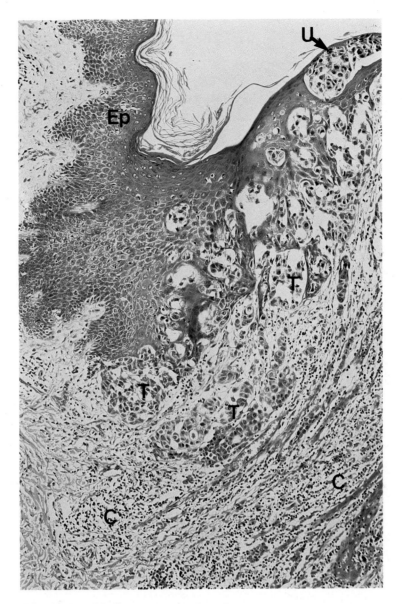

## Fig. 20.14 Malignant melanoma (HP)

This highly malignant tumour of melanocytes occurs most commonly in the skin, although it may rarely occur in the eye and other sites. In the skin, the tumour appears as a pigmented nodular lesion which may become ulcerated. The tumour is presumed to originate in naevus cells in the region of the dermo-epidermal junction and quickly invades downwards into the dermis. In this specimen, note the incipient surface ulceration **U** and adjacent normal epithelium **Ep.** The tumour cells **T** exhibit marked nuclear and cytoplasmic pleomorphism and frequent mitoses; many cells contain melanin pigment, although *malignant melanomas* may sometimes be *amelanotic.* There is frequently a chronic inflammatory cell infiltrate **C** around the margins of the tumour. The tumour spreads via dermal lymphatics to the surrounding skin forming *satellite lesions* and metastazes early to regional lymph nodes and thence via the bloodstream to many organs.

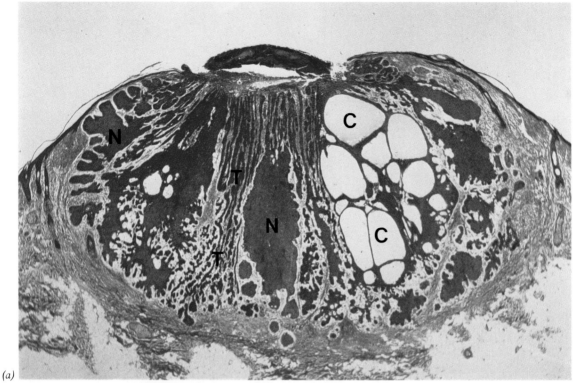

(a)

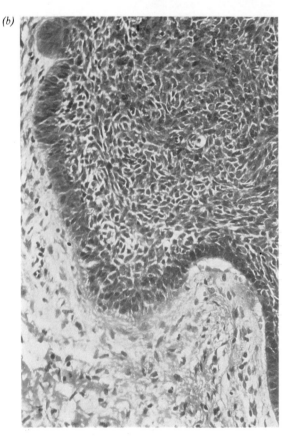

(b)

### Fig. 20.15  Basal cell carcinoma
**(a)** LP
**(b)** HP

*Basal cell carcinoma* is a common tumour composed of cells with deep blue staining nuclei centrally located in sparse, poorly defined cytoplasm. As seen in micrograph (b), the cells at the periphery of the tumour clumps are characteristically arranged in a *palisade pattern*, whereas the central cells are more haphazardly arranged. Micrograph (a) shows the typical growth pattern of the tumour; a nodular pattern **N** is most common but trabecular **T** and cystic **C** patterns are also seen often in the same lesion as in this example.

Basal cell carcinoma arises from the basal cells of the epidermis or epidermal appendages; it behaves as a malignant tumour in that it invades dermis and any deeper underlying structures, but almost never metastasizes. Basal cell carcinomas occur most frequently on the light-exposed areas of skin, particularly the face, and present as nodular lesions which may undergo ragged ulceration giving rise to the colloquial term *rodent ulcer*.

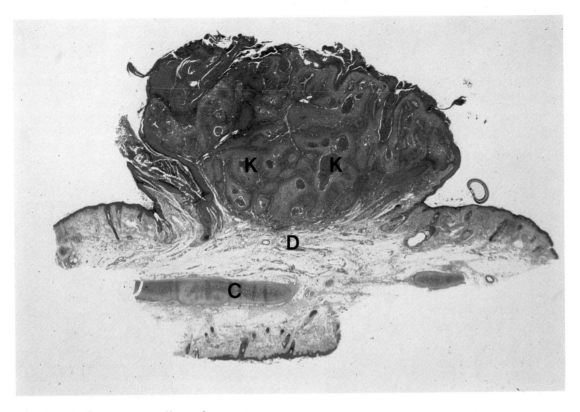

## Fig. 20.16 Squamous cell carcinoma (LP)

Squamous cell carcinomas of the skin histologically resemble squamous cell carcinomas in many other sites (see Fig. 6.11), but the skin tumours are usually very well differentiated and highly keratinizing, containing numerous keratin pearls **K**. The tumour may invade the dermis **D** and underlying structures, and may spread via the lymphatics to regional lymph nodes. Invasive squamous cell carcinoma of the skin may develop from intra-epidermal carcinoma, the skin equivalent of carcinoma in situ, (see Fig. 20.17). In this micrograph the tumour has arisen on the pinna of the ear, but has not yet invaded underlying cartilage **C**.

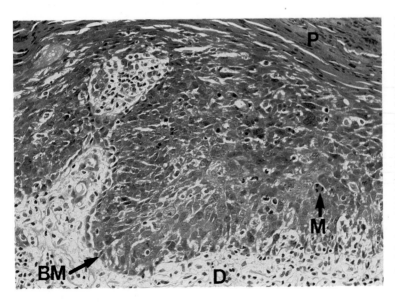

## Fig. 20.17 Intraepidermal carcinoma ( HP)

Invasive squamous carcinoma may be preceded by a variable degree of epidermal dysplasia. When the dysplasia is severe and involves the full thickness of the epidermis, it is termed *intra-epidermal carcinoma*. In this micrograph, note the severe dysplasia extending through the whole epidermis with the loss of normal organisation and stratification; the surface layer exhibits parakeratosis **P**. Note a tripolar mitotic figure **M**. The basement membrane **BM** is intact with no invasion of the dermis **D**.

When the degree of epidermal dysplasia is more moderate, the condition is known as *actinic (solar) keratosis*; in this case the most marked dysplasia is confined to the lower levels of the epidermis (see Fig. 5.6 d).

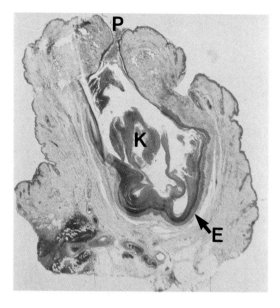

### Fig. 20.18 Epidermal cyst (LP)

These common lesions were formerly known as *sebaceous cysts* although they contain no sebaceous material. They occur in the dermis and hypodermis and may open to the exterior through a punctum **P**. The cyst contains masses of degenerating keratin **K**, and is lined by flattened, stratified squamous epithelium **E**. Trauma to the cyst may lead to escape of keratin into surrounding tissues exciting a giant cell inflammatory reaction with swelling, tenderness and redness around the cyst. Clinically this change is inaccurately referred to as infected sebaceous cyst.

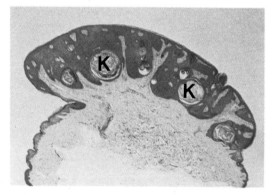

### Fig. 20.19 Seborrhoeic keratosis (LP)

*Seborrhoeic keratosis* is a common lesion of the elderly composed of a localized proliferation of basal cells forming a raised warty lesion. Such outgrowths are vulnerable to chronic trauma leading to overlying hyperkeratosis and formation of keratin nests **K** in the lesion. The aetiology of seborrhoeic keratosis is unknown, although in the past it has been regarded as a benign skin tumour (*basal cell papilloma*).

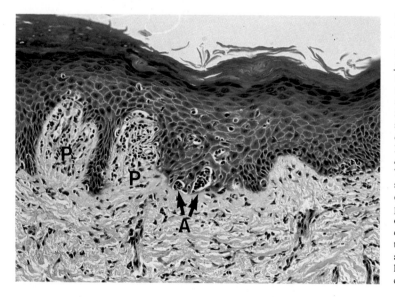

### Fig. 20.20 Mycosis fungoides (HP)

Despite its traditional name, *mycosis fungoides* is not an infective lesion but rather a form of lymphoma in which the skin is the primary site of involvement although other tissues may later become involved. The typical skin lesion may show acanthosis of the epidermis which contains small aggregates of atypical lymphoid cells, known as *Pautrier abscesses* **A,** and scattered abnormal cells. There is also a heavy infiltrate of dark staining lymphoma cells in the upper dermis, most obvious in the dermal papillae **P** in this micrograph. The cellular infiltrate includes large abnormal cells identical to those seen scattered in the epidermis and in the Pautrier abscesses. The abnormal lymphoid cells have been found to be almost always T cell in type.

# 21. Skeletal system

## Introduction

Bone is a highly specialized type of connective tissue formed by the deposition of calcium salts within a dense matrix comprising collagen fibres and ground substance; the unmineralized matrix is known as *osteoid*. Osteocytes maintain the integrity of bone structure and participate in calcium homeostasis by mediating the continuous turnover of matrix and mineral constituents. On a wider scale, bone is being constantly remodelled by the resorptive activity of osteoclasts and redeposition by osteoblasts so as to reinforce bone architecture in response to changing functional demands. In normal bone, dynamic balance thus maintains total bone mass at a relatively constant level whilst providing a potentially large calcium pool which can be drawn upon to maintain serum calcium homeostasis.

*Osteoporosis (osteopaenia)* is a condition in which total bone mass is decreased by reduction of bone trabeculae in number or size (usually both) and thinning of cortical bone; nevertheless the bone otherwise appears structurally normal. In contrast, *osteomalacia* is a disease in which osteoid fails to undergo normal mineralization, usually due to deficiency of vitamin D, although other causes of total body calcium depletion may also be responsible; *rickets* is the childhood equivalent of osteomalacia. The appearance of normal bone, osteoporosis and osteomalacia are compared in Fig. 21.1.

*Paget's disease* of bone (Fig. 21.2) is a condition of unknown aetiology occurring in the elderly, characterized by haphazard inappropriate osteoclastic erosion of formed bone and concurrent osteoblastic deposition of new bone. *Hyperparathyroidism* may cause somewhat similar haphazard osteoclastic erosion of bone; this condition is rare and therefore not illustrated in this chapter.

*Bone fracture* is a common and important result of trauma, although where there is some underlying bone abnormality (e.g. osteoporosis, osteomalacia, Paget's disease, metastatic tumour), the trauma or extra stress required to produce bone fracture may be minimal; this condition is termed *pathological fracture*. The healing of a bone fracture is briefly outlined in Fig. 2.11 as an example of a specialized form of tissue repair. Torn ligaments and tendons and sprained joints are even more commonplace sequelae of accidents and sporting injuries; repair of such tissues occurs by the usual method of scar formation (see Figs 2.8 to 2.11).

Infections of the bone are now comparatively uncommon, though bacterial osteomyelitis, both pyogenic and tuberculous, were formerly important crippling diseases. *Acute osteomyelitis* caused by pyogenic bacteria (usually *Staphylococcus aureus*) usually occurs in infants and young children, the bacteria gaining access to the marrow cavity via the blood stream, but it may also follow penetrating trauma in people of any age, e.g. compound fracture. Pathologically, acute osteomyelitis represents abscess formation in the medullary space of the bone, but the course of the disease in bone is complicated by two factors. First, increased pressure in the confined space causes infarction of further large areas of bone, and secondly, masses of dead bone (*sequestra*) behave as foreign bodies inhibiting normal repair processes and providing haven for bacteria inaccessible to body defence mechanisms. *Chronic osteomyelitis* may follow if treatment is delayed or inadequate. *Tuberculous osteomyelitis* is illustrated in Fig. 3.16.

Primary tumours of bone may arise from all the cell types found in bone and the essential features of the more important of these tumours are tabulated in Fig. 21.4. In addition, there is a miscellaneous group of tumour-like lesions also found in bone the main features of which are presented in Fig. 21.5. *Osteosarcoma* is of great clinical importance and is shown in Fig. 21.3). Malignant tumours may also arise from lymphoreticular cells of the bone marrow e.g. myeloma, lymphoma, leukaemia etc. (see Chapter 15). Bone is a frequent and important site of metastatic haematogenous spread of malignant epithelial tumours, particularly carcinomas of bronchus, breast, kidney, thyroid and prostate. Metastatic tumour deposits usually destroy bone trabeculae, although carcinoma of the prostate sometimes stimulates excessive new bone formation resulting in *osteosclerotic* rather than the more usual *osteolytic* deposits.

The two most important disorders of joints are *rheumatoid arthritis* and *osteoarthritis*. Osteoarthritis (Fig. 21.6) is the name given to the wear and tear degenerative changes which occur in some joints with increasing age, and appears to be clearly distinct pathologically from rheumatoid arthritis (Fig. 21.7), a chronic inflammatory synovitis and arthritis of probable immunological origin.

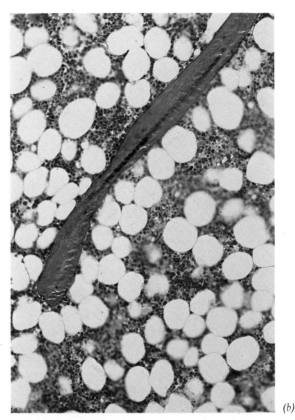

*(a)*

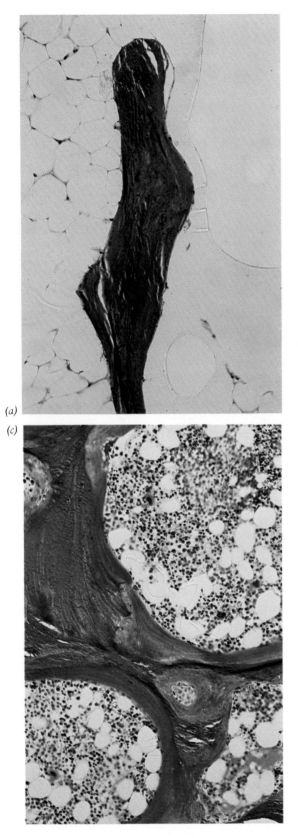

*(c)*

*(b)*

### Fig. 21.1 Osteoporosis and osteomalacia
(undecalcified resin sections; Goldner's trichrome)
**(a) normal bone** (MP)
**(b) osteoporotic bone** (MP)
**(c) osteomalacia** (MP)

In *normal trabecular bone* as shown in micrograph (a), the entire trabeculum is fully calcified (stained green by the Goldner trichrome method).

In *osteoporosis* the bone appears qualitatively normal but its mass is diminished; the trabeculae are reduced in number and size as seen in micrograph (b), although all trabeculae are fully calcified. Osteoporosis is extremely common in the elderly, especially in post-menopausal women, and is exacerbated by immobility. It may also occur in an isolated limb if immobilized for any reason (e.g. postoperatively, or after a fracture). Osteoporosis probably represents disuse atrophy to some degree but can also be the result of endocrine disorders and is particularly seen with iatrogenic steroid excess and in Cushing's syndrome.

In contrast, in *osteomalacia* shown in micrograph (c), the trabeculae are of normal or increased thickness, but there is deficient mineralization so that each trabeculum has a central core of calcified bone (stained green) coated by an outer shell of unmineralized osteoid (stained orange-red). Osteomalacia is usually the result of vitamin D deficiency. Vitamin D deficiency in the growing child causes *rickets*, identical to osteomalacia pathologically but causing gross skeletal deformity by disruption of bone mineralization at growth plates, and distortion of shape in bones too weak to accommodate normal functional stresses.

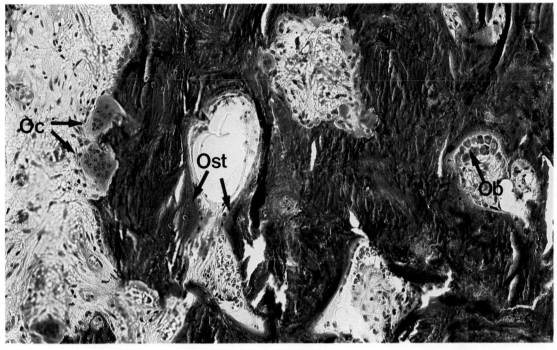

*(a)*

*(b)*

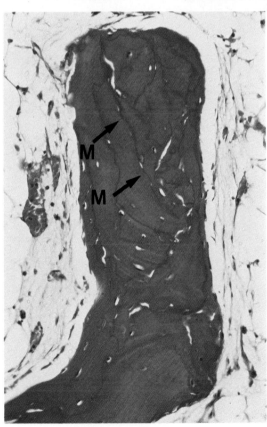

### Fig. 21.2  Paget's disease of bone
**(a) active osteolytic lesion** (undecalcified resin
section, Goldner's trichrome; HP)
**(b) inactive sclerotic lesion** (decalcified paraffin
section, H & E; HP)

In *Paget's disease of bone* there is indiscriminate and
uncontrolled osteoclastic erosion of bone followed by excessive
osteoblastic activity producing excess osteoid which
subsequently becomes mineralized, leading to irregular
trabecular thickening. Micrograph (a) shows typical large
multinucleate osteoclasts **Oc** lying in lacunae formed by active
erosion of bone. Alongside, and in other areas, the trabecular
surface shows a layer of newly deposited red staining osteoid
**Ost** underlying rows of large active cuboidal osteoblasts **Ob**.
When actively synthesizing osteoid, these normally
insignificant spindle-shaped cells become enlarged and cuboidal
in shape. This progressive haphazard erosion of original bone
and formation of new bone results in gross distortion of
trabecular and cortical bone often with marked thickening; the
condition tends to be confined to a relatively small number of
long bones, vertebrae or cranial bones in a symmetrical
fashion. The disruption of normal trabecular architecture
weakens the bone which may become inadequate to withstand
functional stresses leading to severe skeletal deformity, e.g.
bowing of long bones, or even pathological fracture.

 With time, the bone cell activity slowly diminishes, the
initially highly cellular bone becoming progressively sclerotic;
usually the bone is left thicker than before but paradoxically
weaker, as much of the former strong lamellar bone is replaced
by weaker woven bone. The disruption of the optimum
lamellar pattern can be readily viewed by polarizing
microscopy, and in old lesions as in micrograph (b), the limits
of separate episodes of previous bone destruction and irregular
new bone formation is marked by thin dark *mosaic lines* **M**.

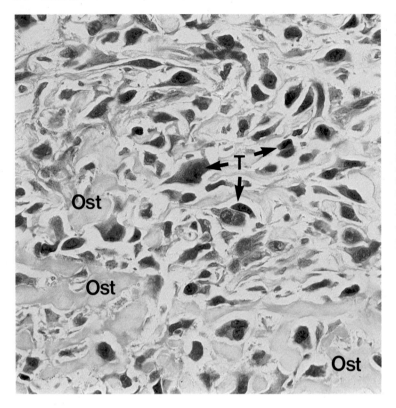

## Fig. 21.3    Osteosarcoma (HP)

This tumour, although relatively uncommon, is nevertheless the most frequently occurring primary malignant tumour of bone. Most cases occur in children and adolescents (usually around the knee), but it may occasionally occur in elderly patients with long standing Paget's disease. Histologically, the tumour has a very variable appearance, but islands of delicately pink stained osteoid **Ost** are usually present although some parts may be irregularly mineralized. The tumour cells **T** which are derived from osteoblasts are usually poorly differentiated and pleomorphic with much mitotic activity. These tumours are generally highly vascular and early bloodstream metastasis to the lungs is common.

## Fig. 21.4    Important primary tumours of bone

| Name | Presumed cell of origin | Age incidence Sex incidence | Common sites | Behaviour |
| --- | --- | --- | --- | --- |
| Osteoid osteoma | Osteoblast | Adolescents M > F | Lower limb | Benign, osteosclerotic painful |
| Nonossifying fibroma | Uncertain | Child/Adol M > F | Long bones of lower limb | Benign, osteolytic, occasionally multiple |
| Chondromyxoid fibroma | Uncertain | Adol/Young adult M > F | Long bones esp. tibia | Benign, osteolytic |
| Enchondroma | Chondrocyte | Young adults M > F | Bones of hands | Usually benign, expansile |
| Giant cell tumour | Osteoclast | 20-40 yrs M > F | Around knee | Mostly benign but with tendency to recur, occasionally metastasize |
| Chordoma | Notochord tissue | 40 + yrs M > F | Sacrum | Extensive local bone destruction, metastasize very rarely |
| Osteosarcoma | Primitive osteoblast | (i) 10–25 yrs (ii) over 65 yrs M > F | (i) Around knee (ii) At site of Paget's disease | Highly malignant, early metastasis to lungs |
| Chondrosarcoma | Chondrocyte | 30–60 yrs M > F | Spine and pelvis | Malignant, extensive local invasion and metastasis |
| Ewing's tumour | Uncertain | Child/Adol M > F | Midshaft of long bones | Malignant, early and extensive metastatic spread |
| Myeloma | Marrow plasma cells | 50 + M > F | Any | Monostotic, multifocal or diffuse marrow involvement |

**Fig. 21.5    Tumour-like lesions in bone**

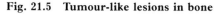

| Name | Age incidence Sex incidence | Common sites | Behaviour |
|---|---|---|---|
| Cartilage-capped exostosis | Child/Adol M > F | Upper tibia Lower fibula | Benign (? hamartomatous) cartilage and bone outgrowth from bone surface, but potential for malignant transformation |
| Aneurysmal bone cyst | Adol/Young adult M > F | Shaft of long bones or spine | Osteolytic, predispose to fracture |
| Fibrous dysplasia | Child/Adol M > F | Femur, tibia, ribs, facial bones | Osteolytic, predispose to fracture |
| 'Brown tumour' of hyperparathyroidism | Adults M > F | Anywhere | Osteolytic lesions, often multiple |

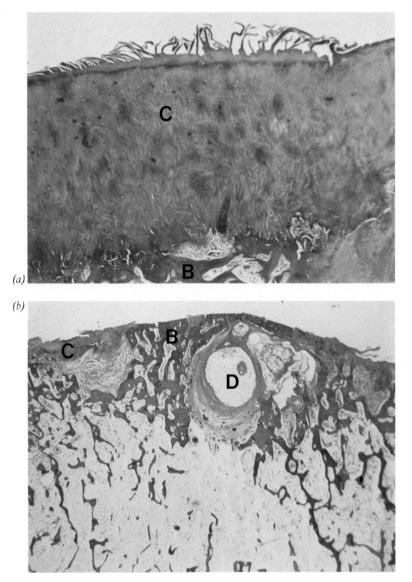

*(a)*

*(b)*

**Fig. 21.6    Osteoarthritis (a) early changes** (LP) **(b) established lesion** (LP)

*Osteoarthritis* is a degenerative disorder of articular cartilage believed to occur as a result of excessive wear and tear although there may be secondary inflammatory changes in the soft tissue components of the joint. In the earliest stages, the articular cartilage **C** loses its smooth appearance and develops surface fibrillations and flaking as shown in micrograph (a). The damaged cartilage is progressively eroded until the underlying cortical bone **B** is exposed. After prolonged articulation of naked bone with the opposing surface, the bone becomes slightly thickened, hard, dense and highly polished, a process known as *eburnation*. At the same time, there is irregular outgrowth of new bone (*osteophytes*) at the articular margins. In the established case shown in micrograph (b), note that only a small amount of cartilage **C** remains and that the exposed bone **B** has undergone eburnation. The bone underlying the traumatized eburnated surface may undergo cystic degeneration **D**.

All of these changes lead to joint pain and progressive limitation of movement at the joint. The hips and knees are most commonly and severely affected.

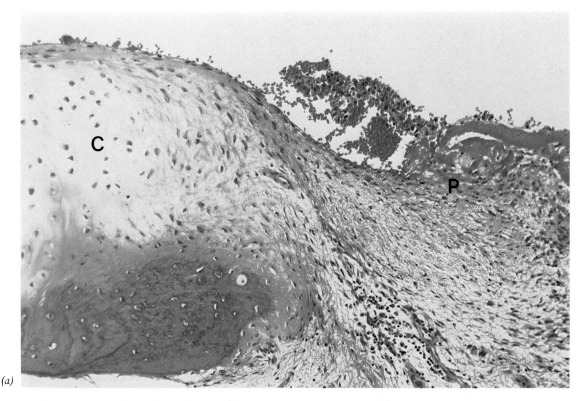

*(a)*

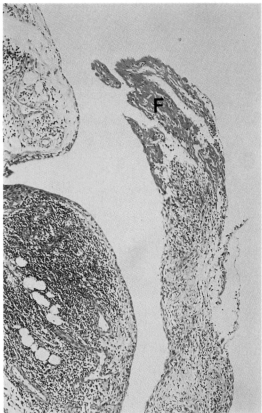

*(b)*

## Fig. 21.7  Rheumatoid arthritis
### (a) articular cartilage changes (HP)
### (b) synovial changes (HP)

*Rheumatoid arthritis* is a systemic disorder, the predominant
feature of which is chronic relapsing inflammation of articular
joints, particularly in the hands and knees. The disease affects
both the synovium lining the joint capsule and the cartilage on
the articular surfaces. The earliest changes occur in the
synovium which becomes thickened, excessively vascular and
thrown up into papillary folds as a result of oedema and heavy
lympho-plasmacytic infiltration; this is seen in micrograph (b).
This is accompanied by exudation of excess fluid into the joint
space with precipitation of fibrin **F** on the synovial surface.
The articular cartilage changes shown in micrograph (a) follow
later and involve localized destruction of cartilage **C** and its
replacement by fibrovascular granulation tissue known as
*pannus* **P** (from the inflamed synovium). Initially, joint
mobility is limited by pain and swelling then later by gross
cartilage and bone destruction and fibrous ankylosis across the
joint space due to fusion of transjacent granulation tissue
pannus.

# 22. The nervous system

## Introduction

Despite its apparently diverse morphological and functional components, the nervous system can be considered to have three main structural elements: neurones, specialized supporting cells and connective tissue. After early infancy, neurones are incapable of cell division and their number thereafter declines slowly as a result of atrophy. Accelerated atrophy occurs in the cerebral cortex in *presenile dementia* (*Alzheimer's disease*) or in response to chronic increased intracranial pressure (*hydrocephalus*) and focal atrophy of neurones in the basal ganglia is responsible for *Parkinson's disease*. Diffuse neurone atrophy may result from the toxic effects of various endogenous or exogenous substances such as alcohol. Neurones may also be overtly destroyed by injurious stimuli including trauma, infections, infarction and neoplasms. From a clinical standpoint, neurones appear to have limited ability to recover from most recognizable pathological stimuli, and neurological function, once lost, is in general irrecoverable. Two important exceptions are the ability of the whole CNS to recover from transient generalized metabolic insults such as hypoxia or hypoglycaemia, and the ability of neuronal axons to 'regrow' after being severed. In addition, the whole system has a degree of plasticity which permits some compensation for functional deficits due to focal damage.

Specialized supporting cells are of four types: astrocytes, oligodendrocytes, ependymal cells and microglia. Astrocytes with their numerous delicate cytoplastic processes form a fibrillary supporting framework for the neurones and other support cells of the CNS; in this sense, their function is somewhat analogous to the reticulin supporting framework in organs such as the liver and lymph nodes. Oligodendrocytes are responsible for axonal myelin sheaths in the CNS and Schwann cells are their counterparts in the peripheral nervous system. Ependymal cells provide a simple lining to the ventricles, choroid plexus and spinal canal and have features in common with simple epithelia lining other body cavities. Microglia are small quiescent phagocytic cells belonging to the macrophage-monocyte system of blood and connective tissue.

In the CNS, connective tissue is confined to the meninges and choroid plexuses where it provides a delicate supporting structure for blood vessels. The lack of connective tissue in the rest of the CNS has important ramifications in respect of responses to injury and repair of damaged tissues as described below. In the peripheral nervous system, connective tissue provides support for individual axons (endoneurium), bundles of axons (perineurium) and peripheral nerves (epineurium).

## Response of CNS tissues to injury

As previously described, neurones have a limited ability to survive significant changes in their metabolic or physical environment. Irreversible neurone damage is recognized histologically by breakdown of Nissl substance, neuronal ribosomal RNA which is strongly basophilic, a process known as *chromolysis*. The neuronal nucleus is also displaced towards the cell periphery. In the absence of connective tissue, central nervous tissue does not respond to injury with the classical sequence of changes from acute inflammation through to granulation tissue formation and fibrous repair. Initially, there is a modified exudative response resulting in accumulation of the appropriate type of leucocyte according to the injurious stimulus, and activation of the microglia to become actively phagocytic. For example, in viral infections, whether diffuse as in *encephalitis* or focal as in *poliomyelitis*, there is a lymphocytic accumulation particularly in the vicinity of blood vessels. In bacterial infections, there is accumulation of neutrophils often to form a *brain abscess*. Exudation of fluid either diffusely or focally tends to increase intracranial pressure which may cause fatal secondary brain damage e.g. by herniation. As time passes, damaged brain tissue undergoes liquifaction and is progressively removed by phagocytosis; however the defect is not filled by development of granulation tissue as in other tissues but rather by proliferation of astrocytes which form a scar-like mass with their numerous cytoplasmic processes. This astrocytic response is known as *gliosis*. If the area of tissue damage is extensive such as following infarction, the gliotic response is insufficient to fill the whole defect and a fluid-filled space lined by gliotic 'scar' remains. In contrast, disease involving the meninges evokes a classical granulation tissue-fibrosis response, examples being acute meningitis (see Fig. 2.4) and tuberculous meningitis (see Fig. 3.17).

## Vascular disorders of the CNS

Vascular disorders account for a large part of neuropathology. Thrombosis, embolism and haemorrhage may all cause infarction of brain or spinal cord; such events are collectively known as cerebrovascular accidents and generalized atherosclerosis is a common predisposing factor. Diffuse atherosclerosis of the CNS vasculature reduces blood supply and predisposes to accelerated neuronal atrophy as well as increasing susceptibility to infarction during sudden hypotensive episodes. Thrombosis also occurs more readily when blood flow is slowed by atherosclerotic narrowing and the vertebrobasilar system is particularly vulnerable. Emboli most commonly arise from the left side of the heart, often from mural thrombosis after myocardial infarction or thrombotic vegetations on the aortic or mitral valves; infective thrombi may also originate from heart valves involved by infective endocarditis. Hypertension strongly predisposes to haemorrhage from vessels within the brain substance, particularly branches of the middle cerebral artery. The changes that occur in CNS infarction are illustrated in Fig. 22.2.

Intracranial haemorrhages may also occur from vessels lying outside the brain substance proper and these are classified according to their relationship to the meninges. *Subarachnoid haemorrhages* arise from vessels lying between the pia and arachnoid layers of the meninges and rupture of a *berry aneurysm* (see Fig. 10.6) is usually responsible. Haemorrhage into the potential space between arachnoid and dura mater is known as *subdural haemorrhage* and is usually due to damage to the small veins which traverse the space to drain into the extradural venous sinuses. Finally, *extradural haemorrhages* arise from vessels such as the middle meningeal artery, lying in dense tissue between the dura mater and skull, becoming torn usually after skull fractures.

## Inflammatory conditions in the CNS

Inflammatory processes involving the CNS are usually divided into those involving either the meninges (*meningitis*) or the CNS substance proper (*encephalitis* in the brain, *myelitis* in the spinal cord); in some conditions there is a mixed *meningo-encephalitis*. Inflammation may be directly due to infections, especially by viruses and bacteria, or may represent immunological phenomena, some of which probably follow earlier subclinical viral infections.

Viral meningitis is common, rarely fatal, and merely involves transient inflammation of the meninges. Bacteria, most notably meningococcus, pneumococcus and *Haemophilus,* cause an acute purulent meningitis (see Fig. 2.5) the sequelae of which may be cranial nerve damage and secondary hydrocephalus due to obstruction of the outflow foramina of the fourth ventricle by fibrous scarring of the meninges. Tuberculosis may cause meningitis which is characterized by a lymphocytic exudate and formation of typical tuberculous meningeal granulomata (see Fig. 3.17); syphilis may also cause a chronic granulomatous meningeal thickening. Encephalitis and myelitis are usually caused by viruses, some types having a predilection for particular types of neurones. For example, the polio virus tends to attack lower motor neurones of the anterior horns of the spinal cord, hence the term poliomyelitis (see Fig. 22.4). In contrast, the herpes virus causes a more diffuse encephalitis (see Fig. 22.3) with temporal lobes and limbic system particularly severely involved.

*Disseminated (multiple) sclerosis* is by far the most common of the CNS disorders thought to be of essentially autoimmune aetiology; its epidemiological characteristics however suggest that infection, probably viral, plays some crucial role in its early pathogenesis. The dominant pathological feature of disseminated sclerosis is focal destruction of myelin associated with accumulation of chronic inflammatory cells; axons, thus denuded of their myelin sheaths, are unable to transmit impulses normally and may be destroyed giving rise to the clinical features of the disease. The histological features of disseminated sclerosis are shown in Fig. 22.5. Other rare disorders of the CNS, such as *Jakob-Creutzfeldt disease,* sub-acute sclerosing panencephalitis following measles, and tertiary neurosyphilis, probably also represent abnormal immunological responses to infection.

There is also a wide spectrum of rare inherited disorders affecting the CNS, including polysaccharide and lipid storage diseases. Most manifest themselves early in life but a few such as Friedreich's ataxia and Huntington's chorea only become evident later on and their pathogenesis is obscure.

## Tumours of the CNS

Primary tumours of the central nervous system may arise from the three major groups of cells: neurones and their precursors, glial cells, and connective tissue and other embryologically associated cells. Their essential features are summarized in tabular form in Fig. 22.1 and the histological features of the clinically more important are shown in Figs 22.6 to 22.11. Primary CNS tumours are rarely malignant in pathophysiological terms and rarely metastasize, however the clinical effects of even small CNS tumours may be devastating when they arise in vital centres. In numerical terms, secondary metastatic lesions are more common in the CNS than primary tumours; bronchus and breast are by far the most common sites of origin of the primary lesion.

## Peripheral nerve disorders

Diseases of the peripheral nerves present as *peripheral neuropathies* and the pathological stimuli may act either upon the nerve cell body, at the axon, or upon the supporting tissues (Schwann cells, connective tissue, blood vessels). Two peripheral nerve tumours, the *Schwannoma* and the *neurofibroma,* are shown in Figs 22.10 and 22.11 respectively. Schwannomas are benign tumours arising from the sheath of Schwann cells responsible for myelination of peripheral nerves. These tumours often arise in the eighth cranial nerve where they are known as *acoustic neuromas*; since they are intracranial in location and often cause CNS symptoms by local pressure effects, they are often classified with CNS tumours. Neurofibromas arise from fibroblasts in the surrounding connective tissue of peripheral nerves. These benign tumours may arise close to the spinal cord in the spinal nerve roots and thus cause clinical symptoms and signs of spinal cord compression identical to those of a similarly located meningioma; thus they too are often classified with CNS tumours. Multiple neurofibromas with a tendency to arise subcutaneously also occur in an inherited disease called *neurofibromatosis* or *von Recklinghausen's disease.* Neurofibromas occasionally undergo malignant transformation into *neurofibrosarcomas.*

## Disorders of skeletal muscle

Diseases of skeletal muscle present as weakness, wasting or pain but since muscle function is utterly dependent on the integrity of the lower motor neurones, these symptoms may equally derive from neurological disorders; hence primary muscle disorders, which are referred to as *myopathies,* are usually considered along with neurological diseases.

Histology often provides the only satisfactory method for distinguishing between myopathies and certain neuropathies. Myopathies can be classified according to aetiology into three groups: genetically determined muscular disorders collectively known as *muscular dystrophies*, inflammatory disorders of skeletal muscle known as *myositis*, and *myopathies secondary to systemic disease.*

The muscular dystrophies are genetically determined disorders of skeletal muscle characterized by degeneration of muscle fibres resulting in muscle wasting and weakness of the affected group. There are several syndromes differing in age and sex incidence, time of onset and clinical course and also differing from one another in that each tends to have a predilection for specific muscle groups. Histologically, there are abnormalities of size, structure and function of the muscle fibres, often associated with atrophy of muscle fibres and fibrosis of the supporting tissue; a typical example is *Duchenne type muscular dystrophy* shown in Fig. 22.12. For comparison, *neurogenic atrophy* is illustrated in Fig. 22.13.

In contrast, myositis is primarily inflammatory, the muscle cells may degenerate and the supporting tissues become infiltrated with inflammatory cells. Finally, the myopathies secondary to systemic diseases such as thyrotoxicosis, Cushing's disease and carcinomatosis represent atrophic changes and diminish the cellular function in most cases.

## Fig. 22.1  Primary tumours of the CNS

| Cell of origin | Tumour | Peak age incidence | Behaviour |
|---|---|---|---|
| Neurones | Neuroblastoma | Commonly childhood | Malignant invasive tumour; rare |
| | Medulloblastoma | Commonly childhood | Malignant invasive tumour; rare |
| Astrocytes | Astrocytoma | Adults + childhood | Infiltrative tumour (adults) Expansile tumour (children) |
| Oligodendrocytes | Oligodendroglioma | 40–50 yrs | Infiltrative tumour |
| Microglia | Microglioma | 50–60 yrs | Primary intra-cerebral lymphoma |
| Ependyma | Ependymoma | Childhood + adolescence | Slow growing infiltrative tumour |
| Arachnoid villi | Meningioma | 30–70 yrs | Compressive effects; may grow rapidly |
| Schwann cell | Schwannoma | 40–50 yrs | Compressive effects on CNS and associated peripheral nerves |
| Fibroblasts in peripheral nerve | Neurofibroma | Any age | Compressive effects |

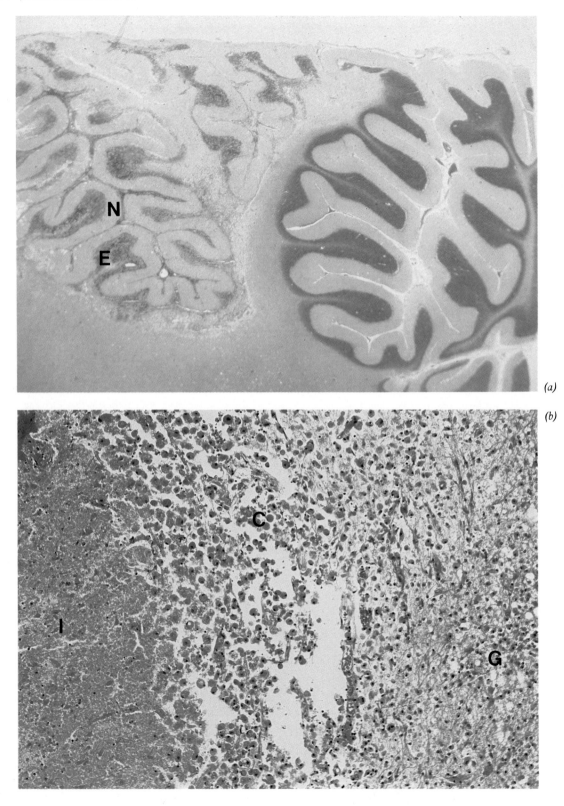

*(a)*

*(b)*

Fig. 22.2 **Infarction of the brain**

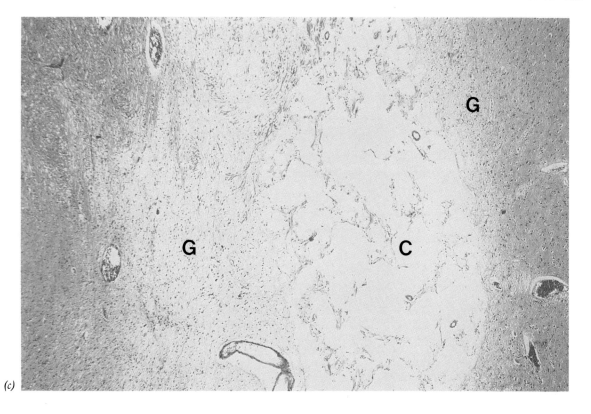

*(c)*

## Fig. 22.2    Infarction of the brain *(illustrations (a) and (b) opposite)*
**(a) early infarct** (LP)
**(b) later infarct** (MP)
**(c) old (cystic) infarct** (LP)

These three micrographs illustrate the typical histological features of CNS infarction.

The earliest histological manifestations become evident about 6 hours after the event when there is loss of neuronal basophilia accompanied by increasing cytoplasmic eosinophilia. The affected brain becomes oedematous and myelin begins to break down. Neutrophils, seen in great numbers in infarcts of other organs, are only a transient feature in brain tissue infarcts and usually appear only in small numbers. During the 2 days post-infarction however, macrophages begin to appear in the infarct territory probably derived both from the blood and by activation of pre-existing microglia. Macroscopically, infarcts may appear pale or *anaemic* or may be *haemorrhagic*. The haemorrhagic pattern is thought to be caused by blood flowing back into capillaries damaged by the initial anoxic episode, nevertheless in anaemic infarcts small areas of extravasated blood can also be seen around blood vessels. Microgaph (a) illustrates a haemorrhagic infarct of the cerebellum, the patient having died about two days post-infarction. The infarcted area is on the left and normal cerebellum on the right. Note the loss of staining in the necrotic tissue **N** and the pallor of the infarcted brain. Note also the extravasation of erythrocytes **E.**

Over successive days the necrotic tissue begins to undergo autolysis and liquifaction. Invading macrophages take up lipid material from the dead cells and myelin forming foamy or clear cells known as *compound granular corpuscles* or *gitter cells*. By about 7 to 10 days post-infarction, the infarct becomes

macroscopically soft and cystic in appearance. Blood pigment degenerates and the infarct may become yellow in colour if there has been significant bleeding into the lesion. Micrograph (b) shows this phase in a cortical cerebral infarct; the infarcted area **I** consists of a homogeneous pink stained mass of necrotic neurones. Surrounding this area is a zone of compound granular cells **C** and beyond this a zone of proliferating glial cells **G** which are small with pale staining nuclei. The glial cell proliferation is analogous to the formation of granulation tissue in infarcts elsewhere in the body. This process, known as *gliosis*, will attempt to fill the whole of the defect in the area of infarction to form a so-called *glial scar* formed not of fibrous tissue but of the cell bodies and numerous cytoplasmic processes (fibres) of the glial cells.

When the infarct is extensive, the process of gliosis appears to be unable to completely fill the defect and a cyst-like cavity remains, lined by dense glial tissue. Micrograph (c) shows such an old cystic infarct in the internal capsule, with the central cystic cavity **C** surrounded by glial tissue **G**. In large infarcts, blood vessels may even be seen traversing the cystic space. Note that there is no neuronal regeneration in an infarct.

Some of the early clinical manifestations of a CNS infarct are due to the pressure effects of oedema occurring in the relatively undamaged tissue bordering the infarct. This oedema gradually resolves as healing proceeds and this explains some of the clinical improvement which the patient often experiences with time.

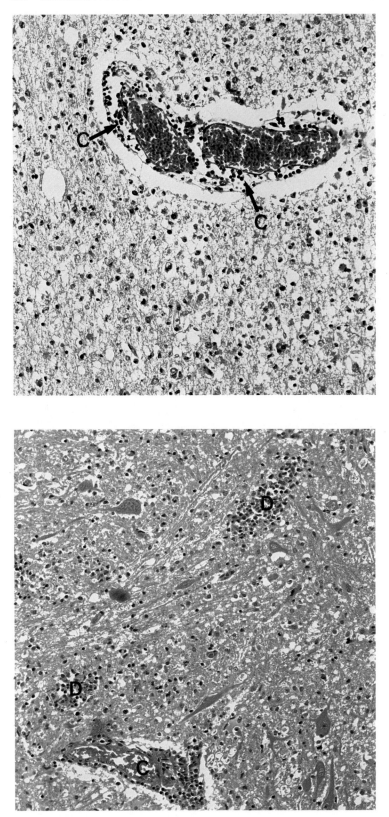

## Fig. 22.3  Herpes encephalitis (HP)

Apart from its more common cutaneous lesions, the herpes simplex virus is capable of causing a severe diffuse necrotizing infection of the brain. The virus spreads to involve particularly the frontal lobes, limbic system and temporal lobes, and in severe cases there may be macroscopic evidence of necrosis in such areas. As shown in this micrograph, the neurones of affected areas undergo necrosis, astrocytes become activated and the area becomes diffusely infiltrated by microglia. The viral infection excites a lymphocytic response which is manifest as characteristic *perivascular cuffing* **C** of the blood vessels. Some neurones which have not been totally destroyed may exhibit small eosinophilic inclusions within their nuclei, probably representing viral particles. *Herpes encephalitis* has a high mortality rate and if the patient survives there is often severe neurological deficit subsequently.

## Fig. 22.4  Poliomyelitis (HP)

Although it may cause a diffuse encephalomyelitis, the polio virus most commonly attacks the anterior horn cells of the spinal cord (cell bodies of lower motor neurones) resulting in skeletal paralysis; it may also affect cranial nerve nuclei and cause bulbar paralysis. Nerve cells are invaded by the viral particles and undergo degeneration as evidenced by loss of basophilia and eventual destruction; the disintegrating cell bodies become surrounded by microglia which engulf the cellular debris **D.** As with other viral infections of the central nervous system, the histological hallmark is perivascular lymphocytic cuffing **C.**

Healing is by gliosis and there is no replacement of the destroyed neurones.

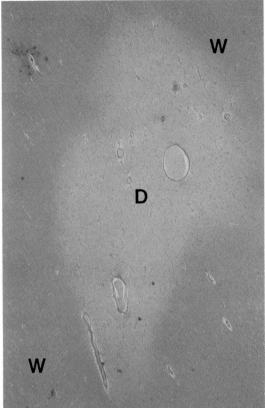

*(a)*

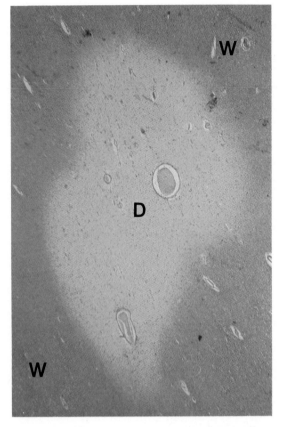

*(b)*

**Fig. 22.5    Disseminated (multiple) sclerosis**
(a) H & E stain; (LP)
(b) Loyez staining method; (LP)

*Disseminated sclerosis* is a demyelinating disease in which the primary defect appears to involve destruction of the myelin surrounding the axons in the central nervous system. It is postulated that the cause is a viral infection which triggers some immunological reaction to myelin. There are three histological stages in the demyelination process. First, during an acute episode, myelin breakdown occurs associated with lymphocytic infiltration around the blood vessels of the affected area; at this stage there is clinical evidence of focal neurological dysfunction. In response to myelin breakdown, there is proliferation of astrocytes which with their cytoplastic 'fibres' form a typical glial scar. With time, the glial scar becomes less cellular and more discrete. Macroscopically the areas of demyelination and glial scarring appear as pale greyish plaques which are commonest in the periventricular white matter and optic tracts.

Micrograph (a) shows the typical H & E appearance of an established focus of demyelination. The pale staining

demyelinated area **D** is easily distinguishable from the more strongly staining white matter **W**; between these areas is a narrow zone of glial tissue which cannot be distinguished at this magnification. Micrograph (b) illustrates the same lesion stained by a method used for demonstrating myelin; the demyelinated area remains unstained whilst the unaffected area of white matter stains blue-grey.

Disseminated sclerosis runs a variable but usually prolonged course characterized by episodes of focal demyelination which are disseminated both in terms of their location in the central nervous system and their time of occurrence. During episodes of active demyelination, focal neurological signs often appear but at times of remission there is usually partial or even complete resolution of the neurological deficit probably due both to the diminution of inflammatory oedema in the nonaffected areas surrounding the primary lesions and also due to neurological compensation.

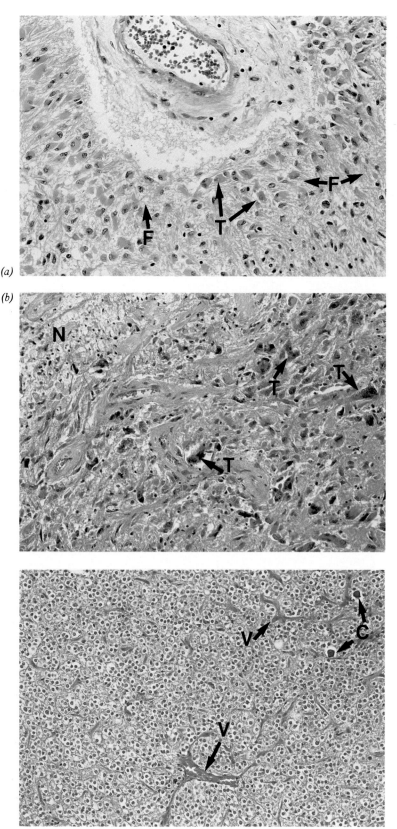

*(a)*

*(b)*

## Fig. 22.6   Tumours derived from astrocytes
**(a) astrocytoma** (HP)
**(b) glioblastoma multiforme** (HP)

Astrocytes give rise to a spectrum of tumours, the less common benign forms being known as *astrocytomas* and the more common malignant form known as *glioblastoma multiforme*. Astrocytomas may be graded from 1 to 4 (most benign to least benign) according to cytological criteria, the presence of necrosis, degree of endothelial proliferation in nearby blood vessels, and degree of infiltration of surrounding tissue.

Micrograph (a) illustrates an astrocytoma grade 2. The tumour cells **T** are large, with abundant pink staining cytoplasm; this form of astrocyte is known as a *gemistocyte*. Astrocyte fibres **F** extend out between the cells.

Glioblastoma multiforme represents the most malignant end of the spectrum of astrocytic tumours; an example is shown in micrograph (b). These tumours grow rapidly and may show areas of necrosis **N** and haemorrhage. The tumour cells **T** have large pleomorphic nuclei and giant cell forms may be seen. Mitotic figures are common. The tumour cells are markedly different from benign glial cells and macroscopically the tumours are well delineated from the surrounding brain tissue. In the low grade astrocytoma, the tumour cells are often indistinguishable from normal astrocytes and the margins of the tumour may be difficult to delineate.

## Fig. 22.7   Oligodendroglioma (HP)

These tumours are derived from oligodendrocytes and are most commonly seen in the cerebral hemispheres. Histologically, the tumour cells form dense homogeneous sheets; they are of uniform appearance with a compact nucleus surrounded by a vacuolated poorly stained cytoplasm. Small blood vessels **V** present in the tumour have a typically branching pattern. Frequently there are foci of calcification **C**. In many *oligodendrogliomas*, foci of astrocytoma-like cells may also be seen.

Unlike astrocytomas, the behaviour and prognosis of oligodendrogliomas cannot be related to the histological appearance of the neoplastic cells and their behaviour is unpredictable.

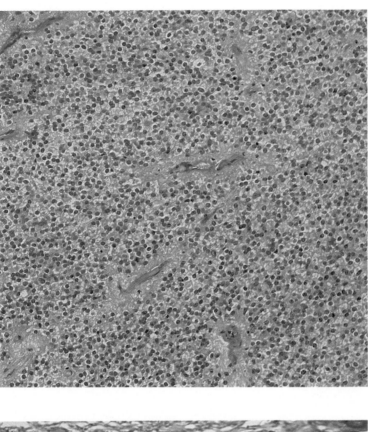

## Fig. 22.8　Ependymoma (MP)

These tumours are derived from the ependymal cells which line the ventricles of the brain and spinal canal. Histologically they are somewhat variable but show several characteristic features. The cells are small and darkly staining and tend to be arranged around blood vessels so as to leave a pink staining nuclear-free perivascular gap, the appearance giving rise to the term *pseudorosette pattern*. Occasionally the tumour cells form tubules which simulate the central canal of the spinal cord in appearance.

*Ependymomas* are most commonly seen in the region of the fourth ventricle but they also account for a large proportion of tumours in the spinal cord. A peculiar variant of this tumour is the *myxopapillary ependymoma* of the filum terminale where the tumour produces large vacuolated cells with a mucinous intercellular matrix.

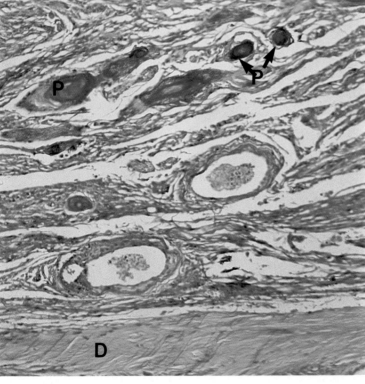

## Fig. 22.9　Meningioma (MP)

The term *meningioma* is applied to tumours arising from the meninges and it is thought that the cells of origin are those of the arachnoid granulations. The tumours are benign and produce their symptoms by compression of the underlying brain or spinal cord. Histologically there are several well recognised patterns.

This micrograph illustrates a meningioma arising from the dura mater **D.** It is composed of spindle shaped cells arranged in sheets and whorls and producing collagen. At the centre of the whorls are foci of lamellar calcification known as *psammoma bodies* **P**. Mitotic figures are not commonly seen but when they are present, there appears to be a greater chance of recurrence after excision.

Occasionally, meningiomas may erode into the overlying bone. These tumours occur most commonly in adults over the age of forty and they usually arise in relation to the sagittal sinus although they may appear anywhere in the meninges of the CNS. Most tumours are amenable to complete surgical excision.

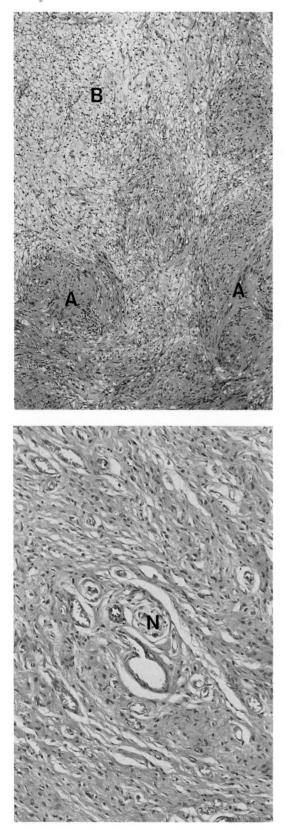

## Fig. 22.10    Schwannoma (MP)

These tumours are derived from sheath of Schwann cells, the cells responsible for myelin formation in the peripheral nervous system. Although they arise in peripheral nerves they also occur in the eighth cranial nerve and in this context are known as *acoustic neuromas*.

There are two typical patterns of growth designated as Antoni type A and B respectively which may coexist in the same tumour. *Antoni type A* has a dense cellular pattern with the cells arranged in palisades and whorls. *Antoni type B* pattern is relatively acellular the tissue being loose and pale stained. In this micrograph both Antoni type A and type B areas are present and labelled accordingly. One feature that distinguishes this tumour from a neurofibroma is the lack of nerve fibres within the tumour.

*Schwannomas* are usually solitary rounded white nodules and arise in relation to nerve bundles. They are benign and usually slow-growing. Schwannomas of the acoustic nerve produce symptoms usually by pressure on adjacent cranial nerves.

## Fig. 22.11    Neurofibroma (MP)

The *neurofibroma* is a tumour of peripheral nerves which is believed to be derived from either Schwann cells or fibroblasts of the supporting connective tissue of the nerve. The tumours may be solitary but are more often multiple and they constitute the skin lesions found in the condition known as *neurofibromatosis (von Recklinghausen's disease)*. The commonest site for these tumours is on peripheral nerves where they form nodules beneath the skin. Tumours may also occur on spinal nerves within the spinal canal thereby giving rise to symptoms of spinal cord compression.

Histologically, the tumour is composed of loosely arranged spindle cells with variable amounts of intervening collagen. A frequent feature is myxoid change producing a grossly gelatinous mass of tissue; the illustrated example is more densely collagenous. In contrast to the Schwannoma, bundles of normal peripheral nerves **N** may be seen running through the tumour. Neurofibromas are usually benign but occasionally they may become malignant when they are termed *neurofibrosarcomas*.

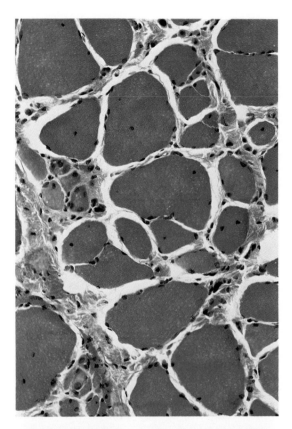

## Fig. 22.12 Muscular dystrophy: Duchenne type (HP)

The commonest of the muscular dystrophies is known as *Duchenne type dystrophy*; the condition is transmitted in an X-linked recessive manner thus affecting boys almost exclusively. The symptom of muscular weakness develops in early childhood and particularly involves the proximal muscles of the lower limbs at an early stage; other muscles then become progressively involved with death occurring usually during the second decade.

Histologically, there is gross variation in size of muscle fibres, with fibres of all sizes being randomly arranged within the muscle fascicle. The morphology of individual fibres is abnormal, the fibres assuming a rounded appearance in cross section and some of the nuclei being displaced from their normal position, immediately underlying the cell membrane, towards the centre of the cytoplasm. Degenerate fibres eventually undergo phagocytosis. As the disease progresses the number of muscle fibres diminishes, however there is concomitant fibrosis and fat accumulation in the muscle and this feature is responsible for the *pseudohypertrophy* seen in the calf muscles of children affected with this disease. Degeneration and death of muscle fibres is reflected in an elevated serum level of creatine phosphokinase. The other forms of muscular dystrophy are also characterized by progressive loss of individual skeletal muscle fibres which may involve the selective destruction of one metabolic type of fibre in preference to another e.g. type 1 fibres as opposed to type 2 fibres.

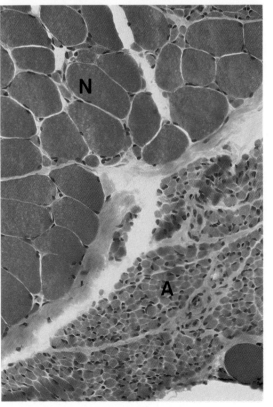

## Fig. 22.13 Neurogenic muscular atrophy (HP)

Weakness and wasting of skeletal muscle may be due not to primary muscle disease but secondary to lower motor neurone damage. Histologically, this can be distinguished from muscular dystrophy since the only fibres affected are those belonging to motor units, the controlling axon of which has been damaged. The fibres supplied by affected motor neurones are small and atrophic and, rather than being scattered randomly amongst the large normal fibres as in muscular dystrophy, they are arranged in groups representing motor units. Note in this micrograph, the bundle of large normal muscle fibres **N** and the discrete bundle of small angulated atrophic fibres **A** belonging to motor units innervated by damaged axons.

# Index